Preventive Cardiology

Preventive Cardiology

Gary E. Fraser

M.B., Ch.B., Ph.D., Dip. Stat., M.P.H., F.R.A.C.P.
Associate Professor of Epidemiology
Associate Professor of Medicine
Loma Linda University

New York   Oxford
OXFORD UNIVERSITY PRESS
1986

Oxford University Press
Oxford   New York   Toronto
Delhi   Bombay   Calcutta   Madras   Karachi
Petaling Jaya   Singapore   Hong Kong   Tokyo
Nairobi   Dar es Salaam   Cape Town
Melbourne   Auckland

and associated companies in
Beirut   Berlin   Ibadan   Nicosia

Published by Oxford University Press
200 Madison Avenue, New York, New York 10016

Library of Congress Cataloging in Publication Data

Fraser, Gary E.
Preventive cardiology.

Includes bibliographies and index.
1. Coronary heart disease—Prevention.   2. Cardiology.
I. Title.   [DNLM: 1. Coronary Disease—prevention & control. WG 300 F841p]
RC685.C6F69   616.1'205   84–29565
ISBN 0–19–503571–2

Printing (last digit):   9 8 7 6 5 4 3 2 1

Printed in the United States of America

Preface

Preventive cardiology, while by no means a new concept, has only recently been considered a separate discipline. It represents a common ground that covers clinical cardiologic practice, cardiovascular epidemiology, and behavioral science. Enormous research efforts in this area over the last 20 to 30 years have produced a body of knowledge that is relevant to students of medicine, nursing, and public health, as well as busy practitioners.

This book is an introduction to preventive cardiology, and it has been written with the following objectives:

To acquaint readers with the present knowledge of the factors contributing to the epidemic of coronary heart disease afflicting most Western or industrialized countries.

To give readers an appreciation of the pitfalls in analyzing even carefully conducted population research.

To introduce readers to the scientific basis of prevention and the methods that can produce behavioral change and affect a patient's health, especially as they relate to primary and secondary prevention of coronary heart disease. Emphasis is placed on the role of the individual clinician as a therapist.

The text is data oriented so that readers can get a clear sense of the issues being discussed. Many of these issues, of course, have been investigated in more than one study. In the interests of space, it was necessary to be selective. Choices of studies to illustrate particular questions were based primarily on methodologic adequacy. Among other considerations were clarity of presentation, characteristics of the population studied, and recency.

The book is built around a central core of chapters on individual risk factors: serum cholesterol, diet, smoking, high blood pressure, psychosocial and socioeconomic variables, physical inactivity, and alcoholic beverage consumption. These chapters deal with the relationship of the risk factors to clinical coronary syndromes and to myocardial and coronary pathology, and they describe the distribution of each factor in the population. Risk factors for subsequent events once ischemic heart disease is established are discussed in a separate chapter. Other chapters cover the epidemiology of hypertension—a disease entity with diverse sequelae—sudden death, and preventive cardiology in childhood. A philosophy of prevention is presented, and the conceptual difficulties arising from the multifactorial etiology of ischemic heart disease are considered.

Another group of chapters reviews strategies of *intervention* to prevent the first onset, or recurrence, of ischemic heart disease. These include attempts to change the life-style of whole communities or large sections of communities as well as intervention on an individual basis. Coronary bypass surgery and cardiac rehabilitation may prevent recurrent events in patients with established disease. Antihypertensive, antiarrhythmic, antiplatelet, hypolipidemic, beta-blocking, calcium-channel-blocking drugs, and female sex hormones are also known or suspected of affecting risk of ischemic heart disease events.

The 34 percent decline in ischemic heart disease mortality between 1968 and 1982 has occurred too rapidly to be explained by genetic influences, thus implying environmental changes as its source. Exactly which environmental factors are responsible is controversial, but it seems very likely that changing health habits in the population have played a major role, while more effective treatment of established disease is probably also important. Whatever the precise causes, this decline points to the strong potential for prevention if we can understand the causal factors at work.

Loma Linda, California   G.E.F.
May 1985

Acknowledgments

I would like to recognize the dedication and expertise of my secretary, Mrs. Hannelore Bennett, who has carefully assembled the several preparatory versions of this manuscript, and also Dr. Leonard Syme, for his valuable comments on Chapter 11. Mr. Jeffrey House, my editor at Oxford University Press, has spent many hours with this manuscript and has given dozens of helpful criticisms and suggestions which have been much appreciated. I wish also to thank Dr. L. D. Watkins, who offered advice and constructive criticism of Chapter 16, and Ms. Pam Reeves and Jean Matthai, for secretarial assistance with the same chapter. Finally, thanks is due to the large number of investigators from many countries who have given permission for their work to be published here. Preparation of this manuscript was largely funded by N.I.H. grant # HL00663.

Contents

Preventive Cardiology

1

The Descriptive Epidemiology of Ischemic Heart Disease

The Scope of the Problem

Although there have been substantial declines in mortality from the cardio-vascular diseases in recent years, these diseases still account for about 985,000 fatalities annually in the United States, about one-half of all deaths. More than 200,000 of these deaths occur before age 65, and another 200,000 premature deaths occur between age 65 and normal life expectancy. Seventy-five percent of all deaths from cardiovascular disease are due to heart disease, and 16 percent are due to cerebrovascular diseases. These are, respectively, the first and third leading causes of death in the United States (Table 1–1). The relationship of age to cardiovascular disease mortality is well known and profound (Fig. 1–1). In the 25–44 age range, heart disease is only the third leading cause of death, and even at ages 45–54 its lead is markedly diminished. This reflects the decline in mortality from ischemic heart disease (IHD) since 1968.

In 1982 there were 554,900 deaths from ischemic heart disease, the most common form of heart disease, and 159,630 deaths from stroke. The sum of fatal and nonfatal heart attacks in the United States is well over 1 million each

Table 1–1 Mortality from the seven leading causes of death, United States, 1982 (provisional results)

Cause of death	Number	Percentage
Total	1,986,000	100.0
1. Ischemic heart disease	554,900	27.9
2. Malignant neoplasms	435,550	21.9
3. Cerebrovascular diseases	159,630	8.0
4. Other cardiovascular causes	270,511	13.6
5. Accidents	95,680	4.8
6. Chronic obstructive pulmonary disease	56,920	2.9
7. Influenza and pneumonia	50,460	2.5
All other causes	362,349	18.2

Source: Adapted from National Heart, Lung and Blood Institute (1983a).

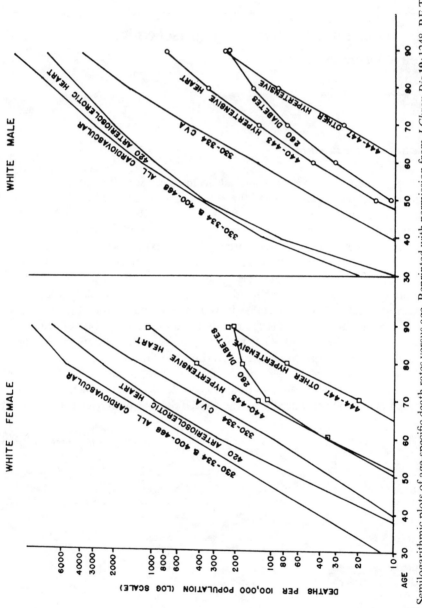

Figure 1–1 Semilogarithmic plots of age-specific death rates versus age. Reprinted with permission from *J Chron Dis* **19**:1248. RE Tracy: Sex difference in coronary disease: Two opposing views, 1966. Pergamon Press, Ltd.

4

year, and in about one-third of these cases the victim dies before reaching a hospital. About one-fourth of all *new* cases of ischemic heart disease are manifested as sudden death. About 4 million persons in the United States have clinically manifest ischemic heart disease, and half of them are under age 65.

Persons who survive to be discharged from hospital after a myocardial infarction (MI) have a first-year mortality between 8 and 15 percent (Kuller, 1979). Each subsequent year, mortality is between 3 and 5 percent, and most of these deaths are sudden. Where stable angina pectoris is the earliest manifestation of IHD, males have a 3–5 percent yearly mortality (Weinblatt, 1973), but by contrast women under age 60 years have a very low death rate (Kannel, 1972). Our ability to predict and explain events following onset of ischemic heart disease is explored in chapter 18.

Between 16 and 25 percent of the adult population have high blood pressure, depending on the definition, substantially increasing the risk of stroke and ischemic heart disease. Cerebrovascular disease has partially or completely disabled more than half of the nearly 2 million persons surviving an acute stroke. Both hypertension and stroke are more prevalent among blacks than whites.

Ateriosclerosis is the underlying cause of an estimated 85 percent of deaths from heart and vascular diseases. *Virtually all adult American males and postmenopausal women are afflicted to some degree.* All health care practitioners should keep in mind that their middle-aged male patients have a 25 percent chance of developing IHD before the age of 65 years. Over the same period, they have a 10 percent chance of dying from heart disease, usually suddenly, so that there is little chance of therapeutic intervention. There is a 20 percent probability that the middle-aged male is hypertensive and at risk of several consequences from this over the next one to two decades.

Of the 4.8 million hospital discharges (alive or dead) of patients with cardiovascular disease in 1978, 9 percent were for acute myocardial infarction, 32 percent for chronic coronary disease, and 14 percent for cerebrovascular diseases. The corresponding days of hospitalization and disability are shown in Table 1–2. Of the 55 million physician office visits for these diseases in 1978, 45 percent were for hypertension and 26 percent for ischemic heart disease. The estimated cost of cardiovascular disease in the United States in 1981 was close to $50 billion (Fig. 1–2). This included the cost of about 150,000 coronary bypass operations. The data to be presented in this book suggest that the greatest contributor to this colossal morbidity and economic cost is the middle-aged American male himself who is either ignorant of the facts or more typically refuses to take responsibility for his own health.

Time Trends in the Frequency of Ischemic Heart Disease

It is interesting to trace the history of IHD as far as records allow. Sandison (1962) documented subintimal accumulations of lipid diagnostic of atherosclerosis in the arteries of Egyptian mummies despite having few specimens to

Table 1–2 Disability days attributed to the atherosclerotic diseases and other major chronic diseases, United States[a]

	Disability days (millions of person-days)			
Disease	Hospital days	Bed days	Work-loss days	Restricted activity days
All atherosclerotic diseases	33	86	21	241
Coronary heart disease	20	61	18	184
Cerebrovascular diseases	8	21	3	47
Other atherosclerotic diseases	5	4	[b]	10
Other leading chronic diseases				
Arthritis	5	95	19	404
Hypertension	2	58	12	235
Back problems	[b]	34	11	127
Cancer	22	[c]	[c]	[c]

Source: From Working Group on Arteriosclerosis of the National Heart, Lung and Blood Institute (1981b), p 40, with permission.

[a] All data in this table are for 1978, except hospital days, which are for 1977. Categories of disability days are not mutually exclusive.

[b] A numerical value is not cited because it was too small to meet standards of reliability or precision.

[c] Data unavailable.

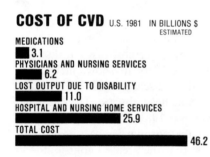

COST OF CVD U.S. 1981 IN BILLIONS $
ESTIMATED
MEDICATIONS
3.1
PHYSICIANS AND NURSING SERVICES
6.2
LOST OUTPUT DUE TO DISABILITY
11.0
HOSPITAL AND NURSING HOME SERVICES
25.9
TOTAL COST
46.2

Figure 1–2 Estimated costs (in billions of dollars) of cardiovascular disease in the United States, 1981. Adapted from *Heart Facts, 1981*, p 11, by permission of the American Heart Association, Inc.

examine. In a single mummy, Long (1931) described a calcified coronary artery with thickened intima, coexisting with what appeared to be fine myocardial scars. Information regarding clinical syndromes is much more vague, but a passage in the Papyrus Ebers (Ebers, 1875, quoted in Leibowitz, 1970) suggests cardiac pain:

When you examine a man for illness in his cardia, he has pains in his arm, in his breast, on the side of his cardia; it is said thereof: this is the w_3d-illness. Then you shall say thereof: it is something which entered his mouth; it is death which approaches him.

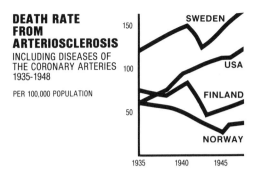

DEATH RATE FROM ARTERIOSCLEROSIS
INCLUDING DISEASES OF THE CORONARY ARTERIES 1935-1948

PER 100,000 POPULATION

Figure 1–3 Death rates from arteriosclerosis in selected Scandinavian countries 1935–1948. Adapted from H Malmros, 1950, with permission.

A complete human body from the second century B.C. was unearthed in China in 1972 (Hall, 1974). The woman had died at approximately 50 years of age and her body was remarkably preserved. A severely occluded left coronary artery was found. Packets of herbal medicines such as cinnamon, magnolia, bark, and peppercorns were also found in the tomb. These are still prescribed today for heart disease by herbal doctors in China, and may indicate that the woman had symptoms of heart disease.

Many individual medical histories highly suggestive of ischemic heart disease have been assembled by Leibowitz (1970) from records of ancient Greece and Rome, the Middle Ages, and the 17th and 18th centuries. While the histories over the last 300 years are generally clearer, this probably reflects advances in physiologic and anatomic knowledge and a more familiar use of language. Heberden in 1772 described with great clarity the clinical syndrome of angina pectoris. He commented that this disorder was not uncommon in his London practice at that time. A definitive statement will probably never be possible, but the above allows speculation that IHD may not be only a 20th-century disease, and such symptoms may have been known since antiquity.

There was a growing realization of the magnitude of the ischemic heart disease problem during the mid-20th century. Serious epidemiologic investigations to find the causes of this major public health problem began in the late 1940s. Around this time Malmros (1950) noted that mortality ascribed to IHD had dropped in Scandinavian countries during the deprivations of the German occupation (Fig. 1–3), in contrast to trends in the United States. Although many life-style variables were changing simultaneously in Scandinavia during this period, several dietary variables do show a temporal change coinciding with the decline in Scandinavian mortality (see Fig. 1–4 for Swedish data as an example). Such data are interesting but cannot prove a cause–effect relationship.

During the 1950s and early 1960s there was fairly consistent evidence of a substantial rise in male heart disease death rates in many different countries (Fig. 1–5). In the United States the upward trend was modest for males and not seen at all in females (Fig. 1–6). Data collected before 1948 are possibly unreliable because of inadequate methods of disease coding for such research. Statistics like these are influenced by the varying accuracy with which death

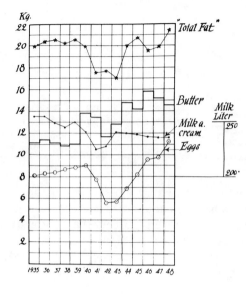

Figure 1–4 Per capita consumption of eggs, dairy products, and total fat in Sweden, 1935–1948. From H Malmros, 1950, with permission.

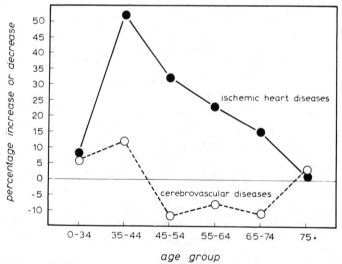

Figure 1–5 Percentage change in male mortality from 1954 to 1964 in 23 countries, by age group: Australia, Austria, Belgium, Canada, Czechoslovakia, Denmark, England and Wales, Federal Republic of Germany, Finland, France, Hungary, Israel, Italy, Japan, Netherlands, New Zealand, Northern Ireland, Norway, Scotland, Sweden, Switzerland, United States, Venezuela. Based on data in *Epidemiol Vital Stat Rep* **20**: 539, 1967. World Health Organization, with permission.

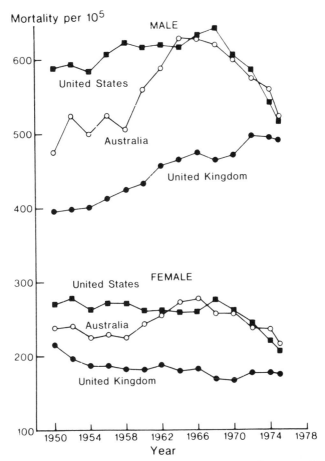

Figure 1–6 Age-standardized ischemic heart disease mortality rates: United States, United Kingdom (England and Wales), Australia, 1950–1975. From T Dwyer and Hetzel, 1980, with permission.

certificates are filled in by physicians, but there is no evidence of recent major shifts in diagnostic or recording practice that could account for the apparent changes in mortality.

The recent decline in ischemic heart disease mortality (IHD) began in the mid-1960s (Fig. 1–6). This is seen in males and females in all age ranges and is occurring in the United States, Australia, and New Zealand, but until the last year or two not in the United Kingdom. The decline continues at an average rate of 2 to 3 percent per year in the United States, resulting in an overall decrease in IHD mortality from 1968 to 1978 of 27 percent (Table 1–3). This decline has continued through until at least 1982 (the lastest available figures) and then represented a 34.3 percent decline since 1968. Between 1960 and 1979, mortality from all cardiovascular diseases in the United States declined by 33

Table 1–3   Trends in mortality from ischemic heart disease, age-adjusted for persons aged 35–74 by sex and color, United States, 1968–1978

| | White | | Nonwhite | | |
Variable	Men	Women	Men	Women	All
All coronary heart disease[a]					
1968	875.5	342.8	868.2	569.3	598.4
1978	651.3	242.2	641.0	366.8	434.6
Change 1968–1978	− 224.2	− 100.6	− 227.2	− 202.5	− 163.8
Percentage change	− 25.6	− 29.3	− 26.2	− 35.6	− 27.4
Slope 1968–1973	− 0.0214	− 0.0254	− 0.0179	− 0.0200	− 0.0214
Standard error	0.0032	0.0026	0.0041	0.0104	0.0016
Slope 1973–1978	− 0.0392	− 0.0422	− 0.0424	− 0.0630	− 0.0412
Standard error	0.0019	0.0032	0.0056	0.0060	0.0027

Source: From Working Groups on Arteriosclerosis of the National Heart, Lung and Blood Institute (1981c), p 178, with permission.

[a] As defined by International Classification of Disease Codes 410–413.

percent, compared to only a 10 percent decline for other causes of death. The reasons for this decline are controversial but are probably related to changes in life-style and in therapeutic practice over the last 20 years.

Sex Differences in Ischemic Heart Disease Rates

Ischemic heart disease is most common in males; mortality for women is only about half that for men. The sex ratio is heavily dependent on age, showing the greatest disparity at younger ages, approaching unity at older ages. Figure 1–7 depicts the sex ratio of IHD mortality according to age in groups of countries where IHD mortality is very low, relatively low, moderate, or high. Where the disease is common (as in phase 4 countries), mortality shows a great comparative excess in younger males. Where the disease is uncommon (as in phase 1 and 2 countries) the sex ratio changes relatively little with age and the male disadvantage at younger ages is much diminished. The reasons for these mortality differences by sex and in particular the differences in the sex ratio with age are not well understood, but are only partly explained by more favorable values for smoking habits, blood pressure (below the age of 50), and high-density lipoprotein (HDL) cholesterol (chapter 4) in females (Wingard et al, 1983).

Ischemic Heart Disease in U.S. Racial Minorities

Within the same geographic area of the United States, different racial groups may experience different rates of disease. Death rates from IHD for black and for white males are quite similar at present, but the trends of increase and then decrease over the past 30 years have been more prominent in blacks (Fig. 1–8 and 1–9). Black females have substantially higher mortality for ischemic heart disease as compared to white females and again have shown more exaggerated trends of rising and falling mortality.

The next largest racial minority in the United States is the Spanish-surnamed population. Information is sparse, but Stern and Gaskill (1978) reported that in Bexar County, Texas, mortality from ischemic heart disease in the Hispanic males and females is about 20 percent and 10 percent lower, respectively, than in other whites. He found that this racial group also shared in the decline in ischemic heart disease mortality over recent years.

International Differences in Ischemic Heart Disease Mortality

Different parts of the world show remarkable differences in IHD mortality (Figs. 1–10 and 1–11). This is a key piece of evidence for the influence of environment on the risk of developing IHD. However, such evidence cannot deny the possibility of major genetic influences in addition. In general, industrialized Western countries with high income levels are those at highest risk. Finland and Scotland usually take top "honors." The Mediterranean countries with slightly lower standards of living and industrialization have comparatively modest IHD mortality rates. Rates in Japan are strikingly low compared to the United States. Very little information concerning IHD rates in Third World countries is available, but it appears they are usually negligible except in the highest socio-economic classes. The major hypotheses that attempt to explain these differences, focus on differences in intake of certain nutrients, the amount of physical activity, and the frequency of hypertension. Cigarette smoking probably contributes to risk, particularly when other suboptimal life-styles coexist.

The Evidence for Environmental Causal Agents in Ischemic Heart Disease

Over the last 200 years there have been several mass migrations of people from one country to another. Often this represents the movement of people of one genetic stock, from a particular environment and associated life-style to a contrasting situation. Since the environment and life-style change while genotype remains constant, these movements can be used as "experiments on the grandest scale" to test the nurture portion of nature–nurture hypotheses. Examples include migrations of the British to British Commonwealth countries, people of diverse origins to the United States, Japanese across the Pacific to Hawaii and the mainland United States, Pacific Islanders to New Zealand, and Jews from many places back to Israel. The latter three are of particular interest as they represent migrations from environments associated with low IHD risk to those associated with high risk. One major study along these lines, the Ni-Hon-San

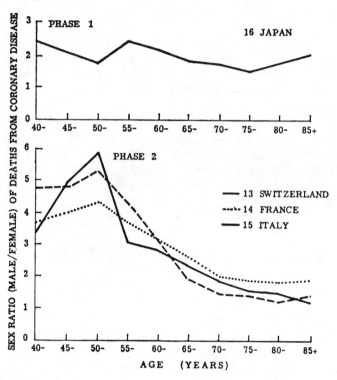

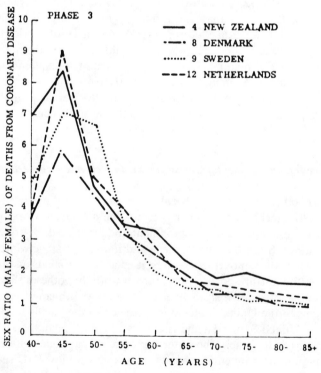

Study, was based on the migration of Japanese across the Pacific. It is described in some detail here because its results will be referred to in several later chapters.

Japanese Migrating Across the Pacific

The Ni-Hon-San Study (Marmot et al, 1975; Worth et al, 1975; Yano et al, 1979) identified three cohorts of Japanese men aged 45–69 years, who lived in southern Japan, Honolulu, or San Francisco. Data collection started in 1965. The group in Japan consisted of 2138 men (an 80 percent response of those eligible) who lived in Hiroshima and Nagasaki and were part of an ongoing epidemiologic investigation of the effects of radiation on health (radiation appears to have no effect on the development of ischemic heart disease). The Honolulu cohort consisted of 8006 men living on the island of Oahu in 1965 (a 72 percent

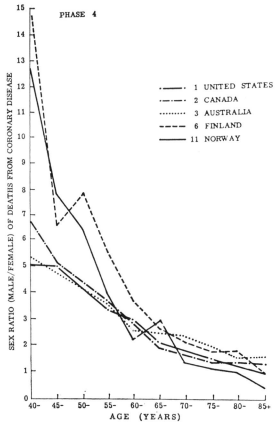

Figure 1-7 Sex ratio (M/F) of death rates from coronary artery disease (1954) by countries grouped according to overall standardized ischemic heart disease mortality. From RM Acheson: The etiology of coronary heart disease. *Yale J Bio Med* **35**:146, 1962, with permission.

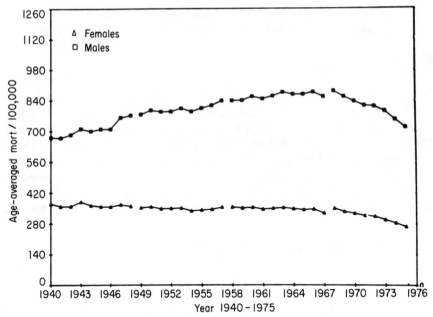

Figure 1–8 Age-adjusted ischemic heart disease mortality, United States: Whites aged 35–74 years. Reprinted with permission from *J Chron Dis* **31**:709. R Cooper et al: The decline in mortality from coronary heart disease, USA 1968–1975, 1978. Pergamon Press, Ltd.

response of those eligible). The San Francisco group was found by a special census in the eight San Francisco Bay Area counties. Of the 2733 Japanese men found, 1842 entered the study (a 68 percent response of those eligible).

At the outset, methods were standardized between cohorts; a central coding lab for electrocardiograms was used as well as common questionnaire and record forms, written in Japanese if necessary. Appropriate baseline measurements were made for each subject, and biennial examinations were performed in the southern Japan and Honolulu cohorts. The Californian cohort was not routinely reexamined (see below). The follow-up of each cohort noted the occurrence of clinical events in men initially free of IHD. As the sample in Japan was small, at each biennial examination younger men were added and older men subtracted to maintain the age of the cohort at risk in the range 45–69 years. In effect, three sequential studies were performed in Japan, each like the one in Honolulu. In Japan, diagnoses were based on researching the circumstances of any deaths and also noting electrocardiographic changes at the 2-year follow-up examination. In Hawaii, the procedures were similar, but in addition, hospital records were surveyed to gain a fuller ascertainment of myocardial infarctions. In California, deaths were researched, and any positive histories of chest pain or hospitalization, as determined by a mail questionnaire, were fully investigated.

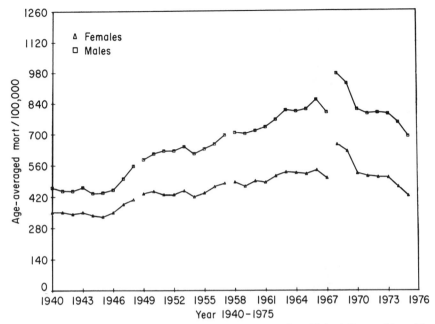

Figure 1–9   Age-adjusted ischemic heart disease mortality, United States: Nonwhites 35–74 years. Reprinted with permission from *J Chron Dis* **31**:709. R Cooper et al: The decline in mortality from coronary heart disease, USA 1968–1975, 1978. Pergamon Press, Ltd.

Thus, follow-up methods were not identical in the three cohorts. Nevertheless, the same criteria for morbidity could be used when comparing either the Japan–Hawaii or Hawaii–California groups. It was possible to compare IHD mortality across all three cohorts simultaneously.

An important question is whether these cohorts were indeed genetically similar. The similarity in the relative proportions of the different blood types gives some evidence to support this (Table 1–4). It is relevant to note that most of the migrants had come from southern Japan, the location of the cohort in Japan.

The *prevalence* of IHD manifestations in each cohort at study baseline is shown in Table 1–5. Definite and possible IHD are ascertained by Minnesota coding (see pp. 25–26) of electrocardiograms and possible infarction and angina pectoris by the Rose questionnaire (see pp. 26–27). There is a consistent trend from Japan to Hawaii to California of increased prevalence for each IHD syndrome defined. However, the interpretation of such prevalence results is complicated by the possibility of differences in survival after developing IHD between the three cohorts. This is because prevalence is dependent on both incidence and survival time.

Ischemic heart disease mortality is an incidence type of measure, and thus mortality trends are easier to interpret (Worth et al, 1975). The same trend for this variable is apparent, but notice the remarkable reverse trend for stroke

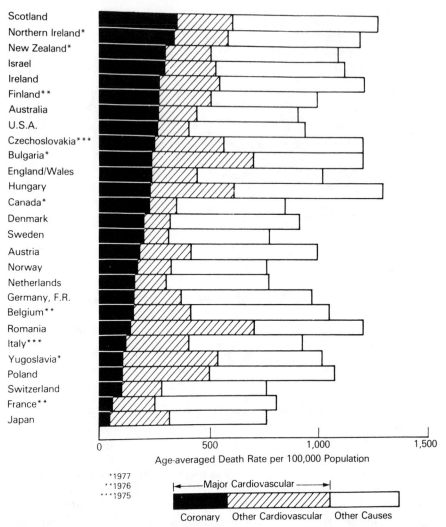

Figure 1–10 Death rates for all causes of death, for coronary heart disease, and for other major cardiovascular diseases: Women, aged 35–74, by country. From Working Group on Arteriosclerosis of the National Heart, Lung and Blood Institute, 1981b, p 514, with permission.

mortality (Table 1–6). These trends for both IHD and stroke are of environmental origin, as there is no evidence of genetic differences or reason to suspect such.

Further evidence of the environmental etiology of these differences in IHD is shown by the following analysis. Japanese in Hawaii show a diversity of Japanese cultural identity. This is manifested by differences in dietary habits, as well as their ability to speak and write the Japanese language. The latter skills are certainly not genetically determined but are probably markers of different

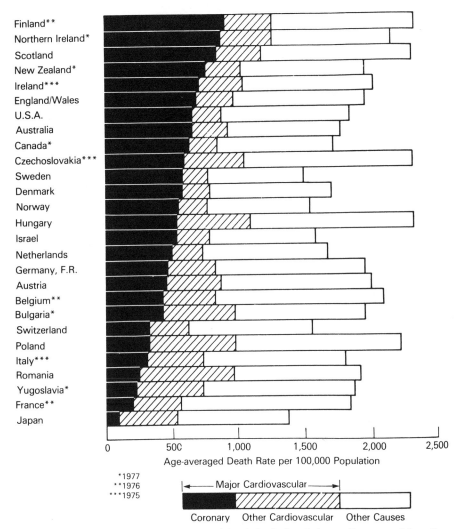

Figure 1–11 Death rates for all causes of death for ischemic heart disease, and for other major cardiovascular diseases: Men, aged 35–74, by country. From Working Group on Arteriosclerosis of the National Heart, Lung and Blood Institute, 1981b, p 514, with permission.

cultural *environments*. Analysis of IHD disease rates according to these variables shows interesting differences favoring those retaining more traditional Japanese ties (Table 1–7).

Jewish Immigrants to Israel

Toor and colleagues (1957) studied Yemenite immigrants to Israel. They divided the Yemenites into "early" immigrants who had arrived in Israel more

Table 1–4 Distribution of ABO blood groups in the three cohorts of the Ni-Hon-San Study

	Distribution (%)		
Blood group	Japan	Hawaii	California
O	29	30	30
A	42	39	40
A	20	21	21
AB	9	10	9

Source: Reprinted with permission from *J Chron Dis* **27**:345. A Kagan et al: Epidemiologic studies of CHD and stroke in Japanese men living in Japan, Hawaii and California, 1974. Pergamon Press, Ltd.

Table 1–5 Prevalence of ischemic heart disease as determined by ECG and standard questionnaire for Japanese males by geographic location

Observational base and diagnosis	Age-adjusted prevalence/1000		
	Japan	Hawaii	California
ECG			
Definite CHD[a]	5.3	5.2	10.8
Definite and possible CHD[b]	25.4	34.7	44.6
Questionnaire			
Angina pectoris[c]	11.2	14.3	25.3
Possible infarction[c]	7.3	13.2	31.4
(Number of men)	(2141)	(8003)	(1834)

Source: From MG Marmot et al: Epidemiologic studies of CHD and stroke in Japanese men living in Japan, Hawaii and California. *Am J Epidemiol* **102**:514, 1975, with permission.

[a] Major Q/QS abnormalities: Minnesota Codes 1-1-1 through 1-1-7.

[b] Definite and possible CHD = major and minor Q/QS abnormalities: Minnesota Codes 1-1-1 through 1-3-6.

[c] Cardiovascular questionnaire (Rose and Blackburn, 1968).

than 20 years before or "late" immigrants who had arrived within the preceding 5 years. These two groups had consequently had very different exposures to a more Western way of life but were from the same racial stock. Although religious and many social customs were similar for both groups, the early

Table 1–6   Mortality from all causes, from strokes, and from ischemic heart disease for the three cohorts of the Ni-Hon-San Study

Age at death	Cause of death	Mortality (%)			
		Japan 1965–1970	Honolulu 1966–1970	San Francisco 1968–1970	P
50–54	All	9.4	4.5	3.3	0.001
	Strokes	1.4	0.5	...	n.s.[a]
	IHD	0.4	1.1	1.3	n.s.
55–59	All	13.9	7.6	13.9	0.001
	Strokes	1.5	0.9	0.5	n.s.
	IHD	1.4	1.7	4.8	0.01
60–64	All	24.5	13.7	14.8	0.001
	Strokes	5.4	1.1	2.5	0.001
	IHD	2.1	3.9	4.9	0.05

Source: From RM Worth et al: Epidemiologic studies of CHD and stroke in Japanese men living in Japan, Hawaii and California. *Am J Epidemiol* **102**:481, 1975, with permission.

[a] n.s., not significant.

migrants ate substantially more animal fat and consumed more calories and were also economically much better off. Mortality from atherosclerosis was about four times higher in the early immigrants on an age- and sex-specific basis. Serum cholesterol levels were also consistently higher in this group.

Pacific Islanders Migrating to New Zealand

The Polynesian peoples also show remarkable differences in IHD mortality apparently associated with different environments, as genetic studies indicate a common genetic stock (Simmons, 1966). Ischemic heart disease is very uncommon in islanders not exposed to European life-styles. An example is the atoll of Pukapuka, Cook Islands. Abnormal Q waves were found in only 0.4 percent of Pukapukan males, but in 3.9 percent of Rarotongan males, who live a less traditional life-style (Prior, 1974). By contrast, the Polynesian Maori of New Zealand have been exposed to strong European influence for more than a century. The New Zealand Maori has a relatively high mortality from IHD (Beaglehole et al, 1978), with the indication that Maori females have the highest female IHD death rates in the world.

Spouse Concordance in Framingham

This question of environmental influences is also illuminated by some information from the Framingham Study, which is a well-known longitudinal study of cardiovascular disease within a single U.S. community (see chapter 4). Kannel

Table 1–7 Six-year incidence of coronary heart disease (CHD) by categories of selected cultural variables: the Honolulu Heart Study

		Incidence rate (per 1000)[b]		
Variable	Population at risk[a]	All CHD	CHD death + MI	Coronary insufficiency + angina pectoris
Birthplace (age 60–68 only)				
Japan (Issei)	729	45.9	28.9	17.0
Other (Nisei)	965	74.7	43.0	31.7
P value (trend)[c]		<0.05	n.s.[d]	n.s.
Read/write Japanese				
None	2697	51.3	31.5	19.8
Very little	2001	46.1	27.0	19.0
Fair	1028	25.5	17.9	7.6
Well	1972	28.3	17.5	10.8
P value (trend)[c]		<0.01	<0.01	<0.01
Speak Japanese				
None	146	57.8	29.5	28.3
Very little	913	30.6	14.0	16.6
Fair	2705	45.4	28.0	17.4
Well	3939	34.9	22.1	12.8
P value (trend)[c]		<0.05	n.s.	<0.01

Source: Adapted from K Yano et al: Childhood cultural experience and the incidence of CHD in Hawaii Japanese men. *Am J. Epidemiol* **109**:440, 1979, with permission.

[a] Sample sizes for different variables differ slightly because of unknown values.

[b] Rates are adjusted for age by direct method.

[c] By the method of Mantel and Haenszel for two categories, and the method of Mantel for more than two categories.

[d] n.s., not significant.

(1976) found that when the husband has developed ischemic heart disease, the wife was also more likely to develop this disorder, and vice versa (Fig. 1–12). When the Framingham cohort were of the usual marrying age, determinants of IHD risk were unknown. Thus, it was unlikely that courting couples would be able to select spouses of higher or lower risk status, even if they had wanted to do so. The most plausible explanation is that spouses share a common environment for many years that influences the likelihood of developing ischemic heart disease.

In summary, there are indications that environmental (both physical and social, including habits such as diet and smoking) influences have a major influence on the risk of developing ischemic heart disease. This highlights the

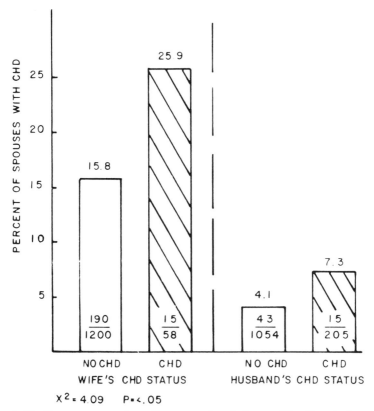

Figure 1–12 Spouse aggregation of coronary heart disease. The Framingham Study. From WB Kannel, 1976, with permission.

need for prevention by manipulation of both personal and community environments.

Summary

1. Ischemic heart disease causes more mortality and probably more serious morbidity than any other disease. This is true in the United States and most other westernized countries.

2. The economic costs of IHD are about $50 billion annually in the United States.

3. Ischemic heart disease has probably existed since antiquity and may not have been uncommon in some classes of ancient society. In the United States and several other countries, recent secular trends include a modest rise in IHD mortality from 1950 to 1968, and subsequently a continuing decline in mortality

(2–3 percent per year) now accounting for a more than 30 percent decline over the high point of 1968.

4. The male/female ratio among ischemic heart disease victims is particularly high in young persons (in countries where the disease is common). With aging the ratio is usually closer to unity.

5. International differences in IHD mortality are striking and demand explanation.

6. Evidence from migration studies (similar genes but differing environments) suggest that environmental influences are an important cause of this disorder. This raises the possibility of prevention by manipulation of both personal and community environments.

2

Defining Ischemic Heart Disease Syndromes

Evaluating medical research usually involves comparisons of results from studies that differ in time and place. A common frustration in such comparisons is the lack of a standardized definition of the disease under investigation. Even more serious, if less common, is the lack of clearly defined diagnostic criteria within individual studies. This is particularly relevant to a disease such as ischemic heart disease, which is manifested in many ways and produces many borderline cases. This chapter deals with IHD diagnostic criteria and two methods (clinical history and electrocardiogram) suitable for assessing these criteria in population studies. Comment is also made on efforts to standardize their application.

Diagnostic Criteria

Several groups have formulated criteria for diagnosing acute MI in epidemiologic research. The World Health Organization published a set of criteria (WHO Working Party Report, 1969) that has been used by several myocardial infarction registers (*Myocardial Infarction Community Registers*, 1976). Recently revised criteria for most categories of IHD have been published by the Joint International Society and Federation of Cardiology/WHO Task Force on Standardization of Clinical Nomenclature (1979). This system divides coronary syndromes into primary cardiac arrest, angina pectoris, MI, heart failure, and arrhythmias resulting from IHD.

1. *Primary cardiac arrest* is usually a sudden event presumed to be the result of electrical instability of the heart.
2. *Angina pectoris* may be of two types. *Angina of effort* is characterized by transient episodes of chest pain precipitated by recognizable circumstances (e.g., exercise). It is subdivided as follows:

- *De novo effort angina* (angina of less than 1 month's duration),
- Stable-effort angina (angina of more than 1 month's duration), and
- *Worsening-effort angina* (a sudden worsening in frequency, severity, or duration of angina, caused by the same effort).

23

Spontaneous angina is angina that has no recognizable provocation. The pain tends to last longer, be more severe, and be less readily relieved by nitroglycerine.

De novo and worsening-effort angina are sometimes grouped with spontaneous angina as different forms of *unstable angina*. Spontaneous angina is sometimes labeled *acute coronary insufficiency*.

3. *Myocardial infarction* is diagnosed by the history of chest pain, the electrocardiogram, and the serum enzymes changes. The history is typical if severe and prolonged anterior chest pain is present. Unequivocal changes in the electrocardiogram include abnormal, persistent Q or QS waves and an evolving injury current (ST elevation) lasting longer than 1 day. Equivocal changes consist of a stationary injury current, a symmetrical inverted T wave, a pathologic Q wave in a single ECG record, or conduction disturbances. Unequivocal changes in serum enzymes consist of a serial change, usually an initial rise and subsequent fall of the serum level. The change must be properly related to the delay between the onset of symptoms and blood sampling for the particular enzyme. Elevated levels of cardio-specific isoenzymes are also an unequivocal change. A diagnosis of *definite acute myocardial infarction* is indicated by unequivocal electrocardiographic changes, unequivocal enzyme changes, or both; the history may be typical or atypical. *Possible acute myocardial infarction* should be considered when serial equivocal electrocardiographic changes persist for more than 24 hours. The history may be typical or atypical, and equivocal enzyme changes may be present. A diagnosis of *old myocardial infarction* is based on current abnormal Q or QS patterns on the electrocardiograph or on earlier typical electrocardiographs or previous enzyme changes if the current electrocardiograph is not diagnostic.

Sudden cardiac death, though not listed in the above classification, is a commonly used term. It includes *primary cardiac arrest* and a portion of both *definite* and *possible myocardial infarction* of the above-listed categories. Sudden death has been defined variously but usually represents deaths within a fixed period after the onset of acute symptoms, for example, 1 hour, 6 hours, or 24 hours. Acute symptoms may include chest pain, collapse, or breathlessness. One set of criteria is as follows (Fraser, 1978a): Sudden cardiac death can be defined as death within 24 hours of some distinct change in the patient's state of health, provided

- The new symptoms were consistent with a primary cardiac cause for the change in health status.
- The patient had not been bedridden during the 24 hours before the symptomatic change.
- The new symptoms may have constituted the fatal event.
- A postmortem examination reveals no pathologic changes indicating that IHD was *not* the primary cause of death.
- There was no history or antemortem physical findings of severe valvular

dysfunction or other nonischemic cardiac disease that may have caused the death.

Diagnostic Methods Used in Population Studies

It is necessary to study disease in a whole community to gain a representative view of the disease process. The combination of the broad perspective of epidemiologic work in the community and the more detailed research of basic and clinical sciences inevitably develops further insights into the disease process. For field and population work, expensive, invasive tests involving heavy nontransportable equipment are impractical. We need easily understood, repeatable tests and convenient equipment. Ideally data should be suitable for collection (but not necessarily interpretation) by nonprofessionals.

One diagnostic criterion suitable for community studies is the history. This use of the history has been extensively explored by Geoffrey Rose, who developed a simple questionnaire (the London School of Hygiene questionnaire) of seven items (Fig. 2–1) to screen for angina pectoris. Rose compared the questionnaire results with the opinions of a small group of expert physicians and also the agreement *between* physicians making this diagnosis (Rose, 1962). His conclusions were somewhat unsettling. The study subjects were 57 men who reported during a medical interview that they sometimes had chest pain. The men were between 40 and 55 years old and had no other evidence of IHD. They were recalled for an interview with each of the three experienced physicians, who had no information about the patients except that which they gathered in the interview. Their task was to decide whether the patients had angina or not. They did not discuss results among themselves. The physicians agreed unanimously on only 43 of the 57 cases (75 percent). For comparability between studies, diagnostic methods ideally need better repeatability than this. Of the 26 unanimous physician-negative cases, all were also classified as negative by the questionnaire. Of the 17 unanimous physician-positive cases, 14 were similarly classified by the questionnaire. Thus, as compared to the physicians, the questionnaire showed reasonable sensitivity (83 percent) and very high specificity. It identified almost the same cases as those the physicians selected unanimously.

These findings encouraged the wide use of the London School of Hygiene Questionnaire in population studies (Rose et al, 1982). Although its ability to distinguish between angina and esophageal pain has been questioned (Areskog, 1981; Tibbling, 1981), Rose has shown that the questionnaire can separate a population into groups with higher and lower subsequent IHD mortality (Rose et al, 1977). Of 938 men in this study, 3.8 percent died of myocardial infarction over the follow-up period. However, of those who initially scored positive for angina or possible myocardial infarction on the London School of Hygiene questionnaire, 17 percent died of myocardial infarction during the follow-up. Even for "all cause" mortality, Rose found a clear difference between mortality for the total group (7.1 percent) and mortality for those who scored positively

(a) **Have you ever had any pain or discomfort in your chest?**
    1. ☐ Yes   2. ☐ No (Go to C)

(b) **Do you get this pain or discomfort when you walk uphill or hurry?**
    1. ☐ Yes   2. ☐ No (Go to B)

(c) **Do you get it when you walk at an ordinary pace on the level?**
    1. ☐ Yes   2. ☐ No

(d) **When you get any pain or discomfort in your chest what do you do?**
    1. ☐ Stop
    2. ☐ Slow down
    3. ☐ Continue at the same pace

(e) **Does it go away when you stand still?**
    1. ☐ Yes   2. ☐ No

(f) **How soon?**
    1. ☐ 10 minutes or less
    2. ☐ More than 10 minutes

(g) **Where do you get this pain or discomfort?**
Mark the place(s) with X on the diagram.

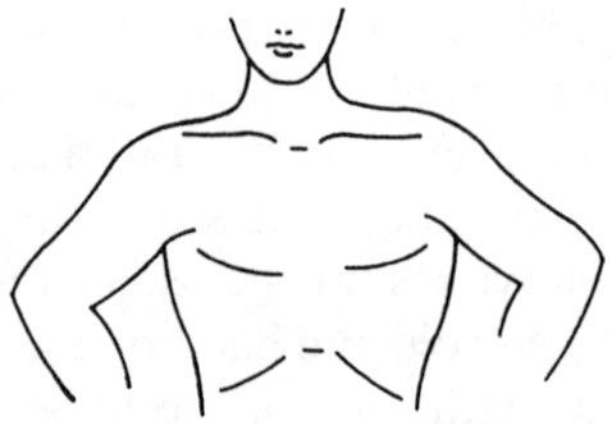

DEFINITION OF POSITIVE CLASSIFICATION

Angina 'Yes' to a and b, 'stop' or 'slow down' to d, 'yes' to e, '10 minutes or less' to f. Site must include *either* sternum (any level) *or* L. anterior chest and left arm. GRADE 1='no' to c, GRADE 2='yes' to c.

Figure 2–1   London School of Hygiene questionnaire for angina pectoris. Adapted from GA Rose et al: Self-administration of a questionnaire on chest pain and intermittent claudication. *Br J Prev Soc Med* **31**:42, 1977, with permission.

on the questionnaire (21 percent). A similar study of 1428 Welsh *women* (Campbell et al, 1984) has demonstrated that angina as determined by the questionnaire predicts higher subsequent cardiovascular and overall mortality also in women, particularly for the 45–54 age group. The general validity of this questionnaire has been demonstrated by correlation with the unanimous opinions of a small group of expert physicians and by its capacity to predict subsequent mortality.

The electrocardiogram is another important diagnostic tool in population research of IHD. It is cheap, noninvasive, and often gives important information. However, it is a complex record, and for consistent interpretation and comparability, measurement and coding techniques must be standardized.

The standardized coding scheme in widest use is the Minnesota Code (Prineas et al, 1982; Rose et al, 1982). It describes any electrocardiogram in terms of a number of discrete numerical codes.. These codes pertain to most aspects of the 12-lead electrocardiogram, including the P wave, QRS complex, ST segment, T wave, and arrhythmias. Measurements are carefully made with a magnifying lens. For instance, an electrocardiogram showing a P–R interval of 0.23 seconds in lead I, a Q-wave duration of 0.04 seconds in lead V_2, a Q/R ratio greater than one-third, an ST (J point) depression of 1.5 mm with a horizontal ST segment, and a negative T wave of 2 mm in lead I, would be coded 6-3; 1-1-2; 4-1-2; 5-2. The Minnesota Code was not originally designed to diagnose new myocardial infarction. However, diagnostic criteria for acute infarction based only on acute changes in the Minnesota Codes for Q, ST, and T items are highly sensitive though somewhat lacking in specificity (Smitherman et al, 1981), when compared to usual clinical criteria. Of course, electrocardiographic Q waves are most specific but need to be backed by symptoms and enzyme values. Uusitupa et al (1983) examined the records of 1194 patients who died but had an ECG recorded shortly before death, and found that of recent and old infarctions diagnosed at autopsy, 71 percent and 49 percent, respectively, are also found by Minnesota Code Q-wave or T-wave abnormalities. Conversely, of persons with no infarction at autopsy, 12 percent had Q waves. Reasons for these inconsistencies include disappearance of acute ECG changes of infarction with time, absence of Q waves in a substantial proportion of both transmural and subendocardial infarctions, and other conditions being associated with Q waves such as cardiomyopathy or pulmonary disease.

Another computerized multivariate scoring system, based on the 12-lead electrocardiogram, permits the diagnosis of new and old myocardial infarction with high sensitivity and specificity (Rautaharju et al, 1981). Rautaharju and colleagues claim that the index would be a useful instrument in following persons with established coronary disease for evidence of further, possibly subclinical, progression of cardiac damage. The resting electrocardiogram can also predict survival of postmyocardial infarction patients over the succeeding 3 years (Bounous et al, 1981; Wagner et al, 1982).

Summary

1. Standardized nomenclature and diagnostic criteria are essential for comparisons across different studies.

2. Ischemic heart disease is manifested in several different ways, each syndrome needing quite complex diagnostic criteria.

3. A standardized questionnaire for angina pectoris suitable for population studies is available.

4. Electrocardiograms are an important part of the diagnostic criteria for IHD. They are a complex record, and the Minnesota coding is a standardized technique for reading them.

3

The Pathologic Basis of Ischemic Heart Disease— Clues from Comparative Pathology

Atherosclerotic coronary artery obstruction and the expression of clinical IHD seem to have a cause–effect relationship. Indeed in the eyes of some this is virtually a one-to-one correspondence, so that coronary artery pathologic findings are often regarded as the disease, and treatment is directed only to this aspect of the problem. Obstructed coronary arteries can also be seen as a risk factor for IHD, albeit an important one, as the correspondence between obstructive pathologic findings and clinical disease is not complete. Ischemic heart disease syndromes in the absence of important atherosclerotic obstructive abnormality are well documented. Conversely, one frequently sees at autopsy severe obstructive disease with no antemortem history of a clinical syndrome. The same degree of obstructive abnormality in different individuals produces different results, probably depending on the individual coronary anatomy and autonomic nervous system reactivity, blood pressure, collateral blood supply, left ventricular hypertrophy, platelet aggregability, coronary artery diameter, tendency to coronary artery spasm, and perhaps blood coagulability. This chapter will discuss the origins of the atherosclerotic plaque and explore the evidence on the relationship between obstructive coronary pathology and the clinical expression of this disease.

The Origins of the Atherosclerotic Plaque

Atherosclerosis affects large and medium-sized muscular arteries, also large elastic arteries. The atherosclerotic plaque is a raised lesion present on the luminal surface of the affected artery, and consists of an inner core of lipids and a covering fibrous cap. The plaque becomes clinically significant when as a result of continued increases in size it causes obstruction of the vessel, or when it ulcerates and causes the formation of thrombi or emboli. In the aorta it may lead to aneurysm formation (a result of weakening of the vessel's wall at the site of the plaque) (Robbins and Cotran, 1979).

The mechanisms of formation and evolution of the atherosclerotic plaque are not fully understood at this time. The fatty streak may be a precursor of the plaque, but this has not been proven. Fatty streaks are elongated lesions

1–2 mm wide and up to 1 cm long. They are only slightly elevated above the intima of the vessel and are characterized by the deposition of lipid in the intima. Fatty streaks are present in the aortas of all children (this is a worldwide finding) by age 3 years (McGill, 1980). They may be found in the coronary arteries by age 10 years, in selected populations that have an increased incidence of atherosclerotic disease in adults. Fatty streaks tend to increase in number with advancing age. There are similarities between fatty streaks and plaques (e.g., site of occurrence, histologic structure), suggesting that the fatty streak is the forerunner of the plaque. There are, however, arguments against this theory. For example, fatty streaks occur as frequently in some populations with a relatively low incidence of atherosclerosis as in those with a high incidence of atherosclerosis (Robbins and Cotran, 1979). It may be that in populations at greatest risk of atherosclerosis the fatty streak progresses, while in those populations with a low incidence the lesion does not progress.

The many questions concerning the fate of the fatty streak are equaled by those questions concerning the pathogenesis of the fibrofatty plaque. The "response to injury" hypothesis is probably the most accepted of the different theories on its pathogenesis. However, before considering this, we should briefly examine the metabolism of lipoproteins.

Lipids are transported in the blood by lipoproteins as a lipid–lipoprotein complex, with the lipids forming a central core that is surrounded by lipoprotein. Lipoproteins transport both those lipids that are of dietary origin and those that are endogenous. Lipoproteins may be classified in different ways, for example, by electrophoretic mobility or sedimentation on centrifugation. Increased levels of lipoproteins may occur as a result of increased dietary intake or of abnormalities in lipid metabolism that may be inherited (both polygenic and monogenic mechanisms) or acquired abnormalities (e.g., diabetes mellitus) or a combination of both (i.e., increased intake and abnormal metabolism).

Five classes of lipoproteins have been identified: chylomicrons (CM) produced in the intestinal wall, very low-density lipoproteins (VLDL) produced in the liver, intermediate-density lipoproteins (IDL) formed as a result of catabolism of VLDL, low-density lipoproteins (LDL) formed as a result of catabolism of IDL, and high-density lipoproteins (HDL) originating in the liver and intestines. High-density lipoproteins may be further subdivided into HDL_2, the lighter subtype, and HDL_3, a heavier subtype (Gotto, 1982). The protein components of the lipoproteins are called apolipoproteins, and these have been divided into five subgroups: A, B, C, D, and E. The apolipoproteins are bound to the phospholipid component of the lipoprotein and are responsible (when combined with the phospholipid) for making soluble the components (unsterified cholesterol, cholesteryl ester, and triglyceride) of the core of the lipoprotein lipid complex. The apolipoproteins also activate the enzymes lipoprotein lipase (LPL) and lecithin cholesterol acyltransferase (LCAT), which are involved in the metabolism of lipoproteins (Gotto, 1982).

In normal subjects individual cells are thought to control the entry of cholesterol into each cell. When cells become deficient in cholesterol, they are thought to synthesize specific surface receptors for LDL. The greater the need of the cell for cholesterol, the greater the number of receptors synthesized (Goldstein and Brown, 1977). The LDL bind to the receptor and are taken into the cell by endocytosis. The endocytic vesicle migrates through the cytoplasm until it comes in contact with the lysosomes. The lysosomes contain hydrolytic enzymes that will hydrolyze the protein component of LDL to amino acids, and the cholesteryl ester to free cholesterol. Free cholesterol inhibits 3-hydroxy-3-methylglutaryl coenzyme A reductase (HMG CoA reductase), an enzyme that is a component of the cell's own cholesterol-synthesizing system, and suppresses cellular synthesis of cholesterol. Excess cholesterol that has been absorbed is stored as cholesteryl ester droplets after conversion by acyl-CoA: cholesterol acyltransferase (Goldstein and Brown, 1977).

Abnormalities of metabolism may occur at points along the pathway of LDL attachment to externally situated cell surface receptors, to its final metabolism intracellularly. Type II (familial) hypercholesterolemia occurs as a result of a deficiency in the number of receptors, or of a defect in the functioning of the receptors, or of a defect in endocytosis. Subjects who are heterozygous for the disease usually have 40 percent of the normal number of receptors, while homozygous subjects are more severely affected. The resulting inability to metabolize LDL normally causes marked increases in plasma cholesterol levels. In homozygotes, these high cholesterol levels are associated with myocardial infarcts before age 20 years (Goldstein and Brown, 1977).

Ross (1982) postulates that the atherosclerotic plaque develops as a result of chronic injury to the endothelial surface of the vessel. This injury may be a result of shear-stress to the endothelium in areas where blood flow is not laminar or may result from elevated blood pressure, viral infection, hypercholesterolemia, or other chronic insult (Robbins and Cotran, 1979). Permeability to plasma constituents increases at the sites of injury, and this results in the deposition of lipoproteins, platelets, and other plasma constituents at sites of injury. Smooth muscle cells are thought to migrate to and proliferate at sites of injury as a result of factors released by platelets. The smooth muscle cells deposit extracellular collagen, elastic tissue, and proteoglycans. Large amounts of cholesterol and cholesteryl esters accumulate inside the smooth muscle cells. The extracellular lipid may be derived from the plasma or may originate from muscle cells that have necrosed. The end result of these processes is a lesion with a fibrous cap of collagen, fat-laden macrophages, and smooth muscle, enclosing a disorganized central core of lipid, cholesterol, plasma proteins, and cellular debris. This is the atheromatous plaque (Robbins and Cotran, 1979). Regression of the lesion may occur resulting in the formation of a fibrous scar. The alternate course is further progression of the lesion leading to ulceration of the luminal surface with rupture of the lesion and discharge of the debris. Thrombi may form on the atherosclerotic plaque and these may embolize. Hemorrhage may occur into the plaque. An aneurysm may form below the plaque as a result of pressure atrophy affecting the underlying media of the vessel.

The Descriptive Epidemiology of the Atherosclerotic Lesion in Coronary Arteries

A major source of evidence is the International Atherosclerosis Project, which gathered the results of 22,509 unselected autopsies (14,606 males and 7903 females) in 19 different location–race groups. The age range was 10–69 years, and most cases came from large general hospitals, or medical examiners' offices. Unless otherwise indicated, pathologic findings discussed here refer only to persons dying from accidental or other acute causes unrelated to atherosclerosis (basal cases). This is necessary because IHD is a major cause of death, and if the hypothesis of association of IHD syndromes with coronary abnormalities is true, consideration of all deaths would bias autopsy results toward more extensive coronary disease. We are attempting to characterize the disease profile of a whole community, not only those dying. It will also be possible to compare the pathologic characteristics of those with and without diagnosed IHD within a single community from this and other studies.

The pathologic findings of the International Atherosclerosis Project were largely expressed as the percentage of the surface area of the coronary arteries having raised atherosclerotic lesions. The results clearly show that nearly all peoples have *some* underlying coronary atherosclerosis, but with different average severity of involvement (Figs. 3–1 and 3–2). Results are shown for four con-

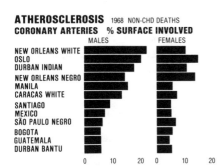

Figure 3–1 Percentage involvement of surface area of the coronary arteries with atherosclerosis in males and females at different geographic locations. Adapted from C Tejada et al, 1968, with permission.

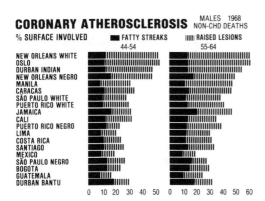

Figure 3–2 Percentage involvement of surface area of coronary arteries with fatty streaks and atherosclerosis in males aged 44–64, at different geographic locations. Adapted from C Tejada et al, 1968, with permission.

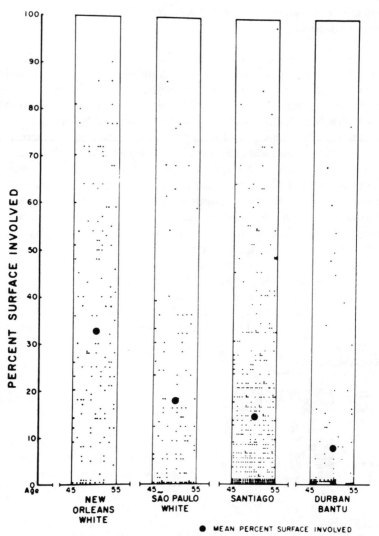

Figure 3–3 Variability of raised atherosclerotic lesions in the left anterior descending coronary arteries of men aged 45–54 years, living in four contrasting geographic locations. From C Tejada et al, 1968, with permission.

trasting communities in Fig. 3–3. This figure displays the diversity of the human organism in responding to what are presumably roughly similar environments, since within each location a wide range of abnormalities was seen. Of the 19 different race–location groups, the highest ranking community had about two to three times the disruption of arterial surface area by raised lesions as the lowest ranking community (Figs. 3–1 and 3–2). These rankings of average surface areas involved with raised lesions roughly follow expectations based on a dietary-acculturation etiologic hypothesis. Among the different communities the ranking of average surface areas involved with raised lesions in women correlates very highly with that in men (Fig. 3–1). In almost all communities, however, men have on average more intimal raised lesions than women. Where disease is uncommon, sex differences for coronary disease tend to be less marked. As the population ages, sex differences in disease incidence also become less marked (Strong et al, 1968). This accords with the characteristics of the clinical disease. Interestingly, there are no consistent sex differences in aortic disease (Tejada et al, 1968), so it seems that atherosclerosis at different anatomic sites does not necessarily have the same epidemiology. Differences in the severity of pathologic changes when comparing blacks with other races at the same location can be seen in New Orleans, Durban, São Paulo, and Puerto Rico. The blacks always rank considerably lower for extent of pathologic involvement, and the sex ratio is usually closer to unity (see Figs. 3–1 and 3–2).

There has been a long-standing debate over the relationship between fatty streaks and subsequent raised coronary lesions. The International Atherosclerosis Project indicates that fatty streaking does not differ systematically between communities within any one age range, but does become more common with advancing age in all communities (Fig. 3–2). By contrast, obstructive coronary lesions vary with age and in a systematic fashion between communities. Thus, it seems unlikely that there is a simple relationship between fatty streaks and the subsequent development of raised lesions. However, cross-sectional studies such as this cannot answer the question with certainty.

As with most other risk factors to be subsequently described in this book, there is evidence of recent apparently beneficial changes in the risk factor of coronary pathology. Strong and coworkers (1984) have very carefully compared the percent of intimal surface involvement of coronary arteries in several hundred autopsies of black and white males in New Orleans during two different time periods. As compared to 1960–64 results, white males showed about 50 percent less average lesion involvement in 1969–78; this was true in each of four different age groups between 25 and 44 years. Results in black males were very different, with the trend being to slight increases in lesional involvement.

The Relationship Between Obstructive Coronary Pathology and Clinical Disease

Probably the most important observation from the International Atherosclerosis Project is that the ranking of arterial surface involvement with raised lesions, between communities, corresponds quite well to the ranking of mortality ascribed to atherosclerotic heart disease (Table 3–1). Of course, in clinical cardiology we are usually more interested in the severity of stenotic lesions than the percentage of arterial surface area showing raised lesions, and there is good

Table 3–1 Ranking of nine cities based on mean percentage of coronary arterial surface involvement with atherosclerosis at autopsy (basal cases), compared with the ranking of IHD mortality, in men aged 45–64 years[a]

	Age group							
	45–54				55–64			
Location-race group	Surface involved with RL (*mean* %)	Rank	Mortality	Rank	Surface involved with RL (*mean* %)	Rank	Mortality	Rank
North American city[b]	29.8	1	310	1	32.0	1	878	1
Caracas	13.3	3	122	2	21.5	2	474	2
São Paulo[c]	14.3	2	120	3	19.8	3	397	3
Cali	13.1	4	92	6	13.8	6	260	7
Lima	10.3	7	94	5	17.0	5	244	8
Santiago	11.5	6	75	8	17.6	4	370	5
Mexico	11.8	5	83	7	12.1	7	281	6
Bogotá	6.8	8	109	4	11.0	8	381	4
Guatemala	5.7	9	43	9	10.5	9	110	9

Source: From C Tejada et al, 1968, with permission.

[a] Mortality per 100,000 from Interamerican Investigation of Mortality, 1966. RL, raised lesions.

[b] Arterial lesions for New Orleans whites; mortality for San Francisco (all races, but predominantly whites).

[c] Arterial lesions for São Paulo whites; mortality for São Paulo (all races, but predominantly whites).

theoretical justification for this. It is true, however, that in general persons with severe stenotic lesions also have rather diffuse involvement of the coronary arteries. Table 3–2 shows the percentage with one or more stenoses of the coronary arteries obliterating at least 50 percent of the lumen. This measure was available only at the locations shown. Again, some correspondence can be seen between this pathologic measure and IHD mortality. However, it seems that of the countries shown, the clearest difference lies between those with low- and mid-range IHD death rates and North America (high IHD death rate).

Keys and colleagues (1958a) reported on 1211 consecutive autopsies obtained from Minnesota, Hawaii, and Fukuoka, Japan. Careful attention was given to comparability of methods and pathologic grading of the severity of coronary atherosclerosis. The results for men aged 50–69 years shows that more than 65 percent of Caucasian men (both Minnesotan and Hawaiian) had severe coronary atherosclerosis (Mayo Clinic grades 3 and 4). Only about 30 percent of Hawaiian Japanese men and 10 percent of Japanese in Japan showed similar pathologic changes. Similar ranking was shown for men aged 30–39 and 40–49

Table 3–2 Nine cities ranked by IHD mortality, showing percentage of basal cases with at least one significantly stenosed coronary artery at autopsy in men aged 45–64 years

			Age group		
	45–54			55–64	
Location	IHD mortality (per 100,000)	More than one vessel stenotic (%)	Location	IHD mortality (per 100,000)	More than one vessel stenotic (%)
North America	310	20	North America	878	32
Caracas	122	8	Caracas	474	7
São Paulo	120	10	São Paulo	397	8
Bogotá	109	0	Bogotá	381	0
Lima	94	3	Santiago	370	13
Cali	92	0	Mexico	281	8
Mexico	83	0	Cali	260	3
Santiago	75	6	Lima	244	6
Guatemala	43	2	Guatemala	110	6

Source: Adapted from C Tejada et al, 1968, with permission.

years. Death rates from IHD are known to follow a similar ranking for these three locations. Tejada et al (1968) reviewed several other studies that either compared coronary pathologic changes between two or more populations or compared two ethnic groups at the same location. He concluded that these studies also supported the hypothesis that severe coronary atherosclerosis is closely related to the frequency of clinical IHD.

It is naturally of interest to know what the coronary artery involvement was in cases diagnosed as having clinical ischemic heart disease. Figure 3–4 illustrates this from the International Atherosclerosis Project in two locations, Santiago and Oslo. In each city, pathologic changes were more severe in the IHD patients than in those not having this diagnosis, but even within the IHD groups there was a great deal of variability of the percentage of surface area having raised lesions. It is interesting to note that even within the groups diagnosed as having IHD, the distribution of coronary lesions differed between the two locations. In the "westernized" communities of this study, most IHD fatalities had some pathologic changes in all three vessels. However, in communities where clinical IHD is uncommon only 50 percent of IHD fatalities showed some pathologic change in all three vessels, and in a significant proportion no vessel had more than 10 percent surface area involvement (Fig. 3–5). Here again the multifactorial nature of the clinical syndrome may be seen.

Diamond and Forrester (1979) reported on the prevalence of coronary abnormalities among the asymptomatic U.S. population, amalgamating results from several studies representing a total of 23,996 autopsies. The prevalence of signi-

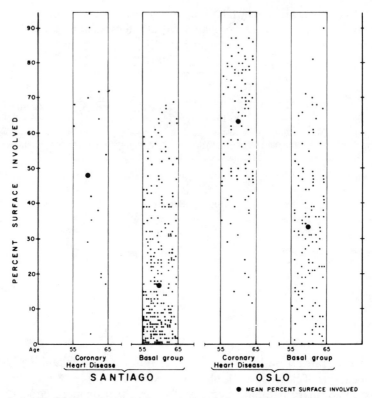

Figure 3–4 Variability of raised atherosclerotic lesions of the coronary arteries of men aged 55–65 experiencing death from IHD or non-IHD (basal group) causes at Oslo and Santiago. From JP Strong et al, 1968, with permission.

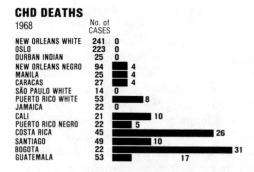

Figure 3–5 Percentage of deaths ascribed to IHD with less than 10 percent atherosclerotic surface involvement of all coronary arteries, at different geographic locations. From JP Strong et al, 1968, with permission.

ficant coronary artery stenosis in men ranged progressively from 1.9 to 12.3 percent as age increased from 30–39 to 60–69 years. Corresponding figures for women were 0.3–7.5 percent. Much more information is available from studies of persons with classical angina pectoris or post-myocardial infarction. Gibson

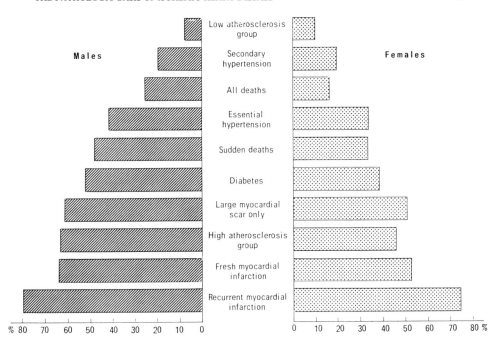

Figure 3-6 Comparison of the percentage of autopsies with coronary stenosis in the low atherosclerosis group, to groups dying of IHD or from causes of death associated with IHD. All towns combined. Age-standardized. From AM Vihert, 1976, with permission of World Health Organization.

and Beller (1983) show the results of five angiographic studies of middle-aged persons with classical angina pectoris or with nonanginal chest pain. The results across studies are quite consistent: 80–96 percent of patients with typical angina have significant coronary obstructions, whereas only 4–16 percent of those with nonanginal pain have such obstructions. Thus, it appears from both angiographic and autopsy studies that about 10 percent of typical angina patients have no significant coronary artery obstructions and that 10–15 percent of middle-aged men have significant coronary artery stenoses, without symptoms.

A study similar to the International Atherosclerosis Project was sponsored by the World Health Organization (Kagan et al, 1976). This compared all autopsied deaths from Malmo (Sweden), Prague (Czechoslovakia), and Ryazan, Yalta, and Tallin (all in the Soviet Union). The average autopsy rate among these communities was 76.8 percent. Figure 3–6 shows the relative frequency of coronary stenoses according to the patient's clinical diagnosis antemortem. The comparison group is a "low atherosclerosis" group of cases dying from causes not related to atherosclerosis or causes not thought to influence its course. Clearly, hypertensives and diabetics have more coronary artery abnormalities than the "low atherosclerosis group." In chapter 9 we will see that hypertension is a well-established risk factor for clinical IHD syndromes. It is also well known that diabetics are commonly prone to the manifestations of ischemic heart disease. Thus, it is not surprising to find that those persons who carried a diagnosis of essential hypertension or diabetes showed an increased prevalence of coronary stenoses at autopsy. In the International Atherosclerosis Project, it was also noted that hypertensives and diabetics had worse disease (Robertson and Strong, 1968). There is concordance between clinical observations and pathology.

We must keep in mind the limitations of studies like these and the possible biases in trying to extrapolate from autopsy data to the pathologic status of living populations. Autopsied cases may not fairly reflect the age, sex, and race distribution of the community. This potential problem was overcome in the International Atherosclerosis Project by analyzing within each of these categories. Autopsied cases may not fairly reflect disease and risk factor distributions of the community, as they have a characteristic—death—not shared by the living community. If they died from some cause that may be correlated with the severity of coronary atherosclerosis, then this creates clear biases. Consequently, analyses of deaths due to accidents, infectious diseases, or other causes unlikely to be related to atherosclerosis are preferable for this purpose.

Summary

1. International comparisons as well as autopsy and angiographic studies show a good but imperfect correlation between obstructive abnormality and disease events.

2. Automatically equating clinical disease with obstructive abnormality may lead to an excessive preoccupation with treating the obstruction when other facets of the total pathogenesis may also be amenable to change. Thus, it is probably best to regard the pathologic change as another risk factor—albeit a powerful one—rather than as the disease itself.

3. The variability in severity of pathologic changes across different communities, within communities, and even within the group dying of IHD, is remarkable.

4. The difference in severity of pathologic involvement between males and females follows expectations based on disease rates. It is also noteworthy that blacks seem to have less pathologic involvement than whites at the same geographic location.

5. Overall, the notion that raised coronary artery lesions are the most important known link in the causal chain leading to IHD seems established by these data.

4

Serum Cholesterol as a Risk Factor for Ischemic Heart Disease

Since the early 19th century, it has been known that cholesterol is a prominent component of arterial atheromatous deposits. A natural question was whether the level of cholesterol in the blood was related to the likelihood of developing excessive deposits of cholesterol and other material in the artery walls, and in turn whether serum cholesterol was related to IHD. The latter question has been answered affirmatively by many studies. Fewer studies have investigated the relationship between serum cholesterol and coronary atherosclerosis, but again it has often been demonstrated. To make clear the consistency of the serum cholesterol–IHD relationship, this chapter will describe three longitudinal studies of contrasting design: a cross-cultural comparison (the Seven Countries Study), then a migration study (the Ni-Hon-San Study), and finally a longitudinal study within one U.S. community (the Framingham Study). The Seven Countries and the Framingham studies are discussed in some detail as they are referred to extensively in subsequent chapters. It should be pointed out that the extent of the evidence on this question extends far beyond these three studies.

Other longitudinal studies from the United States (Chapman and Massey, 1964; Doyle et al, 1957; Keys et al, 1963), Scandinavia (Carlson and Bottiger, 1972; Holme et al, 1980; Wilhelmsen et al, 1973), Britain (Morris et al, 1966; Reid et al, 1976), Australia (Welborn et al, 1969), and Japan (Johnson et al, 1968) form a partial list of those associating these two variables.

The Seven Countries Study

The Seven Countries Study, an ambitious project started in the mid-1950s by Ancel Keys and others, examined populations from different countries with very different IHD rates, cultures, and habits. Men from one to three communities in each of seven countries—Japan, the Netherlands, Yugoslavia, Greece, Italy, Finland, and the United States—were compared. Overall, about 11,000 men aged 40–59 were included in the study. The communities were often small villages, except for the United States and Italian cohorts, which involved railroad workers. Realizing the necessity for standard diagnostic criteria and measurement techniques, since the study was to compare heart disease rates as well as the relationship of these rates to various life-style and physiologic variables, the investigators from the different countries devised common protocols and translated them into the different languages to ensure that they were clearly understood. All blood specimens and electrocardiograms were shipped to the University of Minnesota for analysis.

The project was divided into a prevalence study and an incidence study. They first recorded disease prevalence at the beginning of the study and measured several variables concurrently, such as blood pressure, height, weight, age, serum cholesterol, smoking status, ECG, and skinfold thickness. These variables could at least potentially be linked etiologically to cardiac status or to the atherosclerotic process. The same variables were used in the incidence study.

Results from prevalence studies are often difficult to interpret, because disease and risk factors are measured at the same point in time. Thus, whether the potential risk factor resulted in the disease or vice versa is not always clear. A third possibility is that some other unmeasured and perhaps unthought-of factor produces both the supposed risk factor and the disease. Hence, the importance of incidence studies. In the Seven Countries incidence study, men free of disease were checked for potential risk factors and then followed for up to 10 years to assess the frequency with which *new* disease developed by national group. The national groups received different ratings depending on the mean values of the baseline variables. Results were reported after 5 and after 10 years with similar findings for each time period (Keys, 1970; Keys et al, 1981). As expected, large differences in IHD incidence rates were found between different countries (Fig. 4–1). Serum cholesterol and some related dietary variables were those most consistently associated with IHD rates (Fig. 4–2).

From such a study, however, we must be cautious in drawing any firm causal conclusions. Data comparing single statistics that represent whole communities, states, and countries (often referred to as ecologic data) are peculiarly prone to confounding with other causal variables. For instance, what other variables also differ systematically between these countries, and could they be causally related to IHD? Clearly there are many possibilities—perhaps including socioeconomic, occupational, and dietary factors—although most would not have the theoretical coherence of serum cholesterol as an etiologic factor. The Seven Countries incidence data support a causal hypothesis between serum cholesterol and IHD risk; they do not prove it. We must seek further evidence before asserting the consistency and plausibility of this hypothesis.

Although the Seven Countries Study data are usually used for international comparisons, they also proved to be some of the best available data relating serum cholesterol to IHD for individuals *within* each of several widely differing communities (Keys et al, 1981). Significant positive relationships were found in Finland, Serbia (Velika Krsna, Zrenjanin, and Belgrade), the Netherlands (Zutphen), and Greece (Crete and Corfu). For Italy (Crevalcore, Montegiorgio, and Rome) statistical significance was not achieved, and in Croatia (Dalmatia and Slavonia) there was no discernible relationship. Within several of these

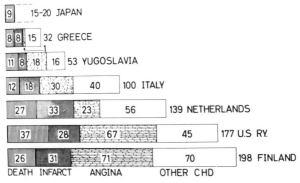

MEN 40-59, CHD-FREE AT ENTRY
CHD INCIDENCE / 10,000 / YEAR

9	15-20 JAPAN
8	8	15	32 GREECE
11	8	18	16	53 YUGOSLAVIA
12	18	30	40	100 ITALY
27	33	23	56	139 NETHERLANDS
37	28	67	45	177 U.S RY.
26	31	71	70	198 FINLAND

DEATH INFARCT ANGINA OTHER CHD

Figure 4–1 Age-standardized average yearly IHD incidence rates per 10,000, of 12,520 men aged 40–59 years, judged to be free of IHD at the outset and followed for 5 years. Nonfatal IHD incidence in Japan is not precisely indicated, as the relevant 5-year clinical and ECG records were not independently reviewed at the University of Minnesota center. From A Keys (ed): Coronary heart disease in seven countries. *Circulation* **41**(suppl 1): I–1, 1970, by permission of the American Heart Association, Inc.

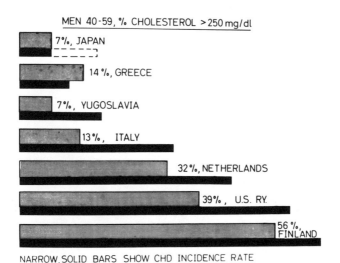

MEN 40-59, % CHOLESTEROL > 250 mg/dl

7%, JAPAN

14%, GREECE

7%, YUGOSLAVIA

13%, ITALY

32%, NETHERLANDS

39%, U.S. RY.

56%, FINLAND

NARROW, SOLID BARS SHOW CHD INCIDENCE RATE

Figure 4–2 Percentage of men with serum cholesterol values over 250 mg/100 ml in seven countries, compared to the IHD incidence rate (narrow solid black bars). From A Keys (ed): Coronary heart disease in seven countries. *Circulation* **41**(suppl 1): I–1, 1970, by permission of the American Heart Association, Inc.

41

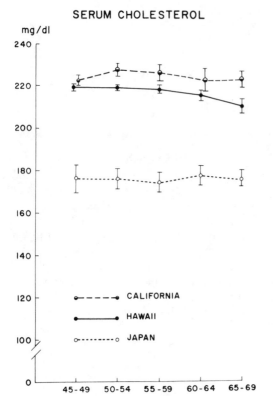

SERUM CHOLESTEROL

Figure 4–3 Serum cholesterol levels by age in three cohorts of male Japanese. The Ni-Hon-San Study. Reprinted with permission from *J Chron Dis* **27**:345. A Kagan et al: Epidemiologic studies of CHD and Stroke in Japanese men living in Japan, Hawaii and California, 1974. Pergamon Press, Ltd.

national study groups numbers of cases were small. In spite of this, there is quite good consistency among these results.

The Ni-Hon-San Study

The design and objectives of the Ni-Hon-San Study were described in chapter 1. Briefly, three cohorts of Japanese men were studied in three different environments: southern Japan, Hawaii, and San Francisco. Mortality from IHD increased consistently from Japan to Honolulu and from Honolulu to San Francisco. This was true for all three age ranges considered. In the two U.S. locations where IHD rates are higher, serum cholesterol levels approximate those of white Americans but are substantially lower in Japan (Fig. 4–3). Thus, these data are consistent with the idea that serum cholesterol levels, or something closely linked to them, are causally related to IHD. This study also investigated the serum cholesterol–IHD relationship within the Hawaiian cohort. A similar positive relationship was shown (Fig. 4–4) among the *individuals* at this location.

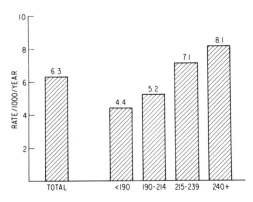

CHD INCIDENCE
BY
SERUM CHOLESTEROL LEVEL

Figure 4-4 The incidence of ischemic heart disease in Hawaiian Japanese males aged 45–64 years, by serum cholesterol level (mg/dl). From A Kagan et al, 1975, with permission.

The Framingham Study

The Framingham Study is probably the classical example of a longitudinal incidence study conducted within one community. After the Second World War there was a great deal of concern over an apparent upswing in mortality from heart disease in the United States. No one understood the cause of this epidemic, although the pathologic process was well known. In 1948, a group of scientists and clinicians began this ambitious undertaking: the first major longitudinal study following a representative sample of a population 30–60 years old, for 20 years. To accumulate enough cases of cardiovascular disease even over this long period required a cohort of about 6000 persons. The researchers chose the town of Framingham, Massachusetts, which at that time had a population of 28,000.

The public, unfortunately, was not fully cooperative. Only about two-thirds of the families in the town participated, so that in the end the sample was not random. Rather, it included anyone eligible who agreed to participate. This raised the question of possible biases and, indeed, mortality statistics over the first 4 years showed that individuals in the study lived longer than those not in the study. After 4 years, however, the death rates of the two groups became comparable. Follow-up was by biennial examination. At the 14th year of follow-up, 4030 of the original cohort were alive, and even after the 20th year of follow-up, only 2 percent had been lost to the study, although attendance at any particular biennial visit was less complete than this. Thus, follow-up has been very thorough. The results of this study, still being reported, are provocative, and with similar studies have formed a basis for extensive clinical, basic science, and epidemiologic research.

As with other studies, many physiologic and life-style variables proved to correlate with the risk of developing coronary disease. Among these was, again,

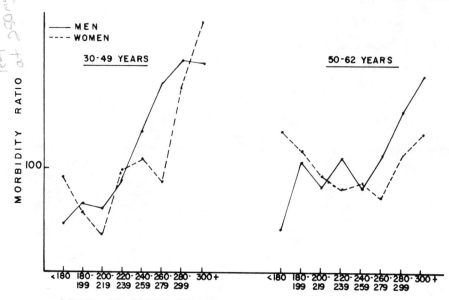

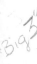

Figure 4–5   Risk of IHD during 14 years follow-up according to serum cholesterol. Men and women aged 30–62 years at entry. The Framingham Study. From WB Kannel et al: Serum cholesterol, lipoproteins, and the risk of coronary heart disease. *Ann Intern Med* **74**:1, 1971, by permission of the American College of Physicians.

serum cholesterol (Fig. 4–5). For both men and younger women at least, those who have moderate to high levels of serum cholesterol are at higher risk for developing IHD. From blood cholesterol levels ranging from 150 to 260 mg/dl there is about a 3-fold increase in risk for men and about a 1.5-fold increase in risk for younger women. This range of cholesterol is below that of type II hyperlipidemic individuals, and these are commonly accepted as "normal" values.

There has been some controversy regarding the optimal level of serum cholesterol and in particular whether there is a moderately low level of serum cholesterol below which risk reduction for IHD does not occur. This seems less likely in view of Framingham Study results (Kannel and Gordon, 1982) and also data from Japan showing gradients of risk within a population with low levels of serum cholesterol (Johnson et al, 1968). Probably, optimum is at least as low as 200 mg/dl and probably lower.

Both the Framingham and the Honolulu Heart studies (the Honolulu cohort of the Ni-Hon-San Study) were consistent in finding two other variables that significantly predicted an increased risk of IHD in persons initially without such a diagnosis. These were cigarette smoking and hypertension. This evidence will be considered in more detail in subsequent chapters.

Prediction Using Different Forms of Serum Cholesterol

In recent years we have been able to measure the individual lipoprotein particles in which blood cholesterol is carried: high-density (HDL), low-density (LDL), and very low-density lipoproteins (VLDL). The Framingham Study (Kannel, 1983a), among others, showed that LDL (the major cholesterol-carrying particle) is the damaging form. Only over the last decade has HDL cholesterol been convincingly shown to be negatively associated with IHD (Fig. 4–6; see also Heiss et al, 1980a).

A powerful predictor of IHD, HDL levels average 10–15 mg/dl higher in women than in men. Total serum cholesterol loses much predictive power in old age, but when it is divided into HDL and LDL cholesterol, both retain individual predictive ability, even in the elderly (Gordon et al, 1977a,b). In this situation, where one factor is apparently protective and the other detrimental, the factors can be combined into a single ratio of LDL to HDL. As this ratio rises by either increased LDL, decreased HDL, or both, IHD risk should rise. As LDL and total cholesterol are highly correlated (LDL makes up most of total cholesterol), the ratio of total cholesterol to HDL predicts just as well, and in terms of laboratory costs, is less expensive to estimate. A recent paper from the Framingham Study shows that total cholesterol/HDL cholesterol ratios correspond to changes in the relative risk of IHD (Castelli et al, 1983). For men, ratios of 3.4, 5.1, 6.8, and 7.8 correspond to half-average, average, twice-average, and triple-average risk of IHD, respectively. For women, ratios of 2.5, 4.4, 6.4, and 7.5 also correspond to the same risks.

The realization that LDL and HDL cholesterol levels are important has focused much attention on their determinants. This issue will be discussed at many points later in this book, but to summarize, LDL cholesterol seems to be determined in part by dietary factors (see chapters 5 and 6), obesity (Caggiula et al, 1981; Garrison et al, 1980; Wolf and Grundy, 1980), age (see below), and heredity (Garrison et al, 1979). The HDL cholesterol levels are determined in part by obesity and exercise level (Gordon et al, 1977a; Krauss et al, 1977; Leon et al, 1979; Lopez et al, 1974; Rhoads et al, 1976; Wood et al, 1974), gender (see below), sex hormones (Heiss et al, 1980a,b), alcohol consumption (Castelli et al, 1977, Fraser et al, 1983a), and cigarette smoking (Garrison et al, 1978; Hames et al, 1978).

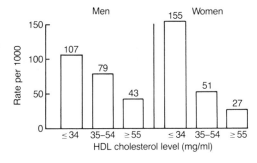

Figure 4–6 Incidence of ischemic heart disease by high-density lipoprotein cholesterol level. Men and women aged 50–79 years from Framingham Study, exam 11. Trends were significant at $P < 0.01$. From WB Kannel: *Am J Cardiol* **52**:93, 1983a, with permission.

Most researchers accept LDL cholesterol as an important risk factor in IHD. It is the major constituent of blood cholesterol and has determinants similar to those of total blood cholesterol. This suggests that evidence from older studies implicating total blood cholesterol as a risk factor can now be largely attributed to LDL cholesterol. However, some do not believe that HDL cholesterol has been established as a causal risk factor for IHD (Keys, 1980a); rather they think the relationship may represent a statistical association in which HDL acts as a surrogate for some other causal variable. This possibility is raised by some inconsistencies found particularly in international comparisons. In general, such comparisons do not clearly relate national average values of HDL cholesterol to IHD rates (Connor et al, 1978; Keys et al, 1958a). The explanation may be that while low fat consumption is usually associated with low HDL cholesterol levels in such groups as vegetarians, Tarahumara Indians, Asians, and the Masai (Barrow et al, 1960; Berkel, 1979; Connor et al, 1978; Kesteloot et al, 1982; Robinson and Williams, 1979; Sacks et al, 1975), it is also associated with a reduction in total cholesterol (due to the effect on LDL). The effect on the total cholesterol/HDL ratio is variable, thus raising the possibility that optimal values of this measure for the United States may not apply universally. Of course, such apparent inconsistencies in international comparisons also occur with the variables of cigarette smoking and exercise, and may only reflect the complex multivariate nature of the disease.

The apolipoproteins are the structural proteins of the lipoprotein particles. Different particles have distinctive proportions of these different apolipoproteins. As the proteins are intimately associated with the lipids and in addition often activate enzymes involved in phases of lipid transport, it is natural to ask whether changes in concentrations of these proteins may affect atherogenesis. Only limited epidemiologic work has been done, but the results indicate that both apolipoprotein A-1 (associated particularly with the HDL particle) and apolipoprotein B (associated with the LDL particle) are significant predictors of disease, perhaps even better than the levels of the associated HDL or LDL cholesterols (Avogaro et al, 1979; De Backer et al, 1982; Ishikawa et al, 1978; Maciejko et al, 1983).

Blood Lipid Levels and Pathologic Coronary Conditions

As obstructed coronary arteries are a causal factor of IHD, several investigators have tried to relate lipid levels directly to the severity of such conditions, using coronary angiography and postmortem examinations. Oalmann et al (1981) related postmortem serum cholesterol levels to the percentage of the intimal surface area showing raised coronary lesions. The relationship was statistically significant for whites, and trends were similar but of lesser magnitude for blacks (Fig. 4–7). Similar studies are reported from both the Framingham (Feinleib et al, 1979) and the Ni-Hon-San (Rhoads et al, 1978) studies. Angiographic studies in Japan (Kambara et al, 1982) and Spain (Coll et al, 1983) have shown a

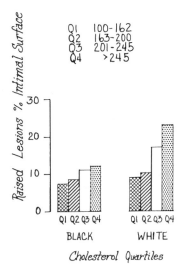

Q1 100-162
Q2 163-200
Q3 201-245
Q4 >245

Figure 4–7 Percentage of coronary artery intimal surface involved with raised lesions in autopsied men, by quartile of serum cholesterol values (in mg/dl) and race. From MC Oalmann et al: Community pathology of atherosclerosis and coronary heart disease. *Am J Epidemiol* **113**:396, 1981, with permission.

positive relationship between the degree of coronary obstruction and serum cholesterol values. Similarly, several studies have found HDL cholesterol levels (Pearson et al, 1979) or the cholesterol of the HDL_2 subfraction (NE Miller et al, 1981) inversely related to coronary atheroma in both men and women. Participants in the latter studies were not representative of the whole population but were biased by a perceived need to undergo coronary arteriography. The data should be interpreted cautiously with this in mind. However, Ramsdale et al (1984) reported on 387 patients, without clinical IHD, who underwent coronary angiography prior to valve surgery. Again, significant relationships were found between a coronary score measuring obstructive lesions and serum total cholesterol, HDL cholesterol, and the ratio total/HDL cholesterol. These patients may more closely represent the general population with regard to coronary disease status. It has also been shown that hyperlipidemic individuals have less fibrinolytic activity (Andersen et al, 1981). This may have implications for coronary thrombosis, although direct evidence is lacking.

Serum Cholesterol Levels and Cancer Risk

In the 3–4 years prior to this writing, several large prospective studies examining risk factors for IHD have shown that low levels of serum cholesterol are associated with higher rates of cancer (Lilienfeld, 1981; Workshop on Cholesterol and Noncardiovascular Disease Mortality, 1981). These include studies from the United States (Kark et al, 1980; Kagan et al, 1981; RR Williams et al, 1980), Puerto Rico (Garcia-Palmieri et al, 1981), United Kingdom (G Rose et al, 1980), Yugoslavia (Kozarevic et al, 1981), France (Cambien et al, 1980), other European countries (Keys, 1980b), and an International Collaborative Group

(1982) reporting on 11 populations in eight countries. The data supporting *some* relationship are impressive. The real question is whether it is *causal* or only correlative.

Problems arise in discerning a causal relationship, because the findings from these studies are not consistent. Rates in different studies are higher for different cancer sites and in different age–sex groupings. It is also well established that American Seventh-Day Adventists have lower serum cholesterol levels than most other Americans (see chapter 6), but they also have lower rates for most cancers, both those associated with cigarette smoking and those that are not (Phillips et al, 1980). Similarly, cancer is not epidemic among the Japanese, although their serum cholesterol levels are much lower than those of Americans. Also, populations with *high* average serum cholesterol levels in general show higher rates for colon cancer (GA Rose et al, 1974).

Some possible explanations of these findings are proposed below:

- Reduced serum cholesterol (from whatever cause) increases cancer risk.
- Persons in the preclinical phase of cancer (which often spans 5–15 years) have low serum cholesterol; that is, existing malignancy or premalignancy causes the low serum cholesterol levels. Some of the above studies support this idea; see GA Rose et al (1974), Cambien et al (1980), and International Collaborative Group (1982).
- A third variable associated with low serum cholesterol levels may be the true causal factor for cancer. For example, low vitamin A consumption is associated with an increased risk of certain common cancers. Kark et al (1980) and Marenah et al (1983) found that low serum cholesterol levels were associated with low serum levels of vitamin A.
- Another possible explanation follows from the observation that genetic as well as dietary variables account for differences of serum cholesterol within a population (see chapter 6). Perhaps a *genetically* low serum cholesterol level represents a marker for neoplastic potential.

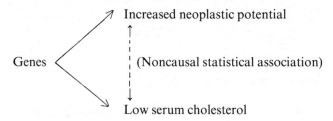

Serum Cholesterol Distribution in the United States

The Lipid Research Clinic Prevalence Study recently reported data on the total cholesterol levels (Fig. 4–8) of 60,502 Americans and the LDL and HDL cholesterol levels of 7733 Americans. Though not a random sample in a statistical sense, subjects came from 10 well-defined U.S. populations across the country. Data were collected between 1972 and 1976, and collection techniques and laboratory procedures were meticulous (Lipid Research Clinics Study Group, 1980).

A characteristic finding is the plateauing of serum total cholesterol in men around age 50 (Fig. 4–8). The data for women show a rather curious crossover phenomenon in which premenopausal women taking sex hormones have higher than average cholesterol levels, whereas in postmenopausal women taking such hormones the reverse is true. The age trends for LDL cholesterol are similar to those for total cholesterol. Figure 4–9 depicts levels of HDL cholesterol by age for both sexes. As compared to trends in LDL cholesterol, HDL levels rise less with age, particularly in males. Sex hormone users show relatively higher levels of HDL cholesterol, which, in combination with the lower postmenopausal total cholesterol values in hormone users, should lower the total cholesterol/ HDL cholesterol ratio in this group. However, the data should not be automatically interpreted to suggest that postmenopausal sex hormone usage is protective for ischemic heart disease (see chapter 20). Women have HDL cholesterol levels 10–15 mg/dl higher than men, the difference first occurring during adolescence. There is a drop in the HDL cholesterol among males during adolescence and the absence of such a trend among females (see chapter 16).

Racial differences within the United States, favor blacks, in that, while serum

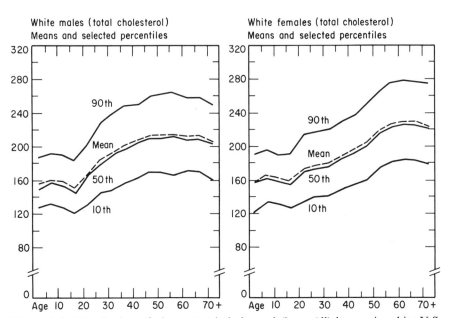

Figure 4–8 Distribution of plasma total cholesterol (in mg/dl) by age in white U.S. males and females. From The Lipid Research Clinics Study Group, 1980, with permission.

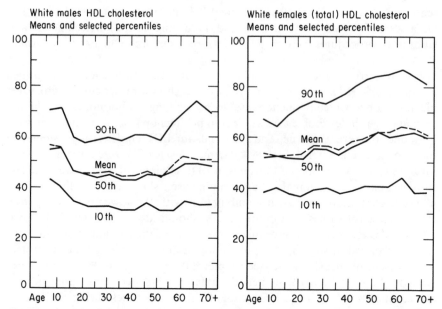

Figure 4-9 Distribution of plasma high-density lipoprotein cholesterol (in mg/dl) by age in white U.S. males and females. From The Lipid Research Clinics Study Group, 1980, with permission.

total cholesterol levels are quite similar for blacks and whites, the lipoprotein cholesterol components are different. Black men and women have higher HDL and lower LDL cholesterol levels than their white similar-aged counterparts (JA Morrison et al, 1981; Tyroler et al, 1975, 1980b). Time trends in serum cholesterol in the United States are of interest because they may relate to trends in disease frequency. Unfortunately, such comparisons are hazardous since laboratory methods for estimating of serum cholesterol are rarely the same a decade apart and, even if they were, different equipment, personnel, and population location are often difficulties. Despite these possible objections, several comparisons have been made where similar methods were used, sometimes even within the same longitudinal study. Beaglehole et al (1979) have compared data from several studies during the years 1960–75, as well as longitudinal data from within one study, the Framingham Study. These comparisons are age adjusted and sex specific, or age and sex specific. Similarly, Gillum and colleagues (1984) have compared data from one suburb of Minneapolis (1973–74) to that of a survey of the entire Minneapolis-St. Paul metropolitan area (1980–81). All of these comparisons suggest a decline in levels of serum cholesterol. The magnitude varies, but it is generally in the range of a 3–10 mg/dl decline over recent decade periods.

Summary

1. Serum cholesterol satisfies most criteria to be considered a causal factor for IHD. The time sequence is established by prospective studies. The relationship is demonstrated in a variety of societies and also consistently on repetition in the same country. A relationship between serum cholesterol levels and coronary atherosclerosis has also often been found. Several mechanisms to explain this relationship have been proposed (chapters 3 and 7).

2. Serum cholesterol can be fractionated to two constituents with opposing influences on IHD risk (LDL and HDL cholesterol).

3. The mean cholesterol value in the United States and many similar societies is 215 mg/dl or higher.

4. Many Mediterranean countries that have average cholesterol values of 200 mg/dl or less have substantially less cardiac disease than other industrialized countries.

5. Communities that have mean cholesterol values of 180 mg/dl or less (e.g., Japan and many primitive tribal communities) experience very few IHD events. The optimal level of serum cholesterol is probably lower than 200 mg/dl.

5

The Relationship Between Diet and Serum Cholesterol

Diet is a very complex variable, yet probably one of the most important in IHD research. Many different foods and nutrients make up our diet, mixed in varying proportions. This produces a vexing measurement problem, particularly in population research (El Lozy, 1983). Perhaps the ideal would be to collect a fixed proportion of all food eaten, for laboratory analysis. However, this is very expensive and does not overcome the problem of subjects consciously or subconsciously changing their diets during the few days of investigation. A related but less accurate way of assessing diet is to have the subjects keep a 3- or 7-day food diary. Again, the possibility that such diaries may not reflect a person's *typical* diet must be considered. A well-known method of measuring diet is the 24-hour recall elicited by a trained interviewer, often using food models. Although the information is probably quite accurate, one day's dietary intake may be quite atypical of the usual diet (Garn et al, 1978; Neaton et al, 1981). A final method of dietary measurement is food frequency recall, which relies heavily on subjects' memory and perception of their diet. The method records only the number of times each day, week, or month (as appropriate) a particular food is eaten, rather than amounts of food, and may seem rather crude. However, it has the advantage of simplicity and of allowing recall over longer time periods. It has also been shown to correlate highly with some of the more detailed methods (Fraser and Swannell, 1981) when published tables of average portion sizes are used as aids to calculate quantities of foods.

Considering the limitations of observational methods, "metabolic ward" or carefully controlled small-group feeding experiments can provide valuable information on the effects of diet. Meals can be provided by the investigators, and the subjects are either institutionalized or selected for the probability of good adherence to a dietary regimen and rewarded for it.

Most of the fat in human diets is in the form of fatty acids either in combination with glycerol (the glyceride fats) or with phosphate-containing molecules (the phospholipids). Acids of chain lengths of 12, 14, 16, and 18 carbons (medium chain length) are the most common, although shorter and longer chains do occur. The discussion below deals with the medium-chain and a few longer chain acids, as those best known to influence serum cholesterol levels or platelet function.

These fatty acids are divided into three groups: those that are completely saturated with hydrogen and thus have no double bonds, those that have one double bond (monounsaturated), and those that have two or more double bonds (polyunsaturated). The major saturated dietary fatty acids are lauric (C_{12}), myristic (C_{14}), palmitic (C_{16}), and stearic (C_{18}). The major dietary monounsaturated acid is oleic (18:1). The major dietary polyunsaturated acids are linoleic (18:2), α-linolenic (18:8), arachidonic (20:4), and eicosapentaenoic (20:5). These polyunsaturated acids are commonly divided into two families according to the configuration of the carbon-terminal structure of the molecule. The n-6 series is based on the parent linoleic acid (found especially in seeds and nuts) and also includes arachidonic acid. The n-3 series is based on α-linolenic acid (found particularly in green leafy vegetables) and also contains eicosapentaenoic acid (found especially in fish and marine oils). Both of these families of polyunsaturated fatty acids are precursors for corresponding families of prostaglandins, which are potent tissue hormones influencing many aspects of human physiology including blood pressure, vascular reactivity, and platelet function.

Experimental Studies Relating Fat Consumption to Serum Cholesterol

In the 1950s and 1960s, Ancel Keys, Joseph Anderson, and Francisco Grande conducted scores of feeding experiments on human male subjects, either in institutional settings or using university students. The men were served all meals for a period of several weeks, and adherence was carefully noted. Usually this was of a high order. The experiments were carefully designed to allow for underlying seasonal trends affecting serum cholesterol. All used at least two diets, each for a minimum of 2 to 3 weeks before blood cholesterol values were estimated. In one study, for example, the stearic acid, providing 10 percent of total dietary calories, was replaced with an equivalent number of calories as palmitic acid (Grande et al, 1970). In all other respects the diets were identical. On average, this dietary change elevated serum cholesterol levels by 24 mg/dl ($P < 0.0001$).

The overall results of the many studies conducted by Keys, Anderson, and Grande can be summarized as follows. The medium-chain saturated fatty acids—lauric (C_{12}), myristic (C_{14}), and palmitic (C_{16})—raised serum cholesterol. Stearic acid, an 18-carbon saturated fatty acid, did not affect serum cholesterol levels (Grande et al, 1970). Likewise, the common monounsaturated oleic acid (found particularly in olive oil) was neutral in effect (Keys et al, 1958b). Hydrogenated vegetable fats acted as saturated fatty acids (JT Anderson et al, 1961) by raising serum cholesterol to a similar degree as the naturally occurring saturated fatty acids. Medium-chain polyunsaturated acids of the n-6 family (mainly linoleic and linolenic) depressed serum cholesterol levels to half the extent that equivalent quantities of the saturated fatty acids mentioned above raised these levels (Grande et al, 1972; Keys et al, 1957). Thus, it is clear that foods with similar quantities but differing qualities of fat can affect serum cholesterol very differently, but predictably.

The same group also investigated the effect of dietary cholesterol on serum

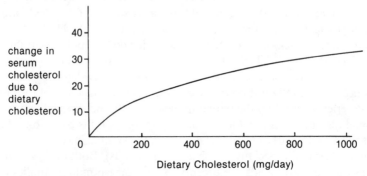

Figure 5–1   The effect of dietary cholesterol on serum cholesterol as predicted by the Keys equation (total calories = 2000 in this example).

cholesterol levels, using similar study designs. They found that dietary cholesterol affects serum cholesterol in a curvilinear fashion (Fig. 5–1), adding to the above effects of fatty acids in the diet (JT Anderson et al, 1976; Keys et al, 1965a). In most situations, dietary cholesterol had less effect on serum cholesterol than fatty acids did. The curvilinear relationship implies that where the initial cholesterol consumption is very low, the effect of adding a fixed amount of cholesterol to the diet will be greater than if the baseline diet contains large amounts of cholesterol.

Keys summarized his many studies in a now-famous equation (JT Anderson et al, 1979; Keys et al, 1965b)

$$\text{serum cholesterol} = 164 + 1.3(2S - P) + 1.5\sqrt{1000DC/E} = 164 + \phi$$

where S is the percentage of calories present as saturated fat, P is the percentage of calories present as polyunsaturated fat, DC is dietary cholesterol in milligrams per day, E is total energy of the diet in calories per day, and ϕ is dietary factor.

This equation is for the average male. It is well known that responsiveness differs among individuals, implying the existence of hyperresponders and hyporesponders in the population (Keys at al, 1965c). The equation implies that if there were no fat or cholesterol in the diet, the average male's serum cholesterol would be 164 mg/dl. The $2S - P$ term predicts that the magnitude of the effect of the saturated acids is double that of the polyunsaturated acids but in the opposite direction. The fatty acids are expressed as a proportion of total calories, with the dietary cholesterol also being related to total calories, showing that the effect of these nutrients is not absolute, but must be related to the total diet. The equation's ability to make predictions is shown in Fig. 5–2. The coefficient for $(2S - P)$ of 1.2 in Fig. 5–2 is an older version of Keys' equation. The agree-

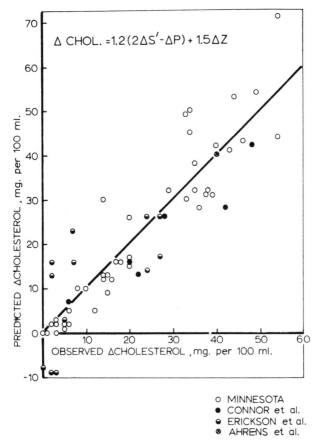

$$\Delta \text{CHOL.} = 1.2(2\Delta S' - \Delta P) + 1.5\Delta Z$$

○ MINNESOTA
● CONNOR et al.
◒ ERICKSON et al.
⊗ AHRENS et al.

Figure 5–2 Predicted versus observed changes in serum cholesterol, using the Keys equation and several different sources of dietary experimental data. From A Keys et al, 1965c, with permission.

ment between observation and prediction is good. The scatter that is observed about the line could be explained by differing responsiveness in different individuals and by random day-to-day fluctuations in serum cholesterol levels. Another illustration of the adequacy of prediction comes from an experiment by Grande et al (1972) that used five different diets with markedly different fat contents, three of which (SP-68, OS-23, OS-68) had S and P balanced in such a way that $2S - P$ was very small (1–2 percent of calories) and so approximately equal for each diet. The dietary cholesterol and total calories did not change. The other two diets were a diet high in saturated fat (butter diet, $2S - P = 23$ percent of calories) and a low-fat diet (CHO, $2S - P = 1.5$ percent of calories). The results are summarized in Table 5–1: the serum cholesterol values for the three balanced dietary periods are virtually identical and close to the value for the CHO diet, where simple carbohydrate (shown previously to have no effect on

Table 5–1   Mean serum cholesterol values after five different experimental diets[a]

Diet	Fat content[b]		Mean serum cholesterol after 4 wks of diet (mg/dl)
	S	P	
SP-68	7.2	13.2	227
OS-23	2.4	2.7	228
OS-68	4.0	6.6	225
CHO	1.5	0.6	221
Butter	12.4	1.9	266 ←

Source: Adapted from F Grande et al: *Am J Clin Nutr* **25**:53, 1972, with permission.

[a] See text for detailed description of diets.

[b] S, percentage calories present as saturated fat; P, percentage calories present as polyunsaturated fat.

serum cholesterol) replaced most of the fat calories. Notice the very different effect of the butter diet, containing much more saturated fat. Little is known of any effect of the distribution of dietary fats throughout the day. One study found that a lipid supplement raised both LDL and HDL to a greater extent when taken as a bolus at the evening meal, than if spread throughout the day (Kay et al, 1983). There was no difference in the total/HDL cholesterol ratios.

The mechanisms of action by which dietary fats raise or lower serum cholesterol are poorly understood. Polyunsaturated fatty acids of the n-6 family (vegetable oils) appear to increase sterol excretion transiently (Connor et al, 1969; Grundy, 1975; Nestel, 1975; Nestel et al, 1973), probably representing a loss of cholesterol from the body pool, and then a new equilibrium at this decreased pool size (Table 5–2). Presumably, a decreased total cholesterol pool would be reflected in a lower serum cholesterol level. There is some tentative evidence that polyunsaturates decrease hepatic cholesterol synthesis, but the idea that polyunsaturated fats simply relocate cholesterol from the blood tissues is not supported by recent evidence (Grundy, 1979).

How saturated fatty acids raise serum cholesterol is even less well understood. The action may be on cholesterol absorption, hepatic cholesterol production, or cholesterol excretion from the bowel (Grundy, 1979). Dietary cholesterol is known to influence hepatic cholesterol production via a feedback loop. Less dietary cholesterol provokes increased hepatic production and vice versa. It has also been shown that excess caloric intake and obesity apparently provoke increased endogenous hepatic cholesterol formation (Grundy, 1979).

The Effect of Vegetables and Fruit on Serum Cholesterol Levels

Vegetarians consistently show markedly lower serum cholesterol levels than the general population. This is undoubtedly attributable in part to their lower in-

Table 5-2 Mean values ($\pm$ SD) and significant differences for cholesterol absorption, bile acid, neutral sterol, and net sterol excretion in four dietary periods

Dietary period[a]	Cholesterol absorption	Sterol excretion (mg/day)		
		Neutral	bile acid	Net
HCP	39.6 ± 10.8	1038 ± 339	381 ± 162	624 ± 332
HCS	44.4 ± 5.4	806 ± 192	281 ± 123	299 ± 195
LCP	44.6 ± 12.5	847 ± 257	315 ± 103	642 ± 262
LCS	52.6 ± 7.8	673 ± 171	297 ± 111	477 ± 203
Significant difference[b]		HCP + LCP vs HCS + LCS $P < 0.01$	HCP vs HCS $P < 0.01$	HCP vs HCS $P < 0.02$ LCP vs LCS $P < 0.05$ HCP + LCP vs HCS + LCS $P < 0.01$ LCS vs HCS $P < 0.01$

Source: From PJ Nestel et al: Increased Sterol Excretion with Polyunsaturated Fat High-Cholesterol Diets. *Metabolism* **24**:189, 1975. Reprinted by permission of Grune & Stratton, Inc. and the author.

[a] HCP, high cholesterol, polyunsaturated fat; HCS, high cholesterol, saturated fat; LCP, low cholesterol, polyunsaturated fat; LCS, low cholesterol, saturated fat.

[b] Paired *t*-test analysis.

take of saturated fats and cholesterol. The Keys equation, however, indicates that the differences are greater than can be accounted for by dietary lipid differences alone.

Keys et al (1960) observed that men in Naples, Italy, had lower serum cholesterol levels than men in the state of Minnesota, and that these differences were substantially greater than the dietary lipid differences were calculated to produce. Another experiment involving U.S. men documented that a Neapolitan-style diet with more fruit and vegetables produced lower serum cholesterol levels (by 17 mg/dl) than a more typical American diet even though both diets had a lipid content calculated to have similar effects on serum cholesterol (Keys et al, 1960). Similarly, JT Anderson et al (1973) found that a diet containing a large proportion of vegetables, legumes, and fruit reduced serum cholesterol by about 30 mg/dl more than predicted by fat changes alone. Grande et al (1974) compared different 600-kcal carbohydrate supplements with a sucrose supplement and found that while the effect of white flour, mixed fruit, and legume supplements did not differ from that of the control sucrose supplement, a mixed-vegetable supplement depressed serum cholesterol significantly by 22 mg/dl.

Other research suggests that Bengal gram (a legume) (Mathur et al, 1968) reduces serum cholesterol (Fig. 5–3). De Groot and co-workers (1963) fed men 140 gm of oatmeal per day for 3 weeks and noted a striking change in serum cholesterol (Fig. 5–4). Some of this effect may be mediated by the fat content of

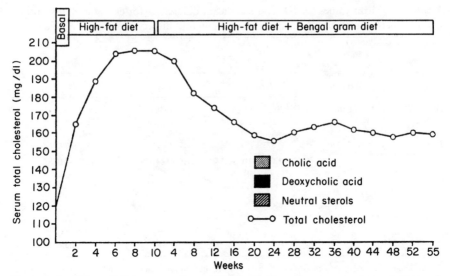

Figure 5–3 Effect of dietary supplementation with Bengal gram on serum cholesterol over 55 weeks. From KS Mathur et al: *Br Med J* **1**:30, 1968, with permission.

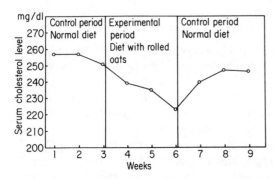

Figure 5–4 Mean serum cholesterol level in 21 male volunteers during three dietary periods, one including rolled oats. From AP De Groot et al, 1963, with permission.

oats. Men fed 200 gm of carrots daily for 3 weeks showed a significant 11 percent decrease in serum cholesterol (J Robertson et al, 1979). In a controlled-feeding experiment we have recently demonstrated that dietary supplements consisting of whole grains (oats, wheat, corn) and vegetable leaves or stalks, added to a fixed basic diet, significantly lower LDL and VLDL cholesterols in comparison to a sucrose supplement (Fraser et al, 1981). These dietary components did not seem to change HDL cholesterol (Table 5–3). Although the magnitude of contrasts with the sucrose supplement shown in Table 5–3 may seem modest, the dietary supplements in this study made up only between 6 and 12 percent of total calories. For a vegetarian, these foods would make up a much larger part of the diet.

Dietary fibers are a heterogenous group of complex plant polysaccharides,

Table 5–3 Observed differences in serum cholesterol levels (mg/dl) comparing three different vegetable supplements to a sucrose supplement

Type of cholesterol	Diet		
	Leafy	Grains	Roots
HDL	− 1.17	− 1.88	− 1.95
LDL	− 5.67	− 8.21[b]	− 1.88
VLDL	− 3.58[a]	1.13	− 0.63
Total	− 10.42[b]	− 9.08[b]	− 4.46
Triglyceride	− 1.17	6.79	1.38

Source: From GE Fraser et al: *Am J Clin Nutr* **34**:1272, 1981, with permission.

[a] $P < 0.05$.

[b] $P < 0.01$.

Table 5–4 Mean changes in serum cholesterol (mg/dl) during sequential 2-week test periods for three different fiber-containing foods

Test results	Wheat fiber (5)[a]	Pectin (7)	Guar (7)
Baseline	224.5	236.0	222.5
Change	− 6.7	− 29.7	− 36.3
P	n.s.[b]	<0.05	<0.002

Source: Adapted from DJA Jenkins et al, 1975, with permission.

[a] Number of volunteers shown in parentheses.

[b] n.s., not significant.

possessing the common feature that they are not absorbed from the bowel lumen. Nevertheless they can affect body metabolism and hence health (Kay and Strasberg, 1978). Of the various dietary fibers (pectin, cellulose, hemicellulose, lignin, gums), pectin and gums clearly lower serum cholesterol (DJA Jenkins et al, 1975; Kay et al, 1977; Trowell, 1973; Truswell, 1977). Jenkins and colleagues supplemented the diet of small groups of normal healthy men with wheat fiber (bran), pectin, or guar gum, and demonstrated substantial lowering of serum cholesterol with the latter two (Table 5–4). The role of bran, a fiber-containing food, in altering serum lipids has also been investigated, but Truswell and Kay (1976) found it had no influence. This is also reflected in the absence of significant change with the wheat fiber supplement in Jenkins' study

(Table 5–4). Although it seems clear that the action of some of the dietary fibers explain much of the serum cholesterol-lowering effect of vegetables, other chemicals also may be active (Beveridge et al, 1958).

The mechanisms by which dietary fibers reduce the serum cholesterol are partially understood. Dietary fibers bind sterols (dietary cholesterol and bile acids) in the gut, increasing their excretion. Fibers also form gels in the small bowel, possibly reducing the surface area of the intestinal contents exposed to the absorptive mucosa (Kay and Strasberg, 1978; Kelsay et al, 1978; Story and Kritchevsky, 1976).

The Effect of Milk and Protein on Serum Cholesterol Levels

The question of what effects milk and protein have on serum cholesterol is a controversial one. The fact that milk fats are largely saturated would suggest a serum cholesterol-raising effect, but several studies have demonstrated that low-fat or skimmed milk reduces serum cholesterol (Hepner et al, 1979; Howard and Marks 1977; Rossouw et al, 1981). These investigators, along with GV Mann (1977), report conflicting findings for yogurt or whole milk. Probably the most that should be concluded at present is that skimmed milk lowers serum cholesterol, whereas yogurt and whole milk at least do not seem to raise blood cholesterol, which is contrary to expectations based on fat content. This may imply the presence of an unidentified cholesterol-lowering substance in milk products.

The evidence that dietary proteins affect serum cholesterol is conflicting. Some studies indicate that vegetable proteins yield lower serum cholesterol values than animal proteins, when dietary fat and calories are held constant (Carrol et al, 1978). However, other well-designed studies do not show any change in serum cholesterol levels when the quality of the protein is altered (JT Anderson et al, 1971). Possibly the specific proteins are important.

Diet and Serum Cholesterol in Population Studies

We next review the evidence relating diet to serum cholesterol in free-living individuals, rather than in the carefully controlled experiments described above. There is an obvious loss of control in that many variables vary simultaneously among different individuals. Investigators either ignore this or take a multivariate analytic approach. What is potentially gained is the ability to generalize findings to large segments of the population, and also to observe interactions between different predictor variables. In addition, both cross-cultural and intra-cultural comparisons are possible.

Cross-Cultural Studies

In the Seven Countries Study the dietary information was obtained from a personal survey. In many communities participants kept a duplicate of meals eaten

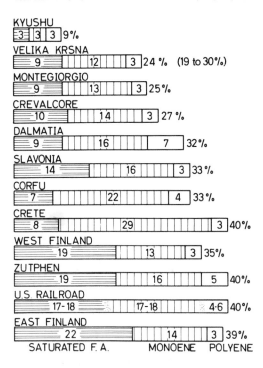

Figure 5–5 Average percentage calories from fats in seven countries. Men aged 40–59 years. From A Keys (ed): Coronary heart disease in seven countries. *Circulation* **41**(suppl 1):I–1, 1970, by permission of the American Heart Association, Inc.

over 7 days, and these were chemically analyzed. The communities of the Seven Countries Study showed wide variation in saturated-fat consumptions (Fig. 5–5), but since the proportion of calories from polyunsaturated fats varies little, it was difficult to investigate this variable in this study. For saturated fat, Keys was able to show a clear relationship with serum cholesterol (Fig. 5–6; note that in Figs. 5–6 and 5–7 each dot represents the mean value for a *community*). The percentage of calories from monounsaturated fat showed no significant relationship with serum cholesterol (Fig. 5–7), as expected.

Using values of dietary saturated and polyunsaturated fat in the various communities, the Keys equation ranks the communities quite accurately as compared to *observed* values of serum cholesterol (Fig. 5–8). Differences in the predicted versus observed values of serum cholesterol are partially explained by the omission of dietary cholesterol from the prediction (it was not accurately estimated in this study) and also the effect of other dietary or nondietary factors on serum cholesterol.

The three cohorts of the Ni-Hon-San Study have different mean values of serum cholesterol (p. 42), and we now see that the dietary differences are generally in accord with the observed cholesterol values (Table 5–5). The dietary information in this study was collected by 24-hour recall. Using the Keys equation, J Stamler (quoted in Keys, 1980b) found excellent agreement between predicted and observed values of serum cholesterol (in milligrams per deciliter) in the three different locations (California versus Hawaii difference: observed =

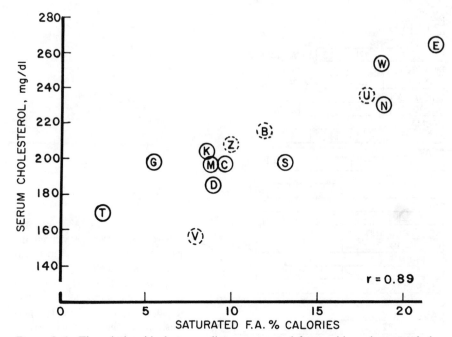

Figure 5–6 The relationship between dietary saturated fatty acids and serum cholesterol, comparing communities from seven countries—5-year follow-up. Abbreviations: B, Belgrade; C, Crevalcore; D, Dalmatia; E, east Finland; G, Corfu; J, Ushibuka; K, Crete; M, Montegiorgio; N, Zutphen; R, Rome railroad; S, Slavonia; T, Tanushimaru; U, American railroad; V, Velika Krsna; W, west Finland; Z, Zrenjanin. Data were not available from some communities. Solid circles have nutrients estimated by chemical analysis, interrupted circles, by dietary recall. From A Keys (ed): Coronary heart disease in seven countries. *Circulation* **41**(suppl 1):I–1, 1970, by permission of the American Heart Association, Inc.

9.9, predicted = 8.8; California versus Japan difference: observed = 47.1, predicted = 54).

With data comparing communities in different countries, we must consider what other important differences apart from diet may account for the differences in serum cholesterol before drawing conclusions. However, these cross-cultural comparisons are very much in agreement with the findings of the carefully controlled experiments of preceding sections.

Studies Within One Culture

Studies conducted within one community use the individual as the unit of measurement rather than the mean of a whole community and should be somewhat less subject to confounding because individuals in a community are more homogeneous with regard to other possibly important variables. Several such studies

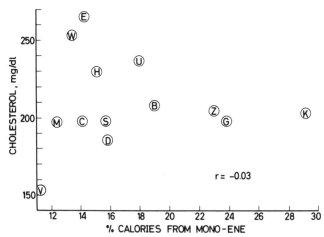

Figure 5-7 The relationship between dietary monounsaturated fatty acids and serum cholesterol, comparing communities from seven countries 5-year follow-up. For key to communities, see Fig. 5–6. From A Keys (ed): *Seven Countries. A Multivariate Analysis of Death and Coronary Heart Disease.* Harvard Univ Press, 1980b, reprinted by permission.

have been reported, including some of the largest and most carefully designed epidemiologic investigations. The results, as they relate diet to serum cholesterol, have been disappointingly difficult to interpret. They represent one of the main sources of "ammunition" for those who disbelieve the diet–heart hypothesis.

A cross-sectional analysis in the Framingham Study failed to relate dietary fats to serum cholesterol at all (Kannel and Gordon, 1970). Investigators obtained a careful dietary history (GV Mann et al, 1962) using the method of Burke (food frequency plus an estimate of portion size). Men and women were placed in one of three categories according to the level of serum cholesterol, and the mean values of virtually all dietary variables showed no consistent trends across the various groups (Table 5–6). Similarly, a longitudinal study of cardiovascular disease in Tecumseh, Michigan showed no relation between food frequency dietary history and serum cholesterol values (Nichols et al, 1976). In a British study (Morris et al, 1963), detailed records were obtained and amounts of food eaten by 99 male bank employees were weighed over a period of 1 to 2 weeks. Serum cholesterol was measured, but unfortunately at a variable time in relation to the dietary measurements. No clear relationships were found.

However, not all epidemiologic studies within a single community have yielded such results. In the Ni-Hon-San Study significant correlations between diet and serum cholesterol were found *within* the cohorts of Japanese in Japan and Hawaii (Kato et al, 1973) (Table 5–7). In California, very little significance was found—perhaps because of the lower numbers of participants at this location. With respect to dietary cholesterol, saturated fat, and complex carbo-

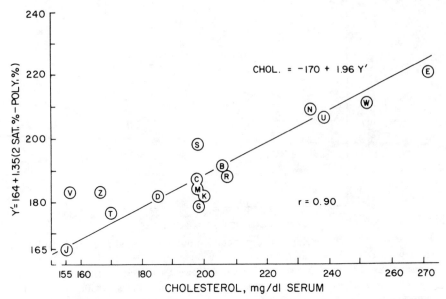

Figure 5–8 The relationship of mean serum cholesterol concentration of the Seven Countries Study cohorts to fat composition of the diet expressed as the Keys equation—10-year follow-up. For key to communities, see Fig. 5–6. From A Keys (ed): *Seven Countries. A Multivariate Analysis of Death and Coronary Heart Disease.* Harvard Univ Press, 1980b, reprinted by permission.

Table 5–5 Mean dietary values from the Japan, Hawaii, and California cohorts of the Ni-Hon-San Study, using 24-hour recalls

Dietary Components	Japan	Hawaii	California
Calories	2132	2274	2268
Total protein (gm)	76	94	89
Total fat (gm)	36	85	95
Fats (gm)			
Mostly saturated	16	59	66
Mostly unsaturated	21	26	29
Dietary cholesterol (mg)	457	545	536
Total carbohydrate (gm)	335	260	251
Simple carbohydrate (gm)	61	92	96
Complex carbohydrate (gm)	278	169	155

Source: Adapted from A Kagan et al: Epidemiologic studies of coronary heart disease and stroke in Japanese men living in Japan, Hawaii and California. *J Chron Dis* **27**:345, 1974, with permission from Pergamon Press, Ltd.

Table 5–6 Mean dietary intake of nutrients from individuals in different ranges of the serum cholesterol distribution: the Framingham Study

	Serum cholesterol range (mg/dl)					
	Men			Women		
Nutrient intake	<180	180–299	⩾300	<180	180–299	⩾300
Number of persons	51	329	51	28	369	45
Fat (gm)						
Animal	94	99	94	63	66	64
Plant	36	39	36	32	30	28
Cholesterol (mg)	669	714	676	499	491	484
Carbohydrates (gm)						
Simple	189	168	153	118	124	127
Complex	166	156	149	106	105	96

Source: Adapted from WB Kannel and T Gordon: *The Framingham Study*, 1970. US Dept of Health, Education and Welfare, with permission.

Table 5–7 Correlation coefficients comparing dietary variables to serum cholesterol levels within each of the three cohorts of the Ni-Hon-San Study[a]

Nutrients	Japan	Hawaii	California
Total calories	−0.018 (n.s.)	−0.015 (n.s.)	−0.073 (n.s.)
Cal/weight	−0.115 (0.01)	−0.063 (0.01)	−0.068 (n.s.)
Cholesterol	0.116 (0.01)	0.038 (0.01)	0.140 (n.s.)
Percent calories from			
Protein	0.110 (0.01)	0.091 (0.01)	0.139 (n.s.)
Fat	0.128 (0.01)	0.122 (0.01)	0.119 (n.s.)
Carbohydrate	−0.067 (0.01)	−0.074 (0.01)	−0.191 (0.05)
Alcohol	−0.048 (0.05)	−0.086 (0.01)	0.050 (n.s.)
Animal protein	0.101 (0.01)	0.101 (0.01)	0.168 (0.05)
Vegetable protein	0.002 (n.s.)	−0.042 (0.01)	−0.110 (n.s.)
Saturated fat	0.147 (0.01)	0.099 (0.01)	0.168 (0.05)
Unsaturated fat	0.023 (n.s.)	0.029 (0.05)	−0.091 (n.s.)
Simple carbohydrate	0.128 (0.01)	−0.023 (0.05)	−0.116 (n.s.)
Complex carbohydrate	−0.127 (0.01)	−0.059 (0.01)	−0.118 (n.s.)
Number of subjects	1717	7949	178

Source: From H Kato et al: Epidemiologic studies of coronary heart disease and stroke in Japanese men living in Japan, Hawaii and California. *Am J Epidemiol* **97**:372, 1973, with permission.

[a] Significance: 0.01, significant at 1% level; 0.05, significant at 5% level; n.s., not significant.

Table 5–8 Regression coefficients, Z scores, and corresponding P values from multiple regressions relating dietary variables to serum cholesterol: the Western Electric Study[a]

Regressor	Diet variables only			All variables		
	Coefficient[b]	Z[c]	P	Coefficient[b]	Z[c]	P
Dietary variables summarized by Keys–Anderson–Grande dietary score						
Keys et al dietary score	0.512	3.407	<0.001	0.537	3.570	<0.001
Body mass index (kg/m²)	—			1.148	2.959	0.003
Age at entry (yr)	—			0.382	1.368	0.171
Constant	216.890			167.901		
Correlation (R)	0.078		<0.001	0.109		<0.001
Saturated fatty acids, polyunsaturated fatty acids, and dietary cholesterol entered directly						
Saturated fatty acids (% of calories)	1.104	2.190	0.014	1.348	2.651	0.004
Polyunsaturated fatty acids (% of calories)	−2.096	−1.524	0.064	−1.699	−1.230	0.109
Dietary cholesterol (mg/1000 kcal)	0.034	1.700	0.044	0.025	1.239	0.108
Body mass index (kg/m²)	—			1.134	2.900	0.004
Age at entry (yr)	—			0.365	1.292	0.196
Constant	229.405			179.552		
Correlation (R)	0.082		0.006	0.110		<0.001

Source: From RB Shekelle et al. Reprinted by permission, *N Eng J Med* **304**:65, 1981.

[a] Note that the results are given adjusted and unadjusted for nondietary covariates.

[b] To convert regression values to millimoles of cholesterol per liter of serum, multiply each coefficient by 0.02586.

[c] Z is the ratio of the regression coefficient to its standard error.

hydrates, the relationships are in the directions anticipated from the small-group experiments. The magnitudes of the correlation coefficients shown in Table 5–7 are small despite frequently being statistically signifcant, but as discussed below, this does not necessarily detract from the hypotheses being tested. A study of 10,000 Israeli men also found small but statistically significant correlations between diet and serum cholesterol (Kahn et al, 1969).

The Chicago Western Electric Company Study (Shekelle et al, 1981) followed 1900 middle-aged men over 19 years to ascertain disease events. Dietary histories were obtained, using the method of Burke on two occasions during the first year of the study. The means of these two estimates were used, as dietary estimates at one point in time (particularly a 24-hour recall) may give a poor estimate of a person's usual diet. The results were analyzed according to individual lipid variables (lower half of Table 5–8) or by the dietary score of Keys' equation (upper half of Table 5–8). Some analyses also included adjustments for nondietary factors (right side of Table 5–8). A statistically significant relationship is found between Keys' dietary score, also the percentage of calories from saturated fatty acids and serum cholesterol levels. This persists when adjusted for non-dietary covariates. There were also significant relationships between *change* in diet and *changes* in serum cholesterol comparing the data collected at the two points 1 year apart. Several studies of vegetarians have also documented significant relationships between diet and serum cholesterol in individuals (pp. 78–81).

Thus, we have an interesting problem. On the one hand, closely controlled experimental work clearly shows that dietary fats influence serum cholesterol in a predictable fashion and international comparisons support this. On the other hand, while some single-community studies of free-living individuals demonstrate such a relationship, other large, well-designed studies do not. In my view, this could have been anticipated and can be explained on the basis of available information (see below).

Analytic Problems in Relating Diet to Serum Cholesterol
in Population Studies

If it is assumed that there is a perfect linear relationship between some combination of dietary variables and serum cholesterol for each individual, then it can be argued that the practicalities of epidemiologic work and the characteristics of a single-community population are such that the observed correlation coefficient will commonly be close to zero. The reasons for this involve measurement errors, the multivariate nature of the relationship, differences in individual responsiveness to diet, and the relative homogeneity of habits within a single population.

Errors occur in measuring both serum cholesterol and dietary variables (Block, 1982; Jacobs and Barrett-Connor, 1982; Jacobs et al. 1979). In addition, there is marked day-to-day "physiologic" variation in serum cholesterol levels within an individual, unrelated to laboratory error. If the relationship between diet and serum cholesterol were identical for everybody, in practice we would *not* find research data falling exactly on a straight line but rather within an ellipse, because of these measurement errors and physiologic variations (inner ellipse, Fig. 5–9).

Factors other than diet affect serum cholesterol levels and need to be adjusted for in any analysis. If this is not done, the apparent correlation is further reduced. As an example, consider the additional effect of obesity on serum cholesterol. Consider two individuals (one thin and one fat) who, as a result of physiologic variations and measurement errors, were thrown far off the true line in either a positive or a negative direction. If the error was in a positive direction (*situation A*, Fig. 5–9), the fat individual would have an even higher cholesterol level because of his fatness and would consequently expand the "shell" of the ellipse in a positive direction. The opposite effect is seen with a negative error (*situation B*, Fig. 5–9) and a thin individual. Consequently, if there is no adjustment for obesity, the correlation coefficient and thus the evidence for a diet–serum cholesterol relationship is reduced—even though we started with the premise of a precise linear relationship. Therefore, other important determi-

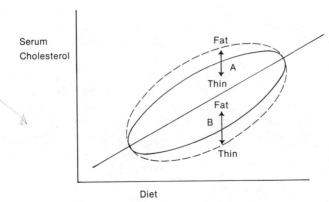

Figure 5–9   Schematic representation of the potential effect of measurement errors and confounding variables on the observed univariate relationship.

nants of serum cholesterol should be measured and adjusted for. A difficulty is that some determinants are probably not known and so cannot be adjusted for.

The problem is aggravated further by differences in individual responsiveness of serum cholesterol to diet. Nearly all individuals do respond to diet with changes in serum cholesterol, but with different linear slopes (Keys et al, 1965c). Keys' equation (p. 54) was for the *average* American male. Adding this complication of heterogeneity of response to our previous diagrammatic representation, we obtain Fig. 5–10. This represents six hypothetical groups, individuals within each group having identical responsiveness to diet. Group C represents the average. Clearly, the magnitude of the overall correlation coefficient has suffered further, and the linearity is difficult to determine when looking at the total data set.

The final complication is that the dietary practices of a population tend to fall within a relatively narrow range. This gives little scope for the relationship to be displayed (Jacobs et al, 1979).

We originally assumed that all individuals respond according to their unique linear relationship, but we end with the prospect of a very small *observed* correlation coefficient when using population data. Population studies need to be carefully designed to overcome some of these problems. Steps that can be taken include

- Assessing diet with great care and using the average of several assessments,
- Taking repeated measurement of serum cholesterol, drawing blood on different days,
- Measuring and adjusting for other factors that may affect serum cholesterol levels,
- Choosing a population with a wide range of dietary habits, and
- Using large numbers of participants to allow the greatest possibility of statistical significance for a given value of the correlation coefficient.

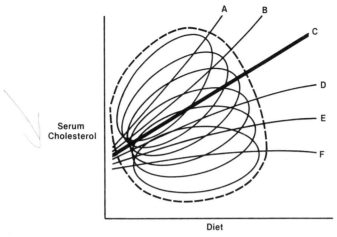

Figure 5–10 A schematic representation of the effect of differences in serum cholesterol responsiveness to diet on the scattergram relating diet to serum cholesterol.

The Western Electric Company Study addresses many of these issues more effectively than most and provides some of the most supportive evidence for the diet–serum cholesterol relationship in a single-community study. If a causal relationship is present, it is the *regression* coefficient not the correlation coefficient that describes the *practical* significance of the relationship by estimating the slope of the regression line. Errors in the estimation of the independent variable, diet, also result in a biased estimate of this regression coefficient to a value lower than the truth (J Berkson, 1950).

A Model and Its Implications for Change

The following two hypotheses concerning reality seem compatible with all the data:

1. Dietary fats are *importantly* and causally related to serum cholesterol levels at both an individual and a community level. The evidence is consistent within studies properly designed to test this hypothesis.
2. Obesity status, heredity, and other unknown factors account for the large majority of the variance in serum cholesterol levels between individuals of a population *within one culture*, not diet.

Note that the truth of this second hypothesis in no way diminishes the validity of the first hypothesis. It is often assumed that where the factor under investigation accounts for only a small percentage of the variance of the outcome variable, the relationship probably has little practical importance. However, in the present context, other explanations are more plausible. Where the *naturally* occurring variability in dietary habits is small and measurement and other

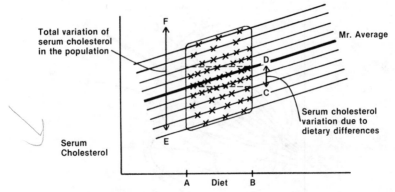

Figure 5–11   A schematic representation of the variation of serum cholesterol ascribable to diet in a single community.

errors are large, the variability in serum cholesterol ascribable to diet can only be small. Such populations are not well suited to test the dietary hypothesis, and this is the situation within the American culture where the standard deviation of Keys' dietary factor (p. 54) is estimated at only 10 (Jacobs et al, 1979). Hypothesis (2) has little relevance to the *individual* in whom obesity, heredity, and other causal factors may be relatively constant. Changes in diet may often be the easiest way to lower serum cholesterol levels, but this may require change to nontraditional dietary habits considering the relatively narrow range of traditional habits when expressed as nutrient intake. *For an individual,* dietary influences may account for a much greater percentage of the week-to-week variability in serum cholesterol. Figure 5–11 depicts this situation, ignoring differences in the slope of responsiveness that may exist between individuals and also ignoring measurement errors. Each straight line in the figure represents a different diet–cholesterol "response track," the differences depending on nondietary factors. As the diet changes from A to B on the abscissa (the community extremes), the ascribable change in serum cholesterol is given by $D - C$. The proportion of the total variability ($F - E$) of serum cholesterol ascribable to diet is roughly represented by the ratio σ_D/σ_T, where σ_T is the standard deviation of serum cholesterol levels across the population, and σ_D is the standard deviation of the serum cholesterol levels that can be ascribed to dietary differences within the population. Figure 5–11 is drawn so that this ratio equals about 0.25, which has been found in practice (Fraser et al, 1981a). The square of this ratio then represents the proportion of variance due to dietary factors and would have a value here of about 6 percent. As the figure shows, however, this in no way denies that each individual will be located on one of the diet–cholesterol "response tracks." Much of the total variability in the community is represented by nondietary differences between individuals that cannot be readily altered.

It follows from this model that cross-cultural comparisons will attribute a higher proportion of the variance of serum cholesterol to diet. This is because

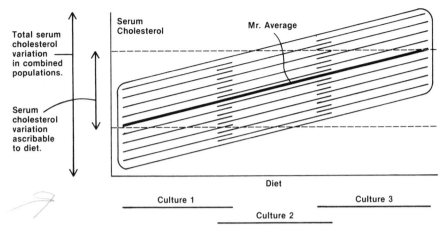

Figure 5–12 A schematic representation of the variation of serum cholesterol ascribable to diet across three communities representing different cultures.

dietary differences are larger across cultures, whereas apparently the variation ascribable to other determinants of serum cholesterol tends to remain fairly constant. Figure 5–12 is schematically similar to Fig. 5–11, but it includes data from three cultures with overlapping dietary habits. As can be seen, the ratio of changes ascribable to diet as compared to the total variability of serum cholesterol implies that diet accounts for about 25 percent of the variance of serum cholesterol.

Serum cholesterol distributions of one country may barely overlap those of a second country. It is often reasonable to ascribe most of this difference to the influence of dietary habits, as in the case of Japan and Finland. Figure 5–13 illustrates this example, using approximate data. Serum cholesterol distributions for Japan and Finland are plotted along the ordinate, and the figure then hypothetically dissects these distributions into dietary and nondietary determinants. The rhomboids schematically represent the boundaries of a scattergram containing 90 percent of individuals in each community. They are positioned according to known values of Keys' diet score and variance of serum cholesterol. Notice that these rhomboids representing the boundaries of each population will collapse back along the ordinate distributions. Consequently, the figure illustrates that using known information, the difference in the distributions of serum cholesterol between these two countries can be explained. A recent report from Finland directly demonstrates that at least a major portion of the hypercholesterolemia here is diet related. Fifty-four middle-aged free-living Finns followed a prudent diet for 6 weeks as part of a switchback study design. Serum cholesterol dropped 62 mg/dl ($P < 0.0001$) in men and 52 mg/dl ($P < 0.0001$) in women during the diet, returning to the previous high values after the diet ended (Ehnholm et al, 1982).

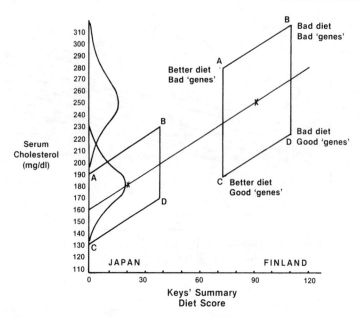

Figure 5–13 A dietary explanation of the widely differing serum cholesterol distributions of Japan and Finland. The term "genes" is used loosely here to refer to nondietary determinants of serum cholesterol.

Obesity and Serum Cholesterol

Although we recognize that diet is not the only contributor to obesity, it seemed appropriate to consider the evidence that obesity affects serum cholesterol levels in this chapter. Many epidemiologic studies have found relatively weak but definite cross-sectional relationships between obesity and serum total cholesterol (Gillum et al, 1982; Kannel and Gordon, 1968; Thelle et al, 1983). Matter et al (1980) performed underwater weighing on 112 sedentary middle-aged men and were able to relate body fat directly to levels of serum total cholesterol. The epidemiologic evidence is even clearer for the relationship between obesity and HDL cholesterol (Avogaro et al, 1978; Glueck et al, 1980), although there is still some discussion regarding whether the inverse cross-sectional relationship is due directly to obesity or to the decreased physical activity generally characterizing obese persons.

The Framingham offspring study showed in 4260 young adult men and women, that as metropolitan relative weight (MRW) increased, so did LDL and VLDL cholesterol, but HDL cholesterol decreased (Garrison et al, 1980). These effects were stronger in males and were particularly demonstrated in the 20–29 age range. Figure 5–14 demonstrates an impressive difference in the total cholesterol/HDL cholesterol ratio between lean (MRW < 100) and obese (MRW > 140) individuals.

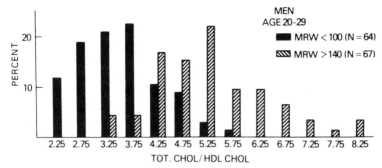

Figure 5–14 Distribution of TCHOL/HDL in 20- to 29-year-old men who are lean (MRW < 140) and obese (MRW > 140). The Framingham Offspring Study. From RJ Garrison et al: Obesity and Liproprotein Cholesterol in the Framingham Offspring Study. *Metabolism* **29**:1053, 1980. Reprinted by permission of Grune & Stratton, Inc. and the author.

The evidence shows that although current obesity status cannot predict future *changes* in serum cholesterol, change in obesity is a potent predictor of change in serum cholesterol (FW Ashley and Kannel, 1974; Gillum et al, 1982). Framingham data suggest that this is independent of age and more pronounced in males. Each 10-unit change in Framingham relative weight was associated with an 11.3 and a 6.3-mg/dl change in serum cholesterol for men and women, respectively. Framingham relative weight was a subject's weight expressed as a percentage of the median weight for his or her particular sex–height group at the first examination of this study population.

Several small experimental studies have investigated the effects of change in weight on serum cholesterol and have generally found similar trends to the epidemiologic work (JT Anderson et al, 1957; Galbraith et al, 1964; Walker, 1953; Wolf and Grundy, 1983). These studies suggest that the effect of weight change on serum cholesterol is probably independent of the quality of fat in the diet.

Summary

1. Measurement of diet for research purposes presents a considerable challenge, hence the value of closely controlled small-group studies.

2. The effects of dietary fatty acids and dietary cholesterol on serum cholesterol have been extensively investigated. The Keys equation describes this relationship for the average male.

3. Medium-chain saturated fatty acids raise serum cholesterol to twice the extent that equivalent amounts of polyunsaturated fatty acids lower serum cholesterol.

4. Stearic (C_{18} saturated) and oleic (C_{18} monounsaturated) acids do not affect serum cholesterol values.

5. Dietary cholesterol consumption affects serum cholesterol in a curvilinear fashion.

6. Certain dietary fibers (pectins, gums) lower serum cholesterol, but wheat bran does not.

7. Skim milk and vegetable protein may lower serum cholesterol, but both of these contentions are controversial.

8. The result of epidemiologic studies seeking to relate diet to serum cholesterol are superficially conflicting. International comparisons find a relationship, but only some studies *within* one culture are positive.

9. Consideration of measurement and analytic problems would lead one to predict such problems in studies within one culture. Sources of error and difficulty include (a) errors in measuring both diet and serum cholesterol, (b) differing individual responsiveness of serum cholesterol to the diet, (c) the effect of nondietary variables on serum cholesterol, and (d) the relative homogeneity of dietary habits within one population.

10. These problems make it difficult to rank individuals within a population appropriately with regard to either serum cholesterol or dietary habits, but much easier to rank appropriately means of whole countries where the intercultural differences are much greater.

11. Within one population, the majority of the interindividual variance of serum cholesterol is nondietary in cause, with much of it probably genetic. This does not contradict the hypothesis that diet is an important determinant of serum cholesterol.

12. A consequence of item 9(d) above is that for some individuals to achieve optimal levels of serum cholesterol, it may be necessary to become nontraditional in dietary habits.

13. Dietary and other habits leading to obesity will elevate serum cholesterol. Studies of weight loss have shown this effect to be reversible.

6

Blood Lipids and Ischemic Heart Disease in Vegetarians

A natural experiment has been under way in the United States for over a century with regard to the blood lipid levels and cardiovascular health of vegetarians. Vegetarianism is considered by many people to be a fad, though less so than 20–30 years ago. In fact, it has been part of American society for at least 150 years, with vocal adherents and detractors. Most studies of vegetarians have been of Seventh-day Adventists (SDA), although there have been occasional studies of other groups of vegetarians that will be mentioned.

The Dietary Habits and Serum Lipid Levels of Seventh-day Adventists

About 50 percent of Seventh-day Adventists are lacto-ovo vegetarians; that is, they eat no meat but may consume eggs and dairy products. Most of the others consume little meat. Adventists also neither smoke cigarettes nor drink alcohol. In most other respects they are typical citizens, integrated with society. One difference is a distinct bias toward upper socioeconomic status and above-average education. Consequently, explanations of differences in health status need to consider more factors than simply dietary differences. Perhaps the most interesting investigations are those that consider health differences within the Adventist population, comparing vegetarians with nonvegetarians.

Several studies have described the dietary habits of Adventists. Wynder et al (1959) interviewed about 950 Adventists and about 820 control non-Adventists to assess dietary habits. The majority of these persons were patients in hospitals, although there were no important differences in the dietary results when compared with the 10 percent or so in each group of cases who were not hospital patients. As can be seen in Fig. 6–1, the Adventists differ sharply in the proportion that do not consume meat, fish, coffee, or tea. Walden et al (1964) compared 145 Californian Adventists with 433 New York non-Adventists (Table 6–1), but did not specify the method of estimating fat, protein, and carbohydrate intake. Nonetheless, it is interesting to compare the figures for the Adventists with the recommendations of the U.S. Senate Select Committee (pp. 103–5), for they virtually coincide. Similar findings on the Adventist diet have been reported by Hardinge et al (1954) and by Fraser and Swannell (1981).

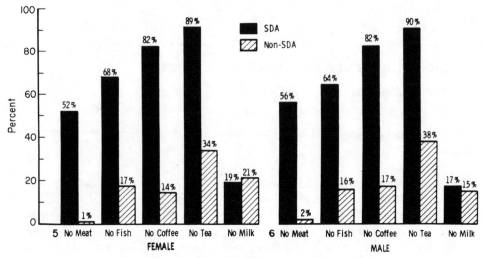

Figure 6–1 Dietary habits of male and female Seventh-day Adventists and non-Seventh-day Adventists. From EL Wynder et al, 1959, with permission.

Table 6–1 Dietary and other habits in Seventh-day Adventists and New Yorkers

	Population group	
Habits	SDA	NYC adults
Calories per day supplied by		
Saturated fat	297 (11%)	540 (18%)
Monounsaturated fat	243 (9%)	510 (17%)
Polyunsaturated fat	270 (10%)	180 (6%)
Protein	405 (15%)	390 (13%)
Carbohydrate	1485 (55%)	1380 (46%)
Total calories	2700	3000
Other factors		
Number of cigarettes per day	0	16
Amount of alcoholic beverages per day (ml)	0	50
Amount of coffee or tea per day (ml)	0	600
Average weight (lb)		
Males	160	177
Females	136	129

Source: Adapted from RT Walden et al: *Am J Med* **36**:269, 1964, with permission.

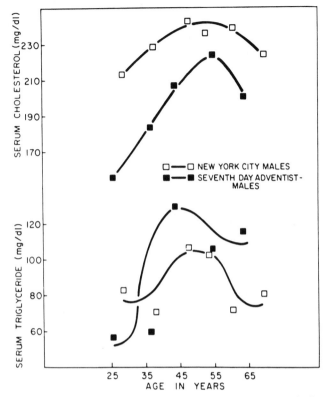

Figure 6–2 Age-specific lipid levels in male New Yorkers and Seventh-day Adventists. From RT Walden et al: *Am J Med* **36**:269, 1964, with permission.

Walden and co-workers also compared serum cholesterol levels between the Californian Adventists and New York non-Adventist adults. Although the age match was rather approximate, the lipid differences are of interest (Figs. 6–2 and 6–3). The Adventists appear to have a clear advantage in serum cholesterol levels, but the serum triglyceride levels are closer. Fraser and Swannell (1981) found that in New Zealand Adventists, serum cholesterol levels were 50 mg/dl lower than a non-Adventist age- and sex-matched New Zealand population. Hardinge et al (1954) reported similar findings in a small group of Californian vegetarians who were mainly Seventh-day Adventists. Lower blood cholesterol levels have also been found in Seventh-day Adventist adolescents. Ruys and Hickie (1976) compared 183 Australian Seventh-day Adventist adolescents with 1456 non-Adventist adolescents aged 12–17 years. Among Adventist children eating no meat, fish, or fowl, the average serum cholesterol was 154.4 mg/dl; for those consuming some meat, fish, or fowl, it was 169.8 mg/dl, and for the non-Adventist adolescents, 200.7 mg/dl. These differences were statistically significant.

The assumption is that these contrasting serum cholesterol values are due to

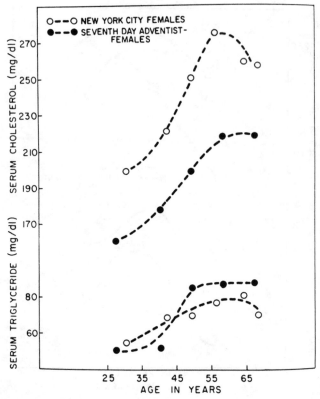

Figure 6–3 Age-specific lipid levels in female New Yorkers and Seventh-day Adventists. From RT Walden et al: *Am J Med* **36**:269, 1964, with permission.

dietary differences. Evidence supporting this comes from three studies that relate diet to serum cholesterol levels *among* Seventh-day Adventists (Fraser et al, 1981a; Hardinge et al, 1962; West and Hayes, 1968). West and Hayes (1968) matched 274 Adventist vegetarians with 274 Adventist non-vegetarians in Washington, D.C. The matching was with respect to the specific church attended, sex, age (within 5 years), marital status, height, weight, and an occupational classification. The results are shown in Table 6–2, where the serum cholesterol levels of the vegetarian member of each pair are compared to those of the nonvegetarian member. The potential confounding effects of all the above-matched variables have been removed, yet the vegetarian Adventists still had an average serum cholesterol level 11 mg/dl lower than the nonvegetarian Adventists. Using multivariate regression techniques, Fraser and Swannell (1981) found significant associations between various foods, nutrients, and serum cholesterol levels in 517 Adventists in New Zealand. Tables 6–3 and 6–4 report the regression coefficients along with their statistical significance. The regression coefficients can be interpreted as the predicted change in the serum

Table 6–2 Differences in serum cholesterol between the vegetarian and nonvegetarian Seventh-day Adventist members of 233 pairs

| Type of nonvegetarian[a] | Number of pairs | Mean serum cholesterol levels (mg/dl) | | P |
		Nonvegetarian	Vegetarian	
MFF less than once each month	61	183	188	>0.20
MFF less than once per week (more than once per month)	47	192	182	>0.05
MFF once or twice per week	48	200	181	<0.01
MFF >3 times per week	77	207	188	<0.01
Total	233	196	185	<0.01

Source: From RO West and OB Hayes, *Am J Clin Nutr* 21:853, 1968, with permission.

[a] MFF, meat, fish, or fowl.

cholesterol for each unit change in the value of the food, nutrient, or other variables, assuming a causal explanation for these associations. At present, little evidence is available concerning lipoprotein profiles in Seventh-day Adventists. Berkel (1979) found lower LDL and HDL cholesterol levels in 190 Dutch Adventist volunteers than 170 of their non-Adventist friends. The trend to lower HDL cholesterol levels in vegetarians is compatible with other reports (pp. 46 and 85–86).

Ischemic Heart Disease Morbidity and Mortality in Seventh-day Adventists

The only investigation of ischemic heart disease morbidity in Adventists was a proportionate morbidity study conducted 25 years ago among eight Seventh-day Adventist Hospitals within the United States (Wynder et al, 1959). Wynder observed that about 10 percent of all patients admitted to these hospitals were Seventh-day Adventists. He hypothesized that if Adventists were particularly protected with respect to IHD, the proportion of patients admitted with this diagnosis who were Adventists would be less than 10 percent. Indeed this was found to be true, especially for males (see Fig. 6–4). However, it was not established that the 10 percent overall Adventist admission proportion applied to both sexes and to all age ranges. Myocardial infarction patients tend to be older and mostly male (at least for the non-Adventists). Nevertheless, the data are impressive and in line with the comparative mortality statistics discussed below. Two other interesting observations emerged. Adventist myocardial infarction

Table 6–3   Multiple regression coefficients showing predicted change in serum cholesterol per unit change of the independent food or other variables[a]

Independent variables	Regression coefficients	P
All cases (constant 318.5 mg/dl; multiple correlation coefficient 0.472)		
Height (cm)	−1.19	<0.001
Age (yr)	2.69	<0.001
(Age)^2	−0.020	<0.005
Only margarine spread (yes = 1, no = 0)	−14.21	<0.001
Ice cream (servings per week)	3.68	<0.05
Cheese (servings per week)	1.55	<0.10
Males (constant 98.30 mg/dl; multiple correlation coefficient 0.508)		
Only margarine spread (yes = 1, no = 0)	−21.37	<0.001
Age (yr)	3.15	<0.001
(Age)^2	−0.025	<0.005
Ice cream (servings per week)	3.97	<0.05
Fried food (servings per week)	2.29	<0.10
Females (constant 417.7 mg/dl; multiple correlation coefficient 0.446)		
Age (yr)	0.58	<0.001
Height (cm)	−1.67	<0.001
Only butter spread (yes = 1, no = 0)	14.24	<0.01
Quetelet's Index (100 × kg/cm^2)	102.11	<0.05
Cheese (servings per week)	2.20	<0.10

Source: Adapted from GE Fraser and RJ Swannell: Diet and serum cholesterol in Seventh-day Adventists. *J Chron Dis* **34**:47, 1981, with permission from Pergamon Press, Ltd.

[a] Under causal hypotheses.

patients were substantially older than non-Adventists, particularly the males, and the sex ratio among the Adventist myocardial infarction patients was close to unity, more in keeping with the pattern of countries where IHD is uncommon (chapter 1).

Three studies comparing IHD mortality in Adventists and non-Adventists have been reported. These are from the United States (Lemon and Walden, 1966; Phillips et al, 1978), the Netherlands (Berkel, 1979), and Norway (Waaler and Hjort, 1981). The U.S. study enrolled in 1958 11,071 Californian Seventh-day Adventist men age 30 years or more and followed them for 4 years, documenting mortality. Death rates among the Adventists for many causes of death, including arteriosclerotic heart disease, were less than 50 percent of those for the general Californian male population at that time (the "expected level" in Fig. 6–5). This is reflected in a changed age distribution for the Adventist male population (Fig. 6–6), which is older than average. The situation for Californian women is quite similar to that of the men. Phillips et al (1978) analyzed this further, reporting also on the 15,850 females who had been included in the

Table 6–4 Multiple regression coefficients showing predicted change in serum cholesterol per unit change of the independent nutrient or other variables[a]

Independent variables	Regression coefficients	P
All cases (constant 218.4 mg/dl; multiple correlation coefficient 0.446)		
Age (yr)	2.79	<0.001
$(Age)^2$	−0.022	<0.005
Height (cm)	−0.84	<0.01
$2S − P$ (gm/wk)	0.044	<0.01
Sex (M = 1, F = 2)	9.34	<0.10
Quetelet's Index ($100 \times kg/cm^2$)	81.36	<0.05
Males (constant 79.47 mg/dl; multiple correlation coefficient 0.434)		
Age (yr)	3.44	<0.001
$(Age)^2$	−0.028	<0.005
$2S − P$ (gm/wk)	0.067	<0.005
Females (constant 389.39 mg/dl; multiple correlation coefficient 0.392)		
Age (yr)	0.62	<0.001
Height (cm)	−1.47	<0.005
Quetelet's Index ($100 kg/cm^2$)	113.41	<0.05
(No lipid variables were significant)		

Source: Adapted from GE Fraser and RJ Swannell: Diet and serum cholesterol in Seventh-day Adventists. *J. Chron Dis* **34**:47, 1981, with permission from Pergamon Press, Ltd.

[a] Under causal hypotheses.

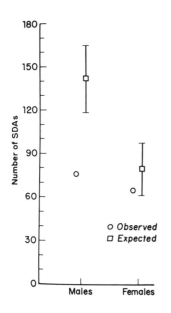

Figure 6–4 Observed and expected numbers of myocardial infarctions in Seventh-day Adventists, based on the proportion of Adventists admitted to these hospitals. From EL Wynder et al, 1959, with permission.

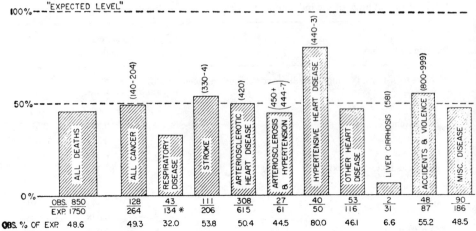

Figure 6–5 Observed and expected cause-specific mortality rates among Californian male Seventh-day Adventists. From FR Lemon and RT Walden: Death from respiratory system disease among Seventh-day Adventist men. *JAMA* **198**:117, 1966. Copyright 1966, American Medical Association.

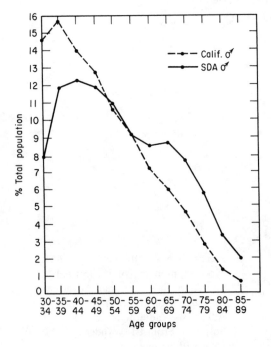

Figure 6–6 Age group distribution of Seventh-day Adventists and California men in 1958 and 1960. From FR Lemon and RT Walden: Death from respiratory system disease among Seventh-day Adventist men. *JAMA* **198**; 117, 1966. Copyright 1966, American Medical Association.

original study. Follow-up was available over 6 years. Compared to a similar population of non-Adventist Californian women, the Adventist women were substantially protected from IHD mortality as standardized mortality ratios were greatly reduced from expectation (the value of 100 in Fig. 6–7 and 6–8). Phillips and colleagues used the data to compare IHD mortality across dietary

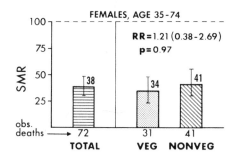

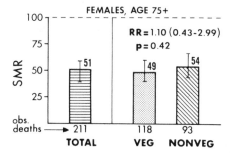

Figure 6–7 Standardized mortality ratios (SMR) for IHD among California SDA females by age and current dietary habits, 1960–1965. Relative risk (RR) = SMR in nonvegetarians: 95% confidence limits are shown in parentheses. From RL Phillips et al: Coronary heart disease mortality among Seventh-day Adventists with differing dietary habits. *Am J Clin Nutr* **31**:S191, 1978, with permission.

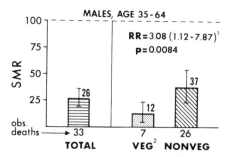

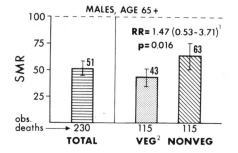

Figure 6–8 Standardized mortality ratios (SMR) for IHD among California SDA males by age and current dietary habits, 1960–1965. From RL Phillips et al: Coronary heart disease mortality among Seventh-day Adventists with differing dietary habits. *Am J Clin Nutr* **31**:S191, 1978, with permission.

categories within the Adventist population for both sexes. In males, clear differences were found between vegetarian and nonvegetarian Adventists with respect to IHD mortality (Fig. 6–8). Females show similar but less impressive differences (Fig. 6–7). The Norwegian study found the male Adventist/non-Adventist mortality ratio to be 64 percent, and the Dutch study found a standardized mortality ratio for ischemic heart disease (males and females combined) of 43 percent. The similar ratio for total mortality in the Netherlands was 45 percent.

Difficulties in Interpreting This Evidence

Seventh-day Adventists are like other Americans in many respects. However, there are differences aside from diet that may be important in influencing risk of IHD. Chief among these is the fact that Adventists do not smoke. However, there is evidence that this alone cannot account for the magnitude of reduction in IHD mortality. Phillips et al (1978) compared the Adventists in the Lemon and Walden (1966) study to Californian male non-Adventists in Hammond's contemporaneous American Cancer Society study (1966). Figure 6–9 shows the standardized mortality ratios for males and females, divided into two age ranges

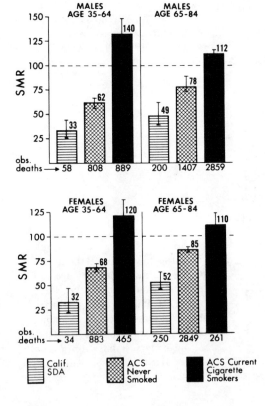

Figure 6–9 Standardized mortality ratios (SMR) for IHD among California SDAs and subjects in the American Cancer Society (ACS) prospective mortality study by smoking habits, sex and age at beginning of study, 1960–1965. From RL Phillips et al: Coronary heart disease mortality among Seventh-day Adventists with differing dietary habits. Am J Clin Nutr 31:S191, 1978, with permission.

and within each age range into Adventists, nonsmoking non-Adventists, and smoking non-Adventists. It is clear that Adventists were substantially protected from IHD mortality even as compared to *nonsmoking* non-Adventist males and females. Another difference is that Adventists generally do not drink alcoholic beverages. The potential effect of this on IHD mortality is controversial (chapter 13). Other differences between Adventists and non-Adventists that may also be important include psychosocial and socioeconomic factors. Adventists are of somewhat higher socioeconomic status than average and probably also have more social support than the average citizen. There are no good comparative data on the incidence or prevalence of hypertension in U.S. Adventists and non-Adventists, but such evidence as exists does not suggest great differences between the two, whether among adults (Fraser et al, unpublished data; JW Kuzma, unpublished data) or among children (RD Harris et al, 1981).

Serum Cholesterol and Ischemic Heart Events in Non-Seventh-day Adventist Vegetarians

Non-Adventist vegetarians show similar trends in blood lipid levels to those of Adventist vegetarians. Barrow et al (1960) compared Trappist and Benedictine monks in the United States. These two Roman Catholic orders are *similar* in most respects apart from their diet: the Trappists are lacto-ovo vegetarians. Levels of total cholesterol, α- and β (closely related to HDL and LDL)-cholesterol were lower in the Trappist monks across all ages (Figs. 6–10 and

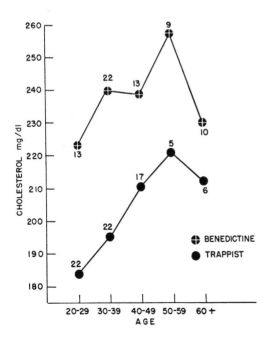

Figure 6–10 The age distribution of total cholesterol in Trappist compared to Benedictine monks. From JG Barrow et al: *Ann Intern Med* **52**:368, 1960, with permission.

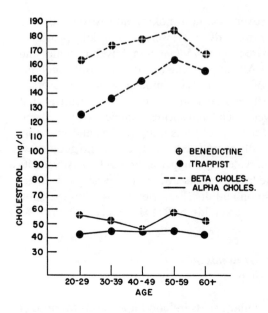

Figure 6–11 The age distribution of α- and β-cholesterol in Trappist compared to Benedictine monks. From JG Barrow et al: *Ann Intern Med* **52**:368, 1960, with permission.

6–11). In a study of young vegetarians who lived in a Boston commune, Sacks et al (1975) matched by age and sex 115 of these persons to a similar number of control nonvegetarians. The lipid differences were dramatic (Table 6–5), as were differences in body weight. Burslem et al (1978) conducted a similar study and published similar findings. Thus, we do not have reason to believe that the results in Seventh-day Adventists are atypical of other vegetarians.

Little information is available on IHD events among the general population of vegetarians. A prospective study of 10,943 British men and women was initiated in 1973 (Burr and Sweetnam, 1982). These persons were eligible because of a special interest in health foods and were recruited as patrons of health food stores, subscribers to certain magazines, or members of appropriate societies. Roughly 42 percent of the men and women were vegetarians. Mortal-

Table 6–5 Lipid differences between 115 vegetarians and matched controls[a]

	Cholesterol (mg/dl)				Triglycerides (mg/dl)	Weight (kg)
	Total	HDL	LDL	VLDL		
Controls	184	49	118	17.2	86	73
Vegetarians	126	43	73	11.8	59	58

Source: From FM Sacks et al. Reprinted by permission, *N Engl J Med* **292**:1148, 1975.

[a] All comparisons significant $P < 0.001$.

Table 6-6 IHD mortality among vegetarian and nonvegetarian British persons interested in health foods, as compared to expectation based on general population rates

Groups studied	Number of deaths		SMR[a]
	Observed	Expected	
Males			
Vegetarians	29	82.8	35.0
Nonvegetarians	58	101.6	57.1
Females			
Vegetarians	28	77.3	36.2
Nonvegetarians	25	59.5	42.0
All subjects			
Vegetarians	57	160.1	35.6
Nonvegetarians	83	161.1	51.5

Source: Adapted from ML Burr and PM Sweetnam: *Am J Clin Nutr* **36**:873, 1982, with permission.

[a] Standardized mortality ratio between study participants and the general population.

ity follow-up was continued for 7 years, and the dietary habits of the vegetarians and nonvegetarians were apparently maintained during this period. The results for IHD mortality significantly favor the vegetarians as compared to the nonvegetarians (Table 6–6). When the authors included cigarette smoking in the analysis, the differences persisted. It was interesting that for the whole group of these persons interested in health foods (vegetarians and nonvegetarians), rates of both IHD (Table 6–6) and overall mortality were 50 percent or less of those pertaining to the general population. A possible healthy volunteer effect should be considered in interpreting this last point.

Summary

1. Seventh-day Adventists and other vegetarians have markedly lower levels of serum cholesterol.

2. It has often proved possible to relate dietary characteristics to serum cholesterol within Seventh-day Adventist populations.

3. Data are sparse regarding IHD morbidity, but one study suggests a considerable morbidity reduction in Adventist males at least, and a sex ratio among Adventist patients more typical of low-risk cultures.

4. It is clear that IHD mortality in Adventists is substantially less than in non-Adventists; also, IHD mortality can clearly be associated with dietary habits within the Adventist group.

5. Possible confounding variables must be considered. Cigarette smoking can

explain only part of the mortality advantage among Seventh-day Adventists. The possible effects of abstinence from alcohol, socioeconomic factors, and social support factors remain to be investigated. It seems unlikely that these could explain the diet–IHD mortality relationships *within* the Adventist population.

6. Non-Adventist vegetarians show similar effects in their blood lipid profiles. One British study shows evidence of lower IHD mortality in an otherwise unselected group of persons interested in health foods, many of whom were vegetarians.

7

Diet and Ischemic Heart Disease

We have seen that diet influences serum cholesterol and that serum cholesterol influences the risk of ischemic heart disease. It would then seem obvious that diet will influence the risk of ischemic heart disease. However, one could argue that the imperfections in the diet–serum cholesterol link and in the serum cholesterol–ischemic heart disease link might add together to make the diet–ischemic heart disease relationship so weak as to have no practical significance. The observation that certain groups of vegetarians have markedly reduced IHD mortality does lend some support to the diet–heart link, and this chapter will further address that relationship by reviewing the evidence directly relating diet to the clinical syndromes of ischemic heart disease. This includes epidemiologic evidence and intervention trials that have mortality and morbidity as end points. We will then discuss the evidence that diet may affect ischemic heart disease by mechanisms other than its influence on serum cholesterol.

Epidemiologic Studies

When the diet–ischemic heart disease relationship is investigated directly, the variables are farther apart in the postulated causal sequence than in the diet–serum cholesterol relationship. Given the difficulties of demonstrating the known diet–serum cholesterol link in some types of epidemiologic studies (pp. 67–71), it is not surprising that the diet–IHD relationship presents similar problems of interpretation.

Ecologic studies that compare whole communities or countries have consistently shown relationships in the expected direction. The abrupt decline in IHD mortality in the Scandinavian countries under German occupation during the Second World War (chapter 1) correlated with dramatic dietary changes but also occurred concurrently with nondietary changes. The Seven Countries Study showed an impressive relationship between saturated-fat consumption and IHD mortality at both 5-year and 10-year follow-ups (Keys, 1980b) (Fig. 7–1). Similar correlations with total fat, monounsaturated fat, and dietary protein were, as expected, much less impressive. As we have seen (chapters 1 and 5), the relationship between dietary variables and IHD mortality in the three locations of the Ni-Hon-San Study is also in the hypothesized direction. The Twenty Countries Study (Byington et al, 1979) also showed a clear correspon-

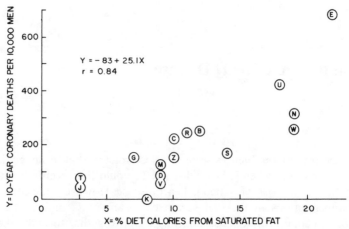

Figure 7–1 The relationship between dietary saturated fat and incidence of IHD in seven countries: 10-year follow-up. For key to communities, see Fig. 5–6 (p. 62). From A Keys: *Seven Countries. A Multivariate Analysis of Death and Coronary Heart Disease.* Harvard Univ Press, 1980b, reprinted by permission.

dence between dietary saturated fatty acids, Keys dietary score, and IHD mortality across different locations.

As with the diet–serum cholesterol relationship, studies within a single population are much harder to interpret. The Framingham Study could find no relationship between diet and IHD (Gordon et al, 1981), except that total calories correlated negatively with risk of MI and IHD death. This may reflect physical activity, in that people who are more physically active consume more calories and physical activity may protect against IHD (chapter 12). In particular, no relationship was found between percentage of calories as fat of any kind, and risk (see Table 7–1). This is hardly surprising in a study that could detect no relationship between dietary fat and serum cholesterol, even though such an effect is established. The Honolulu Heart Study was also unable to relate fat consumption to IHD events within Honolulu males of Japanese descent (Yano et al, 1978), despite documenting some weak but often significant relationships between diet and serum cholesterol (chapter 5). The explanation may be further attenuation introduced by the additional link between serum cholesterol and IHD events that the analysis now includes. Although we expect current diet to relate to current serum cholesterol, it may not relate to present IHD status. If eating habits are altered, the lag between dietary change and change in IHD status may obscure the relationship between diet and IHD.

Some intranational epidemiologic studies do show an important relationship between diet and IHD. In the Western Electric Company Study (chapter 5), as one moves from low to middle to high tertiles of dietary habits within the study population, the IHD death rate changes in the direction expected (Table 7–2). Most of these changes were statistically significant. This study also showed that

Table 7–1 Mean nutrient consumption at baseline according to subsequent CHD status: The Framingham Study[a]

| | | CHD status at end of follow-up | | |
| | | | Developed CHD | |
Nutrient	No CHD ($n = 780$)	Total ($n = 79$)	MI or CHD death ($n = 51$)	Other ($n = 28$)
Percentage of calories from				
Protein	15.7	16.5	16.6	16.6
Fat	38.8	40.2	40.0	40.0
SFA	14.9	15.3	14.8	15.9
MFA	15.8	16.2	16.3	15.9
PFA	5.4	5.8	6.0	5.4
Carbohydrate	38.6	39.7	40.2	38.6
Sugar	11.0	11.8	11.6	11.7
Starch	18.0	19.4	20.4[b]	17.7
Other carbohydrate	9.4	8.4	8.2	9.2
Calories	2622	2488	2369[b]	2651

Source: Adapted from T Gordon et al: Diet and its relation to Coronary Heart Disease and death in three populations. *Circulation* **63**:500, 1981, by permission of the American Heart Asociation, Inc.

[a] Abbreviations: CHD, coronary heart disease; SFA, saturated fatty acids; MFA, monounsaturated fatty acids; PFA, polyunsaturated fatty acids; MI, myocardial infarction.

[b] $P < 0.01$ versus no CHD.

dietary habits were predictive even after adjusting for serum cholesterol levels, which may imply a dietary effect apart from the influence on serum cholesterol levels. Another longitudinal study within one community used 337 male bank employees and London Transport drivers and conductors in a 10- to 20-year mortality follow-up, during which 45 cases of IHD developed (Morris et al, 1977). At baseline, these men had individually weighed dietary records collected for 7 days. As the dietary P/S ratio increased, the incidence of IHD fell. Numbers were small and the relationship did not overall achieve statistical significance, but if real, the magnitude of reduction in events in the highest P/S group was quite marked and reasonably consistent between the subgroups analyzed. In this study population, the dietary P/S ratio varied only between 0.09 and 0.28. As the authors point out, "even this highest ratio is smaller than often regarded as optimal". A case control study reported on the fatty-acid composition of red-cell membrane phosphatidylcholine in 32 men who had recently suffered an acute MI and 32 control men free of IHD (HRC Simpson et al, 1982). This variable reflects long-term dietary fat intake. The patients showed a significantly lower proportion of linoleic acid in their red-cell phosphatidylcholine, indicating that they had eaten less of this substance. Finally,

Table 7–2 Percentage dying from IHD over 19 years, according to baseline tertiles of dietary fat consumption: Western Electric Company Study

Dietary variables[a]	Coronary deaths (%)			Logistic Regression[b]	
	Low third	Middle third	High third	Coefficient	P
Keys et al diet score	9.3	11.2	13.4	0.027	0.010
Saturated fatty acids (% of calories)	10.9	11.2	11.8	0.031	0.144
Polyunsaturated fatty acids (% of calories)	13.5	10.4	10.1	−0.258	0.010
Dietary cholesterol (mg/1000 kcal)	10.9	9.5	13.6	0.003	0.008

Source: Adapted from RB Shekelle et al, by permission, *N Engl J Med* **304**:65, 1981.

[a] The baseline level of each variable in each participant was the mean of the values obtained at the initial examination and at reexamination. The numbers of participants in the low, middle, and high thirds were 631, 636, and 633, respectively, for polyunsaturated fats; they were 633, 634, and 633, respectively, for the other four variables.

[b] Other regressors in each analysis were age, systolic blood pressure, number of cigarettes smoked per day, serum cholesterol concentration, number of alcoholic drinks per month, and body mass index (weight/height^2). Also included were three variables that indicated whether participants or their parents had been born in western or northern Europe, in middle Europe, or in other areas outside the United States. These latter variables were included because ethnicity might have affected diet and risk of coronary heart disease.

two studies involving vegetarians have shown significant relationships between diet and IHD events within single populations (chapter 6).

Clinical Trials of Diet in Ischemic Heart Disease

Intervention trials, particularly when randomized, are one of the best tests of the causal nature of a relationship. They demonstrate the efficacy of the intervention on the disease process, which is the important practical consideration. There is a considerable advantage in using an experimental design, as this allows close control of potentially confounding variables. A disadvantage is expense and the difficulty of obtaining long-term dietary compliance. Consequently, the number of participants in such studies is sometimes relatively small.

Such experimental studies of dietary intervention involve men who do not have clinical signs or symptoms of ischemic heart disease (primary prevention) or in whom ischemic heart disease is already present (secondary prevention). These latter will be considered in chapters 18–19. The end points are the various manifestations of ischemic heart disease. The studies differ in the adequacy of design and in the type of intervention diet. A design where participants were randomized to intervention–nonintervention is preferable. The relevant dietary experiments available with adequate design are compiled in Table 7–3.

Table 7-3 Controlled clinical trials assessing diet as a means of primary prevention of ischemic heart disease

Study and reference	Design	Number of men		Years following	Diet[a]						Serum cholesterol difference (%)	Attack rates		P	Syndrome
		Diet	Control		TF(%) D	C	S(%) D	C	P(%) D	C		Diet	Control		
Finnish Mental Hospital study (Turpeinen et al, 1979)	Crossover	1000	1000	6	31	31	8	17	12	4	18	3.0	6.1/1000 person-years	0.01	Coronary death
												4.2	12.7/1000 person-years	0.001	Major ECG change or coronary death
Anticoronary Club (N.Y.) (Rinzler, 1968)	"Controlled" trial	1473[b]	457	<7	33	40	11	18	11	6	11	5.7	10.25/1000 person-years	?	New IHD events
L.A. Vets (Dayton et al, 1969)	Randomized controlled trial	424	422	8	39	40	7	14	14	4	13	0.28	0.42/8 yr	0.02	Sudden death, definite MI, and CVA
Oslo trial (Hjermann et al, 1981)	Randomized controlled trial (high risk)	604	628	5	28	44	8	18	8	7	13	31.0	57.0/1000/5 yr	0.028	Total coronary events
												26.0	38.0/1000/5 yr	0.246	Total mortality

[a] Abbreviations: D, dieting group; C, control group; TF, total fat; S, saturated fat; P, polyunsaturated fat.

[b] About 40 percent of dieters were "inactive" and are excluded from the "serum cholesterol difference" but included in the event analysis.

Generally the estimated reduction in IHD for the dieting groups is 50 percent or better. The Finnish Mental Hospital Study and the Los Angeles Veterans Administration Study will be described now in more detail. The reader can refer to chapter 17 for a more complete description of the Oslo Study, which had a randomized controlled design, and was based on a community sample.

The Finnish study used two mental hospitals (N and K) in a crossover design (Table 7–4) with 6 years on each limb of the crossover, giving a total study period of 12 years. The intervention diet replaced milk and butter with soybean milk emulsion and a soft margarine. Overall fat content was 31 percent of calories in both the normal and cholesterol-lowering diets. Marked differences in the fatty-acid composition of subcutaneous fat were found during the different dietary periods, indicating good adherence (Table 7–5). There were also marked changes in serum cholesterol levels during the different phases of the study in both hospitals (Fig. 7–2). Clearly defined criteria were developed for the diagnosis of IHD, based on the electrocardiogram or deaths ascribed to ischemic heart disease. Electrocardiograms were classified by Minnesota coding, and patterns were divided into major and intermediate patterns, usually due to IHD. At the beginning of the study, any patients with such changes and so probably having disease, were excluded. The criteria for coronary death were similarly clearly defined to include sudden unexpected death, slower death with objective evidence of IHD, and death with acute changes in the coronary arteries or recent MI at autopsy (Turpeinen et al, 1979). All records were reviewed by three physicians.

The findings are striking. Whether the analysis is stratified by hospital (Table 7–6) or by time period (Table 7–7), the results consistently favor the serum cholesterol-lowering dieters. The differences are often statistically significant. Even among those cases who initially had a diagnosis of ischemic heart disease, and so were excluded from the above incidence analysis, the results were similar, with IHD mortality 32.1 and 52.5, and major ECG change or IHD death 32.3 and 66.1 (per 1000 person-years), respectively, for the dieting and control periods.

This study has been criticized as there was some turnover of participants in each hospital between the different dietary periods, patients being admitted and discharged. Thus, it was not entirely a comparison of the *same* people on different diets. However, the investigators showed that the risk factors of the patients at each hospital during each dietary period were comparable.

The Los Angeles Veterans Administration Study (Dayton et al, 1969), begun in 1959 and completed in 1967, involved 846 veterans with a mean age of 65 years at intake. The men, residents at the Veterans Administration facility, were randomly assigned to the experimental or control groups, with good matching of the important risk factors, and were fed in two different cafeteria lines. The main effort was to replace saturated fat and dietary cholesterol with polyunsaturated fats. Adherence to the diet was only fair, with about 50 percent of the available meals being eaten at the facility by the dieters. That both groups were free to eat elsewhere should decrease the power of the study to show an

Table 7–4 Crossover design of the Finnish Mental Hospital dietary trial[a]

Study period	Hospital N	Hospital K
Period 1 (6 yr)	↑P, ↓S	↓P, ↑S
Period 2 (6 yr)	↓P, ↑S	↑P, ↓S

[a] Abbreviations: P, polyunsaturated fatty acids; S, saturated fatty acids.

Table 7–5 Subcutaneous fatty acid composition (% of total fatty acids) of subjects near end of dietary periods: Finnish Mental Hospital trial

Fatty acid	Near end of period 1		Near end of period 2	
	Hospital N	Hospital K	Hospital N	Hospital K
Myristic	1.54	3.81	4.51	1.43
Palmitic	16.61	22.42	23.19	15.85
Linoleic	26.91	10.25	9.78	32.48

Source: Adapted from O Turpeinen et al, 1979, with permission.

effect, as the dietary differences between the two groups were decreased. Despite this, a substantial drop in serum cholesterol was achieved by the dieters as compared to the control group. Figure 7–3 shows the results for "hard" cardiovascular disease end points over a period of about 8 years. The result clearly favors the dieters to a statistically significant degree. However, there was very little difference in *total* mortality between the two groups. At least a partial explanation for this is that ischemic heart disease deaths account for about 35 percent of total mortality, so that a major difference in IHD mortality would represent a much smaller difference in total mortality. Random fluctuations in non-IHD mortality might then result in even smaller observed differences in total mortality between the groups. It can readily be shown that a study designed with numbers adequate to show a difference in IHD mortality may have inadequate power to detect significant differences in total mortality that are attributable only to reductions in IHD mortality.

The Los Angeles Veterans Administration Study is sometimes cited to support the hypothesis that dietary interventions of this type increase the risk of cancer. Although there were more cancer cases in the dieting group, this difference was not quite statistically significant. A composite of several similar studies (Ederer et al, 1971) gives no suggestion of differences in cancer incidence (Table

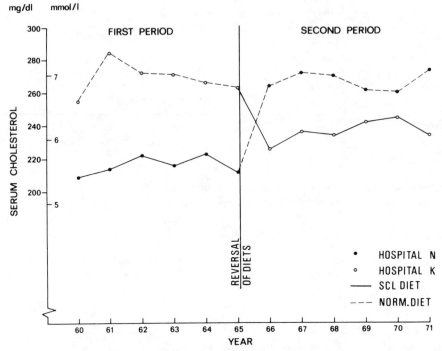

Figure 7–2 Changes in serum cholesterol over time for the two hospitals of the Finnish Mental Hospital dietary trial. From O Turpeinen et al, 1979, with permission.

Table 7–6 Intrahospital comparisons of rates per 1000 person-years between the two dietary periods: Finnish Mental Hospital Study[a]

Hospital	Coronary death		Major ECG change or coronary death		Major or intermediate ECG change or coronary death	
	Diet	Normal	Diet	Normal	Diet	Normal
N	3.7	4.3	3.7	13.9	10.3	20.3
	$P = 0.42$		$P = 0.005$		$P = 0.03$	
K	2.3	8.0	4.7	11.5	16.8	28.3
	$P = 0.06$		$P = 0.06$		$P = 0.06$	

[a] One-tailed P values used.

Table 7–7   Interhospital comparisons of rates per 1000 person-years within each of the two dietary periods: Finnish Mental Hospital Study[a]

Study period	Coronary death		Major ECG change or coronary death		Major or intermediate ECG change or coronary death	
	Hospital N	Hospital K	Hospital N	Hospital K	Hospital N	Hospital K
1	3.7	8.0	3.7	11.5	10.3	28.3
	$P = 0.11$		$P = 0.025$		$P = 0.002$	
2	4.3	2.3	13.9	4.7	20.3	16.8
	$P = 0.25$		$P = 0.02$		$P = 0.29$	

[a] One-tailed P values used. Hospital N on diet in period 1 and vice versa in period 2.

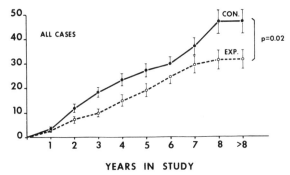

Figure 7–3   Cumulative percentage incidence of hard cardiovascular events in dieters (EXP.) and nondieters (CON.) of the Los Angeles Veterans Administration Dietary Trial. From S Dayton et al: A controlled clinical trial of a diet high in unsaturated fat in preventing complications of atherosclerosis. *Circulation* **40**(suppl 2):1, 1969, by permission of the American Heart Association, Inc.

7–8). Notice that the 95 percent confidence interval for the relative risk (*R*) of cancer in dieters as compared to nondieters always easily includes the null point of 1.0.

In summary, all four primary-prevention experiments cited in Table 7–3 can be interpreted as supporting the effectiveness of diet in primary prevention. In addition, the Coronary Primary Prevention Trial, though a drug trial, has a strong implication that dietary lowering of serum cholesterol will be effective prevention of IHD (chapter 20).

Table 7–8 Tests of significance and estimates of relative risk of cancer in dieters versus nondieters using five studies

	Mantel–Haenszel test (χ_1^2)	Relative risk (R) (Gart) and 95% confidence interval for R
Cancer patients		
Four studies (excluding L.A.)	0.48	0.75 (0.37–1.52)
Five studies (including L.A.)	0.54	1.15 (0.81–1.63)
Cancer deaths		
Four studies (excluding L.A.)	1.25	0.62 (0.28–1.35)
Five studies (including L.A.)	0.08	1.08 (0.71–1.69)

Source: From F Ederer et al, 1971, with permission.

Platelets and Ischemic Heart Disease

The implication to this point has been that any effect of diet on clinical events or atherosclerosis is mediated only by way of serum cholesterol over a long period. In some circumstances, however, the clinical manifestations of ischemic heart disease may be alleviated more rapidly apparently under the influence of marked dietary change, as in the Scandinavian countries during World War II. The short-term controlled studies of Hartley and Ornish (see chapter 18) found important symptomatic improvement in angina patients within a few weeks of a marked dietary intervention. Since it seems unlikely that reduction in serum cholesterol levels could affect such a prompt change by regression of atherosclerotic lesions, there has been much recent interest in a possible second dietary mechanism that involves platelet function.

We now understand that environmental changes can affect both platelet adhesiveness and aggregation (Hammerschmidt, 1982). Good evidence allows us to hypothesize a sequence of events that integrates both platelet function and lipoprotein levels in the production of atherosclerosis. Endothelial damage may have many causes (Ross and Glomset, 1976a,b). In addition to elevated blood cholesterol, these include the mechanical stress of hypertension, the catecholamine response to cigarette smoking, and possibly the effect of carbon monoxide. Such damage usually provokes adherence by platelets to the damaged area, and there is evidence that platelets are more likely to be activated in the presence of elevated blood cholesterol levels (Carvalho et al, 1974; Nordoy and Rodset, 1971). Platelets contain many potent biologically active substances, including platelet growth factor (PGF), which stimulates the proliferation of arterial smooth muscle cells (Ross, 1980). It is postulated that repeated cycles of injury, platelet activation at the site of injury, and release of PGF and other chemicals may lead to a permanent lesion involving mitogenesis and migration of smooth muscle cells into the arterial intima to produce fibrosis. It is likely that endothelial injury from diverse causes allows entrance of lipoprotein complexes through areas of endothelial denudation into the intima, particularly if serum lipoprotein levels are elevated. The role of platelets in atherogenesis was recently reviewed by Haft (1979).

A variety of sources suggest that platelet function not only is important in atherogenesis but is altered in patients with symptomatic IHD and may even be involved in symptom production (J Mehta, 1983). A few investigators have found platelet activation to be enhanced in patients with clinically stable ischemic heart disease (SP Levine et al, 1981; J Mehta and P Mehta, 1981b,c). Evidence of such activation is more consistent when patients are placed under a tachycardic stress, whether by exercise or pacing (LH Green et al, 1980; Kumpuris et al, 1980; J Mehta and P Mehta, 1981c). It seems most probable that platelets are activated as they cross a turbulent and diseased myocardial vascular bed (P Mehta et al, 1979). This may lead to yet worsened atherosclerosis by stimulating the process. Possibly just as important is the documented ability of certain chemicals released by platelets to cause arterial spasm (JB Smith, 1981), which is now known to be associated with many of the clinical events of IHD possibly as an initiating factor (Maseri, 1981). It has also been shown that coronary spasm can increase the tendency to endothelial damage and thus to further platelet activation (Oliva, 1981). So a vicious circle may result. Finally, there is evidence that platelet aggregates themselves may obstruct the coronary microcirculation (Haft, 1979). Some of these platelet-mediated mechanisms such as spasm or formation of obstructing platelet aggregates can change rapidly, hence the potential for rapid reduction in risk.

Two groups of chemicals that affect platelet activation are the prostacyclins and the thromboxanes, both members of the prostaglandin family. Prostacyclins are produced by the endothelium; they inhibit platelet activation and also promote vasodilatation. Thromboxanes are produced by platelets during activation and tend to promote further platelet activation, as well as vascular spasm. The most important members of these prostaglandin families are the prostacyclin PGI_2 and thromboxane A_2. Both are metabolites of arachidonic acid, a long-chain polyunsaturated fatty acid. Dietary linoleic acid can be converted to arachidonic acid, although the conversion is slow and incomplete. The biologic significance of linoleic acid in affecting platelet function is thus difficult to predict, as the formation of both PGI_2 and thromboxane A_2 may be provoked by its conversion to arachidonic acid (Galli et al, 1980; Crawford and Stevens, 1981). There is also some evidence that dietary linoleic acid may directly inhibit the formation of thromboxane A_2 from arachidonic acid, and so be beneficial by altering the balance in favor of prostacyclin PGI_2 (Gerrard et al, 1976).

There exists an analogous pair of prostaglandins, prostacyclin PGI_3 and thromboxane A_3, derived from the n-3 family of polyunsaturated fatty acids (Hamilton et al, 1980). It seems that PGI_3 is normally active, but that throm-

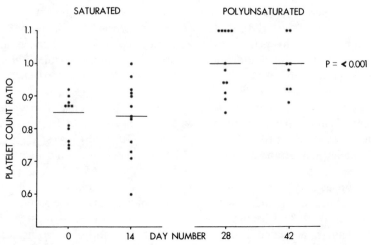

Figure 7–4 An index of the number of blood platelet aggregates during two dietary fat phases of an experiment. (Platelet count ratio has inverse relationship with number of platelet aggregates.) From JA Jakubowski and NG Ardlie, 1978, with permission.

boxane A_3 is relatively inactive. One common precursor to both is the poly-unsaturated eicosapentaenoic acid, found in many fish oils. α-Linolenic acid (found particularly in olive and soybean oils) is also a precursor of eicosapen-taenoic acid in many species, but whether this conversion occurs in humans is controversial. Because of the relative inactivity of thromboxane A_3 yet normal antiaggregatory activity of PGI_3, increased production of this pair may be a beneficial situation.

Diet, Platelet Function, and Ischemic Heart Disease

The theory above has been directly tested, and that diet influences platelet func-tion has been established by studies using saturated fatty acids, linoleic acid, and the longer chain polyunsaturated acids found in marine oils. Small-group feeding experiments with platelet function as the end point consistently show that fats containing linoleic acid reduce platelet aggregability, and saturated fatty acids probably do the reverse (Fleischman et al, 1975, 1979; Hornstra et al, 1973; Jakubowski and Ardlie, 1978; O'Brien et al, 1976). Figure 7–4 depicts the results of an experiment in which 12 healthy male subjects changed from a diet high in butter to one high in polyunsaturated margarine on the 14th day of a 42-day trial. This change reduced the number of circulating platelet aggregates (the platelet count ratio of Fig. 7–4 is an *inverse* measure of circulating platelet aggregates) (Jakubowski and Ardlie, 1978). A few reports suggest that other foods such as onion, garlic, ginger, and an edible Chinese tree fungus may also decrease platelet reactivity (Ariga et al, 1981; Bordia, 1978; Dorso et al, 1980; Hammerschmidt, 1980; Makheja et al, 1979).

Similar experiments have addressed the effect of fish or fish oils. Siess and co-workers (1980) showed that men fed a diet of mackerel had reduced platelet aggregation and reduced thromboxane synthesis. Lorenz et al (1983) supplemented the diet with 40 mg/day of cod liver oil and documented increased bleeding time as well as decreased platelet aggregation and thromboxane formation. Systolic blood pressure also fell significantly by 8 mm Hg. The findings of Hay and co-workers (1982) were essentially the same, but the subjects were persons with established ischemic heart disease. Nagakawa et al (1983) used eicosapentaenoic acid directly (2 gm/day) in an experimental protocol and demonstrated similar changes in platelet function and also significant lowering of serum cholesterol. These results can presumably all be related to increased consumption of the n-3 family of polyunsaturated fatty acids.

A few epidemiologic investigations bear on platelet function. Greenland Eskimos, whose diet is largely carnivorous, have a very low frequency of ischemic heart disease (Bang and Dyerberg, 1972) and despite high fat and protein consumption have relatively low levels of LDL and VLDL cholesterol, and higher levels of HDL cholesterol, as compared to Danes (Bang et al, 1971). In addition, they show prolonged bleeding times and elevated levels of serum eicosapentaenoic acid (Dyerberg et al, 1978; Dyerberg and Bang, 1979). This apparent anomaly in the epidemiologic evidence can probably now be explained. Actually, total fat consumption is not consistently higher than that of many other Western ethnic groups (Bang et al, 1976). Saturated-fat consumption is decidedly less than that of Danes in Denmark, and polyunsaturated-fat consumption is also moderately lower in the Eskimos. A possible explanation for the lower serum cholesterol levels in Eskimos is that most of the fat in the Eskimo diet comes from marine animal sources, whereas most fat in Western diets comes from land animal and dairy sources. The marine sources provide Eskimos with high quantities of monounsaturated fatty acids and, more importantly, with different polyunsaturated fatty acids. Fish oils and to some extent marine mammalian fats from sub-Arctic and Arctic regions contain larger quantities of the n-3 fatty acids, which in addition to their effect on platelet aggregability may also lower VLDL and LDL cholesterols and raise HDL cholesterol (Fehily et al, 1983; Goodnight et al, 1981; Rothrock et al, 1982; Van Lossonczy et al, 1978). However, the evidence for lipid lowering is mixed, and studies often lacked adequate dietary control. The Japanese get much of their protein and fat from fish, and it has been speculated that this may be an additional reason for the protection of Japanese from ischemic heart disease (Hirai et al, 1980; Kobayaski et al, 1981).

Very little epidemiologic evidence is available comparing platelet aggregability within a single population or country. Renaud et al (1981) found that farmers in western Scotland consumed more saturated and less polyunsaturated fats than farmers in eastern Scotland. Platelet reactivity was also significantly greater in the west. Moreover, individual dietary habits and indices of platelet reactivity usually correlated significantly.

The relationships between platelet function, traditional risk factors, patho-

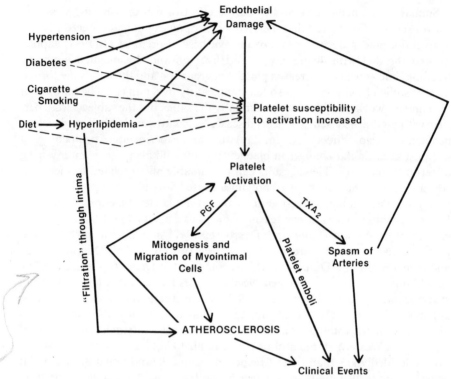

Figure 7–5 A schematic summary of the proposed relationships among diet, platelet function, atherosclerosis, and clinical events. Abbreviations: PGF, platelet growth factor; TXA$_2$, thromboxane A$_2$.

logy, and clinical manifestations are complex; Figure 7–5 attempts to summarize them. Notice that the dietary changes recommended to improve lipid profiles (see U.S. dietary goals below) are those also effective in reducing platelet reactivity. Effects of diet on blood pressure levels are described in chapter 10.

The Prospect of Regression of Atherosclerosis by Dietary Means

The possible resolution of obstructive atherosclerotic coronary artery lesions under the influence of diet has been hotly debated for many years. We should not confuse this question with the prospect of diet-induced improvements in symptoms and the frequency of clinical events. As mentioned in chapter 3, obstructive coronary changes are appropriately considered a risk factor for the clinical disease rather than the disease itself. The majority of the adult population of most western communities have atherosclerotic coronary lesions, and the natural history of these lesions is usually relentless progression (Bruschke et al, 1981). There are 4 million Americans with clinically evident ischemic heart disease. The possibility of regression of lesions should therefore be of vital interest. Is there any evidence that human atherosclerosis might be reversible? Yes, but the evidence, mostly based on sequential contrast angiography, is sparse and difficult to interpret. Malinow (1981) reviewed 11 studies, some of which reported regression in *some* individuals in these studies. The investigators studied either the femoral or coronary arterial beds and used diet, hypolipidemic drugs, or ileal bypass to lower blood cholesterol. Whether it was the diet or other influences that provoked regression is unanswered. This would require a controlled trial to ensure that the frequency of arrest or regression in the intervention group exceeded that of the natural history of the disease as shown by the control group. Most of the studies reviewed by Malinow covered periods of less than 2–3 years. A process that represents accumulation over 40 to 50 years would probably require prolonged dietary intervention to regress.

The Leiden regression trial used a group of angina patients to investigate the effect of a vegetarian diet on coronary artery lesions. Adherence to the diet was excellent over a 2-year follow-up as documented by the linoleic acid content of serum cholesterol esters. Coronary angiography was performed at baseline and at 2 years. The angiograms were read by both a computerized process and also by two independent cardiologists scoring 32 segments of the coronary arteries for each patient. Preliminary reports (Arntzenius et al, 1982, 1983) indicate highly significant associations between changes in serum total/HDL cholesterol ratios and lesion growth with almost identically valued correlation coefficients for both human and computerized coronary artery scoring. About one-third showed increased coronary artery diameters on repeat angiography.

The question of lesion regression has been studied in rhesus monkeys and other primate and nonprimate species (ML Armstrong, 1976; Wissler et al, 1977). ML Armstrong et al (1970) put a group of rhesus monkeys on an atherogenic diet for 17 months, after which a proportion of the monkeys were killed and obstructive coronary atherosclerosis was usually demonstrated. The remaining monkeys were put on a diet low in cholesterol and total fat, or a low-cholesterol, high-corn oil diet for an additional 40 months. These remaining monkeys were then also killed and their coronary arteries inspected. Luminal narrowing, which averaged about 65 percent in the first group, was only 25 percent in the second group (ML Armstrong et al, 1970).

United States Dietary Goals

While not everyone agrees on the detailed interpretation of the data discussed in this chapter, most authorities are impressed with the potential of diet for primary if not secondary prevention. Several organizations have made dietary recommendations in the United States, United Kingdom, Australia, and New Zealand. The U.S. Senate Select Committee on Nutrition and Human Needs (1977) recommends that individuals do the following:

- Avoid overweight, consume only as much energy (calories) as is expended; if overweight, decrease energy intake and increase energy expenditure.
- Increase the consumption of complex carbohydrates and "naturally occurring" sugars from about 28 percent to about 48 percent of energy intake.
- Reduce the consumption of refined and processed sugars by about 45 percent, so that they account for about 10 percent of total energy intake.
- Reduce overall fat consumption from approximately 40 percent to about 30 percent of energy intake.
- Reduce saturated-fat consumption so that it accounts for about 10 percent of total energy intake; and balance that with polyunsaturated and monounsaturated fats, which should account for about 10 percent of energy intake each.
- Reduce cholesterol consumption to about 300 mg/day.
- Limit salt intake to about 5 gm/day.

More recent information on the diet of the average American adult is shown in Fig. 7–6 and compared to the recommendations of the U.S. Senate Select Committee on Nutrition and Human Needs, showing how far apart the two are.

Summary

1. International comparisons support the predicted relationship between diet and IHD. However, intranational epidemiologic studies give mixed results, probably as an extension of the measurement and other analytic difficulties discussed in chapter 5 for the diet–serum cholesterol link.

2. Clinical trials of diet as *primary* prevention give consistent positive results. A reduction in IHD events is seen. However, a reduction in total mortality is not proven, as these studies were generally not designed to adequately investigate this question.

3. Platelet function probably has a major role to play in atherogenesis, the production of angina, infarction, and sudden death.

4. Platelet function is importantly affected by two classes of prostaglandins: the prostacyclins and the thromboxanes. Prostacyclin is antiaggregatory and the thromboxanes are proaggregatory.

5. Platelet function and prostaglandin production are partially under dietary control, with saturated fatty acids being proaggregatory and polyunsaturated vegetable fatty acids being antiaggregatory.

6. Fish oils promote the formation of a particular prostacyclin and thromboxane that appear to favor an antiaggregatory effect. Fish oils may also lower serum cholesterol. This may explain the low IHD status of Eskimos despite a diet high in animal fat.

7. Regression of atherosclerosis by dietary means is unproven; the necessary

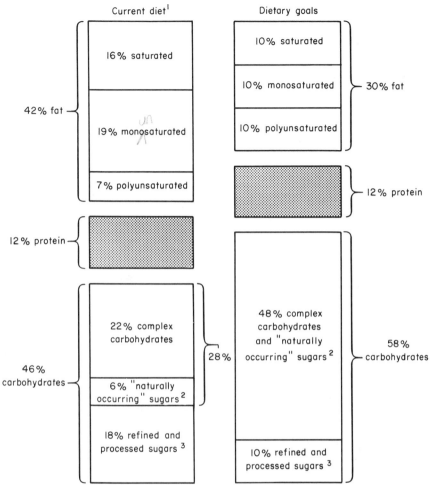

Figure 7–6 Dietary goals for the United States proposed by a Senate select committee, compared to the current U.S. diet. (1) These percentages are based on calories from food and nonalcoholic beverages. Alcohol adds approximately another 210 calories per day to the average diet of drinking-age Americans. (2) "Naturally occurring": Sugars which are indigenous to a food, as opposed to refined (cane and beet) and processed (corn sugar, syrups, molasses, and honey) sugars that may be added to a food product. (3) In many ways alcoholic beverages affect the diet in the same way as refined and other processed sugars. Both add calories (energy) to the total diet but contribute little or no vitamins or minerals. From US Select Committee on Nutrition and Human Needs, US Senate: *Dietary Goals for the United States*, 1977, pp. 4–5.

studies have not been performed. There is suggestive evidence from studies of both human and nonhuman primates.

8. Dietary goals for the United States have been set by an expert committee. Current eating habits are far removed from these.

8

Cigarette Smoking and Ischemic Heart Disease

Cigarette smoking is well known as an important cause of lung, upper respiratory, and oropharyngeal cancers. It is not so widely appreciated that smoking is responsible for more morbidity and mortality from ischemic heart disease than from lung cancer. In the United States, the Office of Cancer Communications, National Cancer Institute (1977), estimated that 25 percent of the 648,540 deaths from IHD in 1975 were attributable to cigarette smoking, whereas the number of lung cancer deaths in the same year was 80,000. In this chapter we will review the evidence for a causal link between cigarette smoking and ischemic heart disease.

An important preliminary issue is the measurement of smoking behavior. Most studies until recently have relied on either questionnaires or interviews to document smoking status. However, there is evidence that up to 20 percent of smokers either lie or at least somewhat distort the truth (Kozlowski et al, 1980).

A search for more objective measures has led to two fairly easily implemented methods. Thiocyanate is a product of the detoxification of trace amounts of hydrogen cyanide in tobacco smoke, and an estimate of serum, salivary, or urinary thiocyanate can serve as a means of distinguishing smokers from non-smokers (Borgers and Junge, 1979; Vogt et al, 1979). An advantage of thiocyanate is the long half-life of metabolism and excretion, around 10–14 days. A disadvantage is that certain common foods such as cabbage, broccoli, cauliflower, turnips, radishes, garlic, mustard, and almonds are also thiocyanate producers. Persons eating relatively large quantities of these may produce false-positive results for smoking.

An alternative method is the measure of exhaled carbon monoxide. Industrial atmospheric pollution and even travel in automobiles can produce false-positive results when this measure is used. The half-life is only about 4 hours, and a smoker need abstain only for a few hours to produce false-negative results. Overall the thiocyanate and carbon monoxide measures have been reported to show a roughly similar sensitivity and specificity of 80–90 percent (JD Cohen and GE Bartsch, 1980). Questionnaires often try to refine the index of exposure by adding such questions as depth of inhalation, amount of the cigarette smoked, and the use of filters. Vogt and colleagues (1979) reported that these questions did not significantly enhance accuracy as assessed by thiocyanate or carbon monoxide analyses.

Studies in Men Linking Cigarette Smoking to Risk of Ischemic Heart Disease

The major longitudinal studies have all analyzed the link between smoking and IHD. The Pooling Project combined the data on men from the Framingham, Albany, Chicago People's Gas Company, Chicago Western Electric Company, and Tecumseh studies, and demonstrated (Table 8–1) that the risk ratio for a first major coronary event, comparing persons who smoke more than a pack per day with nonsmokers, is substantial but *decreases* with age (Pooling Project Research Group, 1978). The dose–response effect is impressive, as can be seen in the right-hand column of Table 8–1. Similar evidence (Kagan et al, 1975) comes from the Honolulu Heart Study (Fig. 8–1). Cigarette smoking is a risk factor for all of the coronary syndromes except possibly angina. This was indicated by the results of the Honolulu Heart Study (Fig. 8–1); the Albany and Framingham studies revealed only a weak relationship between angina and the number of cigarettes smoked (Doyle et al, 1962). These major studies indicated that the risk associated with cigarette smoking is independent of the effects of other major risk factors.

The relationship between cigarette smoking and IHD is probably complex. The Seven Countries Study, for instance, described a fascinating phenomenon (Keys, 1980b). Across these international communities, there was no apparent

Table 8–1 Risk of a first major coronary event in men of stated ages: the Pooling Project

Daily cigarette smoking pattern	Average annual risk by age group (per 1000 person-yrs)					Risk ratio[a]
	40–44	45–49	50–54	55–59	60–64	
Nonsmokers	(1.5)[b]	3.0	3.6	7.3	15.5	0.58
Never smoked	(1.9)	(0.7)	(2.5)	8.7	11.4	0.54
Past smokers	(0.9)	5.5	4.3	6.1	15.5	0.63
~10	(3.1)	(5.0)	(6.2)	15.5	24.3	1.04
~20	3.9	8.4	10.3	13.8	22.0	1.20
>20	4.9	12.2	17.4	22.5	26.8	1.83
Cigar and pipe only	(2.1)	(2.2)	(2.1)	12.1	19.5	0.71
Risk ratio (>20 vs. nonsmokers)	( )	4.1	4.8	3.1	1.7	

Source: Adapted from Pooling Project Research Group: Relationships of blood pressure, serum cholesterol, smoking habit, relative weight and ECG abnormalities to incidence of major coronary events. With permission from *J. Chron Dis* **31**:201, 1978. Pergamon Press, Ltd.

[a] Age standardized. Relates risk for a particular smoking category to average risk for all men.

[b] Figures in parenthesis indicate that less than 10 cases were observed.

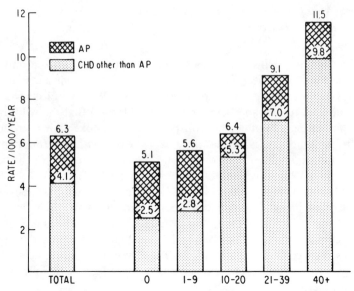

Figure 8–1   Incidence of angina pectoris (AP) and IHD other than AP by number of cigarettes smoked per day. Adapted from A Kagan et al, 1975, with permission.

relationship between cigarette smoking and 10-year incidence of IHD (Fig. 8–2). Within individual cohorts, however, it was found that the influence of smoking on IHD risk was easiest to demonstrate in those communities where IHD was more common, or equivalently where the mean level of serum cholesterol or intake of saturated fats was relatively high. It has thus been suggested that the risk of IHD associated with smoking depends on the level of serum cholesterol, implying an interaction effect (Stamler, 1967). In the Seven Countries Study, the Japanese were the heaviest smokers, but had the lowest IHD risk—perhaps because a relatively elevated serum cholesterol or the associated dietary habits or both are necessary conditions for the development of IHD. If the hypothesized model of atherogenesis and clinical events shown in Fig. 7–5 is correct, this would not be a surprising explanation. Diet and serum cholesterol appear to play a key role, and unfavorable values for these variables may be necessary for the complete expression of other risk factors such as cigarette smoking.

Cigarette Smoking and Myocardial Infarction in Women

Cigarette smoking appears to be a particularly potent risk factor for myocardial infarction in young women. Most studies of women, particularly young women, have used the retrospective case control study design. This is more efficient

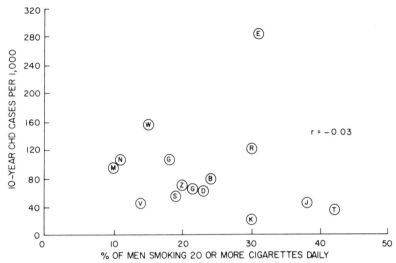

Figure 8–2 Ten-year incidence rate of coronary heart disease in 15 cohorts versus percentage of the men in those cohorts who were smoking 20 or more cigarettes at entry. For key to communities, see Fig. 5–6 (p. 62). From A Keys: *Seven Countries. A Multivariate Analysis of Death and Coronary Heart Disease.* Harvard Univ Press, 1980b, reprinted by permission.

where the disorder is uncommon, which is the case in this subgroup. A retrospective smoking history would seem fairly reliable in this context, at least as compared to the history of a complex variable such as diet. Rosenberg (1980a) studied 318 women who survived a recent first infarction and compared them with 1272 age-matched controls. The relative risks of myocardial infarction between smokers and those who have never smoked are very high (Fig. 8–3), and a consistent dose–response curve is seen. One prospective study of 23,572 white women who were followed for 12 years in Maryland confirmed the importance of cigarette smoking for arteriosclerotic heart disease and especially sudden death (Bush and Comstock, 1983). As for men, no effect was found for older participants.

One can assume that an interaction effect is present if the strength of the effect of one risk factor is modified by the concurrent level of another risk factor. This seems to be the case between cigarette smoking and oral contraceptive use in younger women. Shapiro and colleagues (1979) addressed this question in a case control study of myocardial infarction in women 35–49 years old. Controls were carefully selected to exclude any diagnoses that might introduce bias with regard to cigarette smoking or oral contraceptive use. A group of 234 women aged 25–49 years who had suffered a myocardial infarction were compared to 1742 age-matched controls with regard to various combinations of cigarette smoking and oral contraceptive use. There was a significant increase in risk with both cigarette smoking and oral contraceptive (OC) use (Table 8–2). The extra-

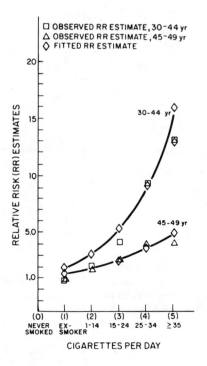

Figure 8–3 Relative risks of myocardial infarction in smokers as
compared to nonsmokers, according to intensity of smoking.
Women aged 30–44 years and 45–
90 years. From L Rosenberg,
1980a, with permission.

ordinary result is the lower right-hand entry, which indicates that women who
are heavy smokers and also use oral contraceptives have a greatly increased risk
of myocardial infarction. Results consistent with these are reported from
Finland (Salonen, 1982b). Stolley's analysis (1980) showed that about 76 percent of myocardial infarctions in young women can be attributed to cigarette
smoking.

Table 8–2 Separate and combined effects of oral
contraceptive use and cigarette smoking on relative risk of MI in young women

Daily cigarette smoking pattern	OC use	
	No	Yes
None	1.0	4.5
1–24	3.4	3.7
≥25	7.0	39.0

Source: From PD Stolley: Epidemiologic studies of coronary
heart disease: Two approaches. *Am J Epidemiol* **112**:217, 1980,
with permission.

Quitting Cigarette Smoking as Primary Prevention of Ischemic Heart Disease

The above findings clearly indicate that cigarette smoking is a factor in the development of IHD, even independently of other risk factors. However, it does not answer the question whether this is a dynamic relationship. Is quitting worthwhile? Based on other evidence, the answer is definitely yes. The Framingham Study examined the incidence of IHD (other than angina pectoris) in the follow-up period after the fourth biennial examination for men who were smokers at baseline (Gordon et al, 1974). Some had quit, while others continued to smoke throughout the follow-up period. Table 8–3 shows that at least in persons under 65, quitters have a substantial advantage. Some have raised the possibility that persons who quit smoking may be different with respect to other factors than those not quitting. If so, it could be the effect of these other risk factors that account for the apparent protective effect of quitting. Gordon and colleagues, however, state that in the Framingham data this did not seem to be the case. GD Friedman et al (1981) investigated this question in the Kaiser-Permanente longitudinal study and found that even after multivariate adjustment for any baseline differences in other risk factors, continuing smokers still had more than double the risk of ischemic heart disease as compared to quitters.

Cigarette Smoking and Coronary Artery Pathology

There is consistent evidence that smokers in Western societies have more extensive coronary atherosclerosis than nonsmokers. Auerbach and colleagues (1965) examined this relationship in 1372 male veterans who came to autopsy. They were able to show (Table 8–4) that among smokers a lesser percentage had no

Table 8–3 Comparative IHD incidence (apart from angina) in men who quit smoking and those who continued to smoke: the Framingham Study

Daily cigarette smoking pattern at previous biennial examination	IHD incidence by age at examination (rate per 1000)		
	45–54[a]	55–64[b]	65–74
None (quit)	3.6	5.7	15.3
<20	7.5	12.0	13.7
20	11.9	19.3	19.0
>20	10.1	15.2	(4.2)[c]

Source: Adapted from T Gordon et al, 1974, with permission.

[a] P (for trend) <0.005.

[b] P (for trend) <0.05.

[c] Based on one event.

Table 8–4 Degree of atherosclerosis in the coronary arteries of 1372 male veterans, according to cigarette smoking status

Daily cigarette smoking pattern[a]	Degree of atherosclerosis (%)				
	Total	None	Slight	Moderate	Advanced
Never smoked regularly	100.0	5.6	57.3	21.8	15.3
Currently smoking cigarettes:					
<20	100.0	2.6	30.9	37.3	29.2
20–39	100.0	0.8	19.7	42.1	37.4
≥40	100.0	0.6	18.1	35.4	45.9

Source: Adapted from O Auerbach et al, by permission, *N Eng J Med* **273**:775, 1965.

[a] Percentages adjusted for age.

atherosclerosis and a greater percentage had moderate or advanced atherosclerosis as compared to nonsmokers. Strong and colleagues (1966; Strong and Richards, 1976) made similar observations and in addition found that smokers had thicker walled, more calcified coronary arteries.

Mechanisms by Which Cigarette Smoking May Cause Ischemic Heart Disease

Many mechanisms have been proposed (McGill, 1979). These include the effect of smoking on HDL cholesterol levels, on platelet function, on blood carboxyhemoglobin levels, and on ventricular premature beats. Several studies have shown that smokers have lower levels of HDL cholesterol than nonsmokers (Criqui et al, 1980a; JA Morrison et al, 1979; Wiklund et al, 1980). Criqui and colleagues studied 2663 men and 2553 women aged 20–69 who were enrolled in the Lipid Research Clinics Prevalence Study at 10 North American locations. Table 8–5 shows there is a consistent dose–response gradient for HDL cholesterol independent of sex hormone consumption and persisting when adjusted for other covariates that may act as confounders. Berg et al (1979) have reported similar changes in apolipoproteins A-1 and A-2, which form the protein portion of the HDL particle. It would be even more convincing if *changes* in smoking habits could be related to *changes* in HDL cholesterol. This minimizes confounding influences in cross-sectional studies as it represents a "before-and-after" situation in the same individuals. If potential confounders remain constant across time, they cancel out. From a public health or medical perspective, such a study would show that HDL can be changed in the same individuals. Hulley et al (1979) has demonstrated such changes in a subgroup of the Multiple Risk Factor Intervention Trial Study population. In this study, serum thiocyanate levels were used as an objective measure of smoking status. A significant

Table 8–5 Mean HDL cholesterol and current cigarette smoking status before and after adjustment for selected covariables

	Men 20–69 yrs (current cigarettes per day)			Women 20–69 yrs not taking hormones (current cigarettes per day)			Women 20–69 yrs taking hormones (current cigarettes per day)		
	0	1–19	≥20	0	1–19	≥20	0	1–19	≥20
HDL cholesterol unadjusted	46.7	45.2	42.7	58.7	56.2	51.9	63.6	59.8	55.6
HDL cholesterol adjusted for age, obesity, alcohol, and exercise	46.2	43.9[a]	40.9[a]	59.7	55.2[a]	51.1[a]	65.0	59.8[a]	55.6[a]
Adjusted difference (0 vs. ≥20 cigarettes/day)		5.3			8.6			9.4	

Source: Adapted from MH Criqui et al: Cigarette smoking and plasma high-density lipoprotein cholesterol. *Circulation* **62**(Suppl 4): 70, 1980a, by permission of the American Heart Association, Inc.

[a] $P < 0.01$ compared with nonsmokers.

negative relationship relating thiocyanate *change* and HDL *change* implied that reductions in smoking were associated with increases in HDL, and vice versa. This is an independent effect, as other variables were simultaneously adjusted for in the multivariate regression analysis.

Platelet function is affected by many environmental factors, one of which is cigarette smoking. Several investigators have found that platelet adhesiveness and aggregability are increased by smoking (Ashby et al, 1965; Fuster et al, 1981; PH Levine, 1973; Murchison and Fyfe, 1966; Mustard and Murphy, 1963). Figure 8–4 is taken from Levine's study and clearly shows the effect of tobacco smoking as compared to sham smoking or smoking lettuce leaves. Another study found that nicotine-containing cigarettes decrease prostacyclin production, one possible explanation for decreased platelet activation (Nadler et al, 1983).

From 2 to 10 percent of the hemoglobin of cigarette smokers is usually in the nonfunctional form carboxyhemoglobin. It is easy to see that this may result in more rapid precipitation of angina in predisposed individuals (Aronow, 1978). Some hypothesize a direct action of carbon monoxide to produce endothelial damage and enhanced atherosclerosis. This is based on animal work, and at present the evidence seems inconclusive (Gori, 1979).

Persons smoking filter cigarettes do not gain any protection with regard to risk of IHD (Castelli et al, 1981). Despite a somewhat lower previous smoking exposure for those 58 percent of smokers using filters in the Framingham Study, their IHD experience was actually slightly worse on follow-up than that of smokers not using filters. This persisted after multivariate adjustment for slight differences in other risk factors, and it implies that the active principle increasing IHD risk may be in the gaseous phase. Carbon monoxide is one such candidate.

There is a little evidence that smokers have a greater tendency to ventricular

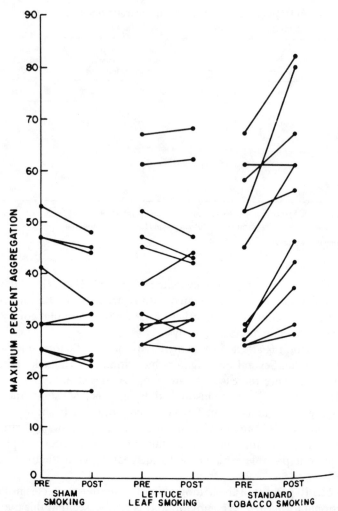

Figure 8–4 Maximum platelet aggregation in response to a fixed amount of ADP. Paired experiments before and after sham smoking, non-nicotine cigarette smoking, and standard cigarette smoking. From PH Levine: An acute effect of cigarette smoking on platelet function. *Circulation* **48**:619, 1973, by permission of the American Heart Association, Inc.

premature beats. Hennekens et al (1980) analyzed data from the Multiple Risk Factor Intervention Trial group and found evidence for a relatively weak relationship of this sort. Overall, there was about a 20 percent increase in the proportion of smokers with ventricular premature beats on the resting electrocardiogram as compared to nonsmokers. The mechanism may be the known abnormal catecholamine release in smokers (RP Lewis and H Boudoulas, 1974).

It is commonly believed that smokers have higher blood pressure levels because of the enhanced catecholamine release and the vasoconstricting action of nicotine. However, it appears that the opposite is true—at least during periods not immediately following the smoking of a cigarette. Seltzer (1974) reports on 318 smoking men, 104 of whom subsequently quit smoking. Blood pressure and weight were measured at baseline before the quitters had quit, and again at 5-year follow-up. The quitters showed a systolic blood pressure *increase* of 4 mm Hg more and a diastolic blood pressure increase of 2.5 mm Hg more as compared to the continuing smokers. These changes were statistically significant even within the same stratum of body weight change. Consequently this effect is probably not due to increased body weight after quitting smoking. Data from the Framingham Study paint a similar picture (Gordon et al, 1975). The explanation for this trend is not known. Such increases in blood pressure can generally be more than counteracted by maintaining optimal weight, moderately reducing salt consumption, engaging in regular physical activity, and reducing alcohol consumption. However, there is evidence that smokers who have hypertension are five times more likely than nonsmokers to progress to a malignant phase. This comes from case control studies in which the smoking habits of malignant hypertensives were compared to those of control hypertensives (Bloxham et al, 1979; Isles et al, 1979).

The Smoking Habits of Americans

In 1978, 37.5 percent of American men and 29.6 percent of American women smoked cigarettes. Over the 13 years from 1965 through 1978 this represented a 26.6 percent decline for men and a 11.1 percent decline for women (Table 8–6).

Table 8–6 Estimated percentage of current regular cigarette smokers among Americans age 17 and over: Health Interview Survey, 1965–1978

Year	Estimated regular smokers (%)		
	All	Men	Women
1965	41.7	51.1	33.3
1970	36.9	43.5	31.1
1974	37.0	42.7	31.9
1976	36.7	41.9	32.0
1978	33.2	37.5	29.6
Decline 1965–1978 (%)	20.4	26.6	11.1

Source: From Working Group on Arteriosclerosis of the National Heart, Lung and Blood Institute, 1981d, p. 359, reprinted with permission.

More detailed analyses (Kleinman et al, 1979) show that both black and white males in all three decades between 35 and 65 years consistently decreased consumption between 1965 and 1976. Trends in females are much less clear and consistent. Younger white females decreased their cigarette use, but those between 54 and 64 actually increased cigarette use moderately. The trends are similar in black females: the decrease in the 35- to 44-year-olds was slight while the increase in the 55- to 64-year-olds represented more than a doubling of cigarette consumption. Over the years 1968 through 1974 there were rapid increases in the smoking behavior of teenage girls. By the mid-1970s, almost as many girls were "regular" smokers as boys (Office of Cancer Communications, 1977).

Summary

1. Objective measures of smoking behaviour are preferable in research and include serum, salivary, and urinary thiocyanate, and also measurement of exhaled carbon monoxide.

2. International comparisons give no good evidence of correlation between smoking habits and IHD. This can be interpreted to suggest that elevated lipids or a high saturated-fat diet may be a necessary factor for expression of the risk of cigarette smoking.

3. Longitudinal studies within westernized communities show clear relationships between smoking and risk of IHD. However, such a relationship is absent or weak for the syndrome of angina pectoris.

4. Cigarette smoking is a particularly important risk factor for myocardial infarction in younger men and women, with the effect apparently tapering with aging. In women the risk of heavy smoking becomes greatly increased with the concurrent use of oral contraceptives.

5. Quitting cigarette smoking does reduce risk; that is, the relation is dynamic.

6. Cigarette smokers have lower HDL levels, increased platelet aggregability, a tendency to more ventricular premature beats, increased levels of carboxyhemoglobin, and probably slightly lower blood pressures. ?/

7. Cigarette smoking rates have been decreasing in U.S. adults, especially in males. Specifically, this is not true in teenage girls and older black women.

9

Hypertension, Left Ventricular Hypertrophy, and Ischemic Heart Disease

Hypertension is one of the most prevalent cardiovascular disorders in American society, and the evidence incriminating hypertension as a risk factor for ischemic heart disease is powerful and consistent. As with imprudent dietary habits and cigarette smoking, its prevalence raises the possibility of remarkable health gains to the community if the problem were controlled.

Blood pressure is an extraordinarily variable measure. This variability consists of true fluctuations and apparent fluctuations. The true fluctuations are actual changes in the blood pressure in an individual from moment to moment. These can result from intrinsic physiologic stimuli (e.g., drowsiness, full bladder, fever, exercise) or from environmental stimuli (e.g., anxiety-producing events, cold). Apparent fluctuations are measurement errors that may result, for instance, from observer inattention or inexperience, poor measurement techniques, or problems with the sphygmomanometer. The aim is to estimate some overall average of blood pressure for an individual—at least as it pertains to normal activities in waking hours. This requires minimizing the true fluctuations as well as the apparent ones. To achieve this, standardization of technique and environmental conditions is important. The observer can control the environment in several ways. The patient should be put at ease. The room temperature should be kept comfortable, and extraneous noise should be minimized. Usually at least two or three measurements will be necessary, as pressures tend to fall on repetition, perhaps reflecting more familiarity of the patient with the procedure. Technical procedures that are helpful include the use of a standard posture, a standard arm height in relation to the axilla, an appropriate cuff size as related to the arm size, and a consistent rate of deflation of the cuff (usually about 2 mm/second). A decision needs to be made whether to use the fourth or fifth Korotkoff sounds for diastolic blood pressure. The American Heart Association has made specific recommendations concerning the measurement of blood pressure (Kirkendall et al, 1976).

Recently, several automated sphygmomanometers have become available. In theory, these have advantages for reliability as they eliminate the "human factor." However, most of these have not been adequately validated against the mercury sphygmomanometer or intraarterial measurements. A few such comparisons have been reported, and they showed fairly good agreement with the human observer, although some machines were inaccurate in some circumstances (DM Berkson et al, 1979; Voors et al, 1976; Whelton et al, 1983). The American Heart Association has established criteria for evaluating such instruments (Feinleib et al, 1974).

Blood Pressure and Ischemic Heart Disease in Longitudinal Studies

The 10-year follow-up of the cohorts of men in the Seven Countries Study revealed a moderate correlation between national blood pressure levels and age-standardized IHD death rates (Fig. 9–1). This analysis compared summary statistics from 16 communities in seven countries. In addition, studies within communities from many different countries consistently show hypertension to be a risk factor for IHD (Holme et al, 1980; Johnson et al, 1968; Keys, 1980b; Reid et al, 1976; Welborn et al, 1969; Wilhelmsen et al, 1973).

The Pooling Project combines the results of five U.S. longitudinal studies of men, and gives some of the best information relating potential risk factors to disease (Pooling Project Research Group, 1978). Its findings on blood (BP) and IHD risk are displayed in Tables 9–1 and 9–2 by age and quintile of blood pressure. It is clear from the final column of each table that as blood pressure increases from the lowest to the highest quintile, there is more than a doubling of risk for ischemic heart disease. The original paper shows that these results

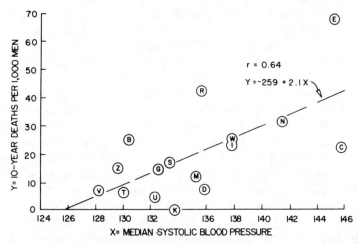

Figure 9–1   The 10-year age-standardized coronary death rates versus the median systolic blood pressures of those cohorts at entry, 16 cohorts of men without evidence of cardiovascular disease at entry. Seven Countries Study. Abbreviations; B, Belgrade; C, Crevalcore; D, Dalmatia; E, east Finland; G, Corfu; I, Italian railroad; K, Crete; M, Montegiorgio; N, Zutphen; R, American railroad; S, Slavonia; T, Tanushimaru; U, Ushibuka; V, Velika Krsna; W, west Finland; Z, Zrenjanin. From A Keys: *Seven Countries. A Multivariate Analysis of Death and Coronary Heart Disease.* Harvard Univ Press, 1980b, reprinted by permission.

Table 9–1 Association between systolic blood pressure and risk of first IHD event, displayed by age

| Quintile of systolic BP[a] | Average annual risk by age at risk (per 1000 person-yrs) | | | | | Risk ratio[b] |
	40–44	45–49	50–54	55–59	60–64	
I	(0.0)[c]	4.7	8.5	7.3	11.1	70
II	(2.1)	6.2	6.3	11.7	16.6	86
III	(2.5)	6.7	7.3	10.5	15.4	87
IV	(3.8)	4.6	7.7	16.1	19.5	102
V	9.6	10.5	11.4	16.7	31.4	150
Risk ratio (V vs. I + II)		1.9	1.5	1.8	2.3	1.9[b]

Source: Adapted from Pooling Research Group: Relationships of blood pressure, serum cholesterol, smoking habit, relative weight and ECG abnormalities to incidence of major coronary events. With permission from *J Chron Dis* **31**:201, 1978. Pergamon Press, Ltd.

[a] Quintiles: I, < 120 mm Hg; II, 120–130 mm Hg; III, 130–138 mm Hg; IV, 138–150 mm Hg; V, > 150 mm Hg.

[b] Age standardized. Relates risk for a particular systolic blood pressure quintile to average risk for all men.

[c] Parentheses imply inadequate numbers of subjects.

Table 9–2 Association between diastolic blood pressure and risk of first IHD event, displayed by age

| Quintile of Diastolic BP[a] | Average annual risk by age at risk (per 1000 person-yrs) | | | | | Risk ratio[b] |
	40–44	45–49	50–54	55–59	60–64	
I	(1.1)[c]	4.2	8.0	8.0	14.1	72
II	(1.3)	4.4	6.9	11.7	(5.1)	69
III	(1.9)	7.3	7.6	10.0	20.9	93
IV	(2.9)	6.0	7.9	16.4	21.5	108
V	9.8	10.4	10.7	17.0	35.8	156
Risk ratio (V vs. I + II)		2.4	1.4	1.7	3.7	2.2

Source: Adapted from Pooling Project Research Group: Relationships of blood pressure, serum cholesterol, smoking habit, relative weight and ECG, abnormalities to incidence of major coronary events. With permission from *J Chron Dis* **31**:201, 1978. Pergamon Press, Ltd.

[a] Quintiles: I, < 76 mm Hg; II, 76–80 mm Hg; III, 80–88 mm Hg; IV, 88–94 mm Hg; V, > 94 mm Hg.

[b] Age standardized. Relates risk ratio for a specific diastolic blood pressure quintile to average risk for all men.

[c] Parentheses imply inadequate numbers of subjects.

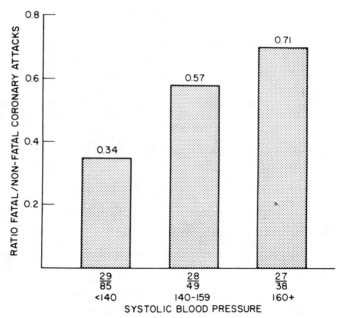

Figure 9–2 Ratio of fatal to nonfatal coronary attacks according to the systolic blood pressure of men aged 30–62 at entry into the Framingham Study: 14-year follow-up. (Note: fatal attack is a death in the same exam period as the CHD event.) From **WB** Kannel, 1975, with permission.

were consistent within the individual studies pooled. In clear contrast to the cigarette smoking data from the same study (chapter 8), the lowest row of each table shows that as the population ages, the risk ratio of the highest to the lowest quintiles, if anything, becomes greater. This suggests that hypertension is most potent as a risk factor in elderly men. That a similar relationship between systolic and diastolic hypertension and IHD holds also for women has been demonstrated by the Framingham Study (Fig. 9–3) (Kannel, 1975; Kannel and Gordon, 1974) and confirmed in Japan and Australia (Johnson et al, 1968; Welborn et al, 1969). Multivariate analyses have shown that the effect of hypertension on IHD is independent of other risk factors such as cigarette smoking and serum cholesterol.

The myocardium may be particularly vulnerable in hypertensives, as Kannel (1975) found in Framingham that not only were hypertensives more likely to have a heart attack, but they were more likely to die from that attack (Fig. 9–2). Hypertension, unlike some of the other risk factors, is associated with increased risk for many other common atherosclerotic manifestations in men and women (Fig. 9–3). Table 9–2 suggests that in males an ideal level of diastolic blood pressure with respect to IHD risk is probably 80 mm Hg or lower, as there appears to be an abrupt increase in risk above this point (see right-hand column of the table). By contrast, the same studies could not show any breakpoint in risk for

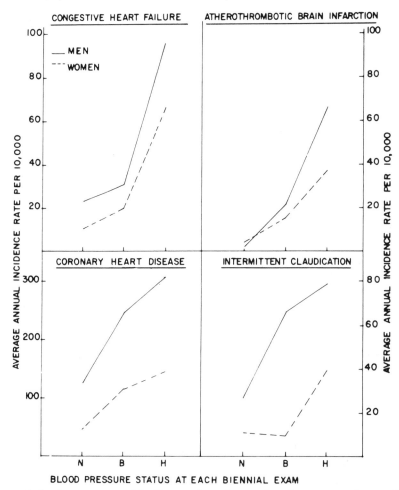

Figure 9–3 Average annual incidence of cardiovascular disease according to blood pressure status at each biennial exam of men and women aged 55–64 at entry into the Framingham Study: 18-year follow-up. N, Normal; B, borderline; H, definite. From WB Kannel, 1975, with permission.

systolic blood pressure (Table 9–1). Rather, there was a change in risk even between the first (< 120 mm Hg) and second (120–130 mm Hg) quintiles.

Thus, elevated blood pressure emerges as a consistent risk factor in both intranational and international comparisons. A common misconception is exposed by these findings. It is not only diastolic blood pressure that predicts risk of ischemic heart disease. Actually, systolic blood pressure (Table 9–1) is equally important. Even isolated systolic hypertension in the elderly has been clearly associated with increased mortality, but not definitely with IHD mortality (Garland et al, 1983; Kannel et al, 1980b; Rowe, 1983).

Despite the high prevalence of hypertension in blacks (chapter 10), the effect of hypertension to cause IHD may not be so pronounced as in whites. Although numbers of events in blacks were small, in the Evans County Study rates of new IHD at every blood pressure level were lower in black than white men, but similar in the women of both races (Tyroler et al, 1971). Similarly blacks in Africa, Latin America, and the Caribbean apparently experience little IHD despite a high prevalence of hypertension (Gillum and Grant, 1982). This finding is even more remarkable considering the increased tendency to left ventricular hypertrophy in blacks for equivalent blood pressure levels (see below). Other sequelae of hypertension such as stroke and congestive heart failure are relatively common. The reasons for this possible relative protection from the tendency of hypertension to cause myocardial ischemia is unknown, but one possibility is the more favorable lipid profile in blacks.

Most atherosclerotic lesions occur at branch points where the arterial tree is weakest. It is likely that intimal damage occurs at these sites most frequently and is aggravated by the increased internal pressures of hypertension that induce more shear and torque within the arterial wall (Ross and Glomset, 1976a,b). Such endothelial damage would be expected to provoke platelet activation, and this has been reported in hypertensives (Coccheri and Fiorentini, 1971; J Mehta and P Mehta, 1981a; Poplawski et al, 1968). Repeated cycles of this sort are hypothesized to result in the formation of atherosclerotic lesions (Fig. 7–5).

Hypertension appears to provoke IHD events in part by accelerating coronary atherosclerosis. Several autopsy studies point to this conclusion (Evans, 1965; Matova and Vihert, 1976; WB Robertson and JP Strong, 1968). The findings from the International Atherosclerosis Project are summarized in Table 9–3 (WB Robertson and JP Strong, 1968). This study investigated men of 13 different location–race groups where a history pertaining to hypertension was available. Excluded are those with an antemortem diagnosis of diabetes or of other diseases associated with atherosclerosis. As can be seen, in virtually all location–race groups for the three age ranges depicted, the hypertensives had greater arterial surface involvement with raised atherosclerotic lesions. These results are for men, but similar findings on women come from this same study.

Blood Pressure and Left Ventricular Hypertrophy

Arterial blood pressure is one important determinant of cardiac work. As for other muscles, cardiac muscle has the capacity to respond to an increased work requirement by hypertrophy. Left ventricular hypertrophy (LVH) as determined by echocardiography (Fig. 9–4) or electrocardiography (Kannel, 1983b) is closely related to blood pressure, particularly systolic pressure. That these two methods of determining LVH are not equivalent is evident as the ECG finds only a small proportion of the LVH detected by the echocardiogram in hypertensives (Savage et al, 1979).

Electrocardiographic criteria for LVH may be voltage alone or include ST–T

Table 9–3   Mean percentage surface involvement with raised atherosclerotic lesions of the coronary arteries at autopsy for 13 location–race groups of men: hypertensives compared to non-hypertensives[a]

| Location–race group | Age group | | | | | |
| | 35–44 | | 45–54 | | 55–64 | |
	HT	No HT	HT	No HT	HT	No HT
New Orleans white	37	17	43	27	41	31
Oslo	38	15	41	25	38	33
Durban Indian	33	9	34	22	28	28
New Orleans black	24	10	34	18	37	24
Manila	21	9	22	15	31	18
Caracas	23	10	22	15	27	23
São Paulo white	12	8	15	14	23	17
Jamaica	13	6	22	8	24	16
Cali	17	6	26	11	22	15
Santiago	11	6	29	11	24	17
Bogota	7	3	21	7	22	10
Guatemala	25	3	15	5	25	9
Durban Bantu	12	4	26	7	14	11
Unweighted mean	21	8	27	14	27	19

Source: Adapted from WB Robertson and JP Strong: *Lab Invest* **18**:538, 1968, with permission.

[a] HT, hypertension.

wave changes. In hypertensives with the latter changes, the hypertension is usually more severe. In Framingham, over 12 years of follow-up, 1 in 13 of the population had some transient or permanent evidence of electrocardiographic LVH. At systolic pressures exceeding 180 mm Hg, some manifestation of electrocardiographic LVH occurred in 50 percent. The relationship between blood pressure and LVH in blacks is particularly strong. Several studies have found higher rates of electrocardiographic LVH in blacks compared to whites with equivalent blood pressures (Hypertension Detection and Follow-up Program Cooperative Group, 1977; McDonough et al, 1964). The reasons for this are not well understood.

It should be remembered that valvular heart disease, cardiomyopathy, and obesity can also result in LVH, although hypertension is the major determinant in the general population. The obese are more likely to be hypertensive (chapter 10), but in addition have an expanded plasma volume and increased cardiac output (Messerli, 1982). This combination of volume overload and increased pressure afterload synergistically burdens the heart and may herald early complications such as increased ventricular mass and congestive heart failure (Alexander and Pettigrove, 1967).

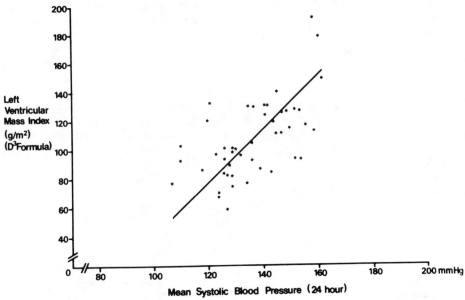

Figure 9–4   Correlation of left ventricular mass index estimated by echocardiography, with mean 24-hour systolic blood pressure ($r=0.5983$; $P<0.001$). From DB Rowlands et al: *Lancet* **1**: 467, 1982, with permission.

Left Ventricular Hypertrophy and Ischemic Heart Disease

Ischemia is the result of an imbalance between oxygen supply and demand. Hypertrophy of myocardial cells is not always accompanied by a compensatory increase in vascular cross-sectional area (Badeer, 1964; Strauer, 1979). This will be particularly true where there are fixed coronary artery stenoses or hypertrophy of the walls of arterioles, both often seen in hypertension. While this may not be important at rest, stress may lead to ischemia. Studies in hypertensive animals and humans have shown reduced coronary circulatory reserve and increased resistance to flow (Marcus et al, 1979; Strauer, 1980). The subendocardial region has the poorest blood supply, perhaps because of the epicardial entry of the coronary arteries to the myocardium, and also the compressive effects of the systolic and diastolic pressures in the immediately adjacent ventricular cavities. Susceptibility to ischemia will be aggravated by the raised systolic and diastolic intracavitary pressures, associated with a noncompliant hypertrophic left ventricle.

It is possible that the ST–T changes seen with more severe hypertension and hypertrophy represent subendocardial ischemia. This may also explain the increase in ventricular ectopy reported with left ventricular hypertrophy (Messerli et al, 1981). Some believe that the isolated increased voltage stage of LVH represents a useful physiologic adaptation but that ST–T changes signal that a critical mass has been reached that is resulting in subendocardial ischemia.

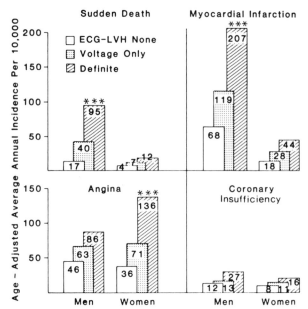

Figure 9–5   Risk of clinical manifestations of coronary disease according to ECG–LVH status, 20-year follow-up. Framingham Study, Subjects 45–74 years of age. *** Trends significant at P <0.001. From WB Kannel: *Am J Med* 75:4, 1983, with permission.

The importance of left ventricular hypertrophy in increasing risk of IHD has been shown by the Framingham Study (Kannel, 1983b). Persons with LVH had greatly increased risk of all major IHD syndromes, as compared to those without LVH (Fig. 9–5). This was true for men and probably for women, with the effect not being diminished in the elderly. It was interesting that adjustment for the concurrent effects of hypertension virtually eliminated the increased IHD risk associated with LVH voltage criteria only—but could not account for the sixfold increased risk associated with LVH diagnosed by both voltage and ST–T changes. This adds further evidence that by this stage LVH has passed from adaptation to disease. Risk of mortality in those with LVH was as high as in persons with established IHD (previous infarction or angina pectoris). Discussion of the reversibility of LVH with drug treatment of hypertension is found in chapter 20.

Summary

1. Blood pressure measurement is subject to considerable fluctuation. Close attention should be given to the environment and technique when measuring it.

2. Consistent evidence for men and women implicates hypertension as an important risk factor for IHD.

3. Both elevated systolic and diastolic pressures carry similar risks. Hypertension retains its importance as a risk factor through to old age.

4. Pathologic studies have demonstrated increased coronary atheroma in hypertensives.

5. Left ventricular hypertrophy is a common result of hypertension and carries a markedly increased risk for development of IHD. This is particularly so where there are ST–T changes on the electrocardiogram, when risk is much elevated beyond that associated with the accompanying hypertension.

10

The Epidemiology of Hypertension

Although hypertension is a risk factor for ischemic heart disease, it is also a disease entity in itself. Our interest in reducing the frequency of hypertension in the community necessitates a knowledge of its distribution and determinants. This chapter, therefore, focuses on hypertension rather than ischemic heart disease.

Even with such a common diagnosis as hypertension, considerable problems arise in defining normal and elevated blood pressure; thus, on occasion the literature can be difficult to interpret. Different investigators have used many different criteria to define blood pressure levels, using varying numbers of measurements to determine these levels. Definitions of hypertension can be based either on percentile levels of population distributions of blood pressure or on the risk of sequelae. For adults, most scientists would probably prefer the latter. This means that blood pressure is elevated if it is at a level shown to be associated with an increased risk of some disease process. Recent intervention studies indicate that an average diastolic blood pressure (usually averaged over two or three occasions) between 90 and 105 mm Hg is higher than optimal, as treatment of such persons reduced subsequent mortality (see chapter 20). Observational studies suggest that optimum may be as low as 80 mm Hg (chapter 9). Criteria for systolic hypertension are more variable—the cutoff line usually in the range of 145 to 160 mm Hg. For children, there usually are no observable sequelae of relatively elevated blood pressures, so less satisfactory criteria such as "exceeding the 95th percentile for that population" are used. Recently recommended standards and nomenclature are shown in Table 10–1.

As mentioned in chapter 9, blood pressure must be measured with standardized techniques under standardized conditions to be meaningful. Three problems in measuring blood pressure are digit preference, systematic changes with repeated measurements, and regression to the mean. The latter is not peculiar to the blood pressure variable. Digit preference refers to the tendency for physicians or technicians to prefer a number ending with a zero (or perhaps a 5), consciously or subconsciously. This has been well demonstrated in the screening results from the Hypertension Detection and Follow-up Program (HDFP Cooperative Group, 1978). Figure 10–1 shows that in the home screen where regular sphygmomanometers were used, there was a distinct tendency to frequency peaks at diastolic values of 100, 110, and 120. In evaluating the frequency of all terminal digits, the investigators found that there were roughly twice as many

Table 10–1 Classification of blood pressure

Range (mm Hg)	Category[a]
Diastolic	
<85	Normal BP
85–89	High normal BP
90–104	Mild hypertension
105–114	Moderate hypertension
≥115	Severe hypertension
Systolic, when diastolic BP is <90	
<140	Normal BP
140–159	Borderline isolated systolic hypertension
≥160	Isolated systolic hypertension

Source: From Joint National Committee on Detection, Evaluation, and Treatment of High Blood Pressure, 1984, with permission.

[a] A classification of borderline isolated systolic hypertension (systolic BP, 140–159 mm Hg) or isolated systolic hypertension (systolic BP, >160 mm Hg) takes precedence over a classification of high normal BP (diastolic BP, 85–89 mm Hg) when both occur in the same person. A classification of high normal BP (diastolic BP, 85–89 mm Hg) takes precedence over a classification of normal BP (systolic BP, <140 mm Hg) when both occur in the same person.

readings with a zero terminal digit as with other possibilities, for both systolic and diastolic blood pressures. The random zero (RZ or zero muddler) mercury sphygmomanometer overcomes the digit preference problem. The blood pressure is measured relative to a random perturbation of the baseline mercury level (a knob is spun or an electronically randomized baseline figure is given). Only *after* the blood pressure is measured is the random baseline also read, and an adjustment made to find the true reading. The screening process in the clinic (Fig. 10–1) did not involve digit preference, because a random zero sphygmomanometer was used.

On repeated blood pressure measurements, values nearly always decrease, apparently as a result of increased familiarity and less apprehension. Investigators should always standardize the number of measurements taken. The third phenomenon of regression to the mean can occur with any variable, subject to measurement error or physiologic variability. It occurs only when a truncated population (such as the group with blood pressure >90 mm Hg in the clinic screening of Fig. 10–1) is reexamined. On reexamination (see the second clinic visit portion of Fig. 10–1), the mean of the truncated population always moves toward the *overall* population mean and the truncated population assumes a more symmetrical form. This is because some persons originally included above the truncation point were there because of a random perturbation and now on reassessment have assumed a more accurate position.

In using blood pressure to predict future events and plan interventions, it is important that we understand the implications of what we measure today for

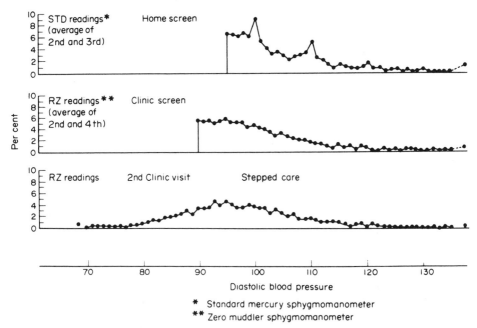

Figure 10–1   Distribution of diastolic blood pressure at three sequential visits of the Hypertension Detection and Follow-up Program. From Hypertension Detection and Follow-up Cooperative Group: Variability of blood pressure and the results of screening in the HDFP program. Reprinted, with permission, from *J Chron Dis* **31**:651, 1978. Pergamon Press, Ltd.

future blood pressure levels. Several sources of information show that the ranking within the population of an individual's blood pressure today will remain relatively similar to that individual's ranking at some later time, so that persons who now have *relatively* high blood pressures will also have *relatively* high blood pressures at future times, despite any upward movement of the whole population's blood pressure such as that associated with aging. This is called *tracking* (Fig. 10–2). Blood pressure tracking is known to occur in children (RS Levine et al, 1979; Paffenbarger et al, 1968; Sneiderman et al, 1976) and adults (Rabkin et al, 1982; Rosner et al, 1977). It is often described by correlation coefficients measuring the association between previous and present blood pressures within a population. It is also true that the amount of *change* in blood pressure over time is positively related to the initial value (Miall and Lovell, 1967; Wu et al, 1980). This means that blood pressure "feeds on itself." In a Welsh longitudinal study, Miall and co-workers (1967) were able to show that persons with higher baseline pressures had greater increases over a 10-year period and vice versa (Fig. 10–3). In terms of treatment, what this emphasizes is the need for early intervention.

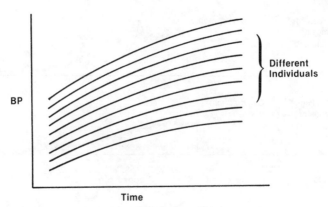

Figure 10–2 A schematic depiction of perfect tracking.

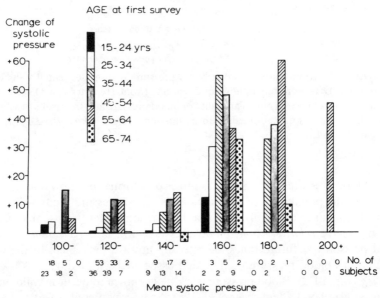

Figure 10–3 Mean change of systolic blood pressure in 10 years according to age and mean systolic pressure at baseline, Rhondda males. From WE Miall, 1969, with permission.

The Consequences of Uncontrolled Hypertension

Uncontrolled hypertension results in a substantial excess of morbidity and mortality from a variety of cardiovascular and renal disorders, as shown in a sobering fashion by the experience of the untreated control group in the Veterans

Administration Cooperative Study (chapter 20) and by community-based studies (chapter 17). The proportion of all deaths that can be ascribed to hypertension is referred to as the population-attributable fraction for hypertension. Reporting from a biracial community study in Georgia, Deubner et al (1980) found that 10 percent of white male deaths, 20 percent of white female deaths, 21 percent of black male deaths, and 37 percent of black female deaths could be attributed to hypertension (systolic blood pressure > 159 mm Hg). Clearly, eradication of hypertension gives promise of substantial health gains, if a causal relationship between hypertension and death from various causes is accepted (and the evidence is very strong). The expected gains would be greatest in black females.

International Comparisons of Blood Pressure

Different societies have different levels of blood pressure. While these differences often are not great in the second and third decades, they become more pronounced in middle and old age. The characteristic finding is that some populations experience a rise in blood pressure with aging and some do not. Almost invariably it is the urbanized, industrialized societies that experience this age-related increase. This gave rise to the now-outdated formula for normality (not optimality) of systolic blood pressure as 100 + age (mm Hg). Joossens (1973) provided some representative examples of societies with virtually no age change in blood pressure (Table 10–2). Many others could be cited, such as Eskimos, Himalayan Indians, Melanesians, Australian Aborigines, other Polynesian examples, Africans, and Amerindians (Page, 1980). Joossens also presented some contrasting data from more urbanized communities (Table 10–3). These

Table 10–2 Populations in which the blood pressure increases little or not at all with age (average of both sexes, in different age groups)

Population	Systolic pressure by age group (mm Hg)			Dietary salt
	20–29	40–49	60–69	
Brazil (Carajas)	107	100	109	No salt: use lyes of vegetable ash (K salts)
New Guinea (Murapins)	126	126	123	0.6 gm (24-hr urine)
Botswana (Kung bushmen)	119	116	122	2.0 gm (24-hr urine)
Cook Islands (Pukapukas)	113	116	125	2.9–4.1 gm (24-hr urine)

Source: From JV Joossens, 1973, with permission.

Table 10–3 Populations in which blood pressure increases markedly with age (average of both sexes, in different age groups)[a]

Population	Systolic pressure by age group (mm Hg)			Dietary salt
	20–29	40–49	60–69	
United States	119	130	149	± 10 gm/24 hr
Portugal	126	134	155	Not measured
Sweden	125	138	159	Not measured
Belgium	132	143	163	4–20 gm (24-hr urine)
Cook Islands (Rarontongas)	124	151	165	7.0–8.2 gm (24-hr urine)
Norway	130	141	167	Not measured
Wales	120	138	169	8.0 gm (24-hr urine)
Bahama Islands (blacks)	129	154	176	15–30 gm (24-hr urine)

Source: From JV Joossens, 1973, with permission.

[a] From more urbanized communities, for comparison with Table 10–2.

two types of populations clearly differ in many ways. The members of tribal communities usually do not gain weight as they age; they remain physically active, and they consume less fat and meat, more vegetables and fiber, as well as more potassium and less sodium.

Observations on blood pressure changes have been made when members of a distinct racial group migrate from one environment to another. One example is the migration of Easter Islanders to Chile (Cruz-Coke et al, 1964). The migrants showed slightly higher blood pressures after migration, but even more importantly showed a highly statistically significant dependence of blood pressure on age. This was not so for those staying on Easter Island. Another migration study traced the effects on blood pressure of relocation of a substantial proportion of the Tokelau Islands population to New Zealand (Prior and Tasman-Jones, 1981; Joseph et al, 1983). Before migration, the Tokelauans showed a rise in blood pressure with age and had higher blood pressures than some other Pacific Islanders (e.g., atoll-dwelling Pukapukans), but notably lower pressures than New Zealand Polynesian Maoris. About 3–5 years after migration, marked differences in blood pressure were seen between migrants and nonmigrants (Fig. 10–4). Beaglehole et al (1977) showed that a scale of social interaction with New Zealand society correlated positively with the blood pressure levels of Tokelauan migrants. The statistical significance was enhanced by controlling for body mass and length of residence in New Zealand. The obvious conclusion from these and similar migration studies is that environmental

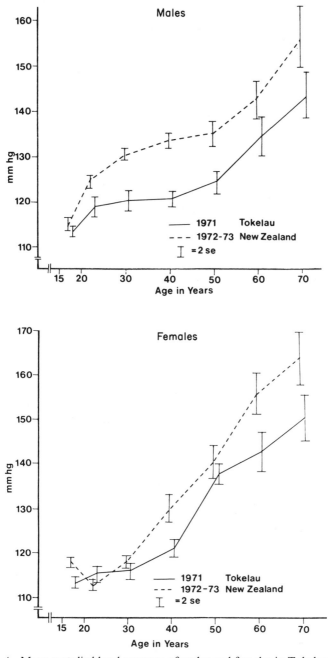

Figure 10–4 Mean systolic blood pressure of males and females in Tokelau, 1971, and migrants to New Zealand in 1972–1973. From I Prior and C Tasman-Jones: New Zealand Maori and Pacific Polynesians, in *Western Diseases, Their Emergence and Prevention*, 1981, p. 227. Reprinted by permission.

influences on blood pressure are strong, and this indicates the possibility of manipulating the environment for prevention and possibly treatment.

Probably the most thoroughly studied racial difference is that between blacks and whites in the United States ("Hypertension in Blacks and Whites," 1980). Blacks have higher blood pressures (Figs. 10–10 and 10–11) and more hypertensive complications, even for the same level of blood pressure (Gillum, 1979). The higher blood pressure levels are found also in black children but are much less pronounced (Voors et al, 1976). Inner-city blacks seem to be at particularly high risk (Harburg et al, 1973). Figures 10–10 and 10–11 show that the important racial difference arises in early adult life.

Stamler and colleagues (1980) have shown that mild hypertension (diastolic pressure $\geqslant 90$ mm Hg) can be improved by attention to diet, body weight, and exercise. The Chicago Coronary Prevention Evaluation Program enrolled 115 men with definite mild hypertension. Appointments with clinic staff were made monthly for the first 2 months and quarterly thereafter. During the first 3 years of follow-up, dropouts amounted to only about 14 percent and the mean reduction in systolic blood pressure was 11.5 mm Hg ($P < 0.001$). The study design virtually ruled out regression to the mean, so this reduction apparently represented a real effect. The next sections in this chapter reinforce the evidence that changes in habits can effectively reduce blood pressure levels.

Age, Body Build, and Hypertension

Virtually every study of blood pressure in westernized communities indicates that certain indices of body build are strongly related to blood pressure levels (Berglund and Wilhelmsen, 1975; Dyer et al, 1982; Kannel et al, 1967b; Sever et al, 1980; Sive et al, 1971). These include obesity, weight, height, and body surface area. Since these are strongly interrelated variables and also are often related to age, it is difficult to know which is primary. The Framingham Study, for example, showed a clear relationship between relative weight and blood pressure for different age–sex groups of adults (Kannel et al, 1967b). Notice the consistency of this relationship across the groups (Fig. 10–5). Another example is the similar relationship shown in adolescents attending two different schools in the Washington, D.C., area (Kotchen et al, 1974).

Some believe that obesity is the most important variable and that the increase in blood pressure with aging simply reflects the increased obesity in an aging population (Miall, 1969; Miall et al, 1968). The role of body fat in adults is emphasized by the findings of Siervogel et al (1980), who subjected 214 individuals (average age 33 years) to underwater weighing and fat biopsy. They were able to show that blood pressure correlated significantly with total body fat mass and fat cell number, but not with lean body mass (non-fatty tissue) or fat cell size. Analysis of information from the first Health and Nutrition Examination Survey (HANES) has suggested that it is centrally located body fat as measured by subscapular skinfolds rather than peripheral fat as measured by

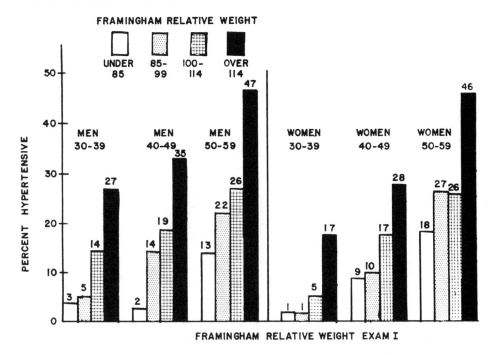

Figure 10–5 Prevalence of definite hypertension by sex and age according to Framingham relative weight. Framingham Heart Study exam 1. All trends significant at 0.05 level. From WB Kannel et al: *Ann Intern Med* **67**:48, 1967a, with permission.

triceps skinfolds that best predicts hypertension (Blair et al, 1984). Of course, central and peripheral fat often coexist. Although the blood pressure rise with age in Western societies may be partially explained by concurrent weight gain, evidence suggests that weight differences cannot entirely explain the different age-related blood pressure trends of different societies (Page et al, 1978; Prior et al, 1968). In children and adolescents, lean body mass may also be important (Voors et al, 1976).

The body weight–blood pressure relationship is probably a dynamic one. Tuck et al (1981) placed 25 obese persons on a 320–kcal diet for 12 weeks. Average weight reduction was 20 lb for each of two groups with constant but differing levels of sodium consumption. Average blood pressure fell about 17 mm Hg in both groups in 12 weeks (Fig.10–6). Reisin et al (1978) found similar effects, also with controlled sodium intake. Analysis of the Framingham Study also suggests a dynamic relationship (Kannel et al, 1967b). All of these studies lacked control for many dietary constituents that may have changed in the weight loss group and may also have been causally important for blood pressure

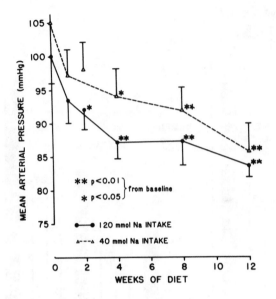

Figure 10–6 Decrements in mean arterial pressure (±SEM) during fasting in obese patients with a constant sodium intake. From ML Tuck et al. Reprinted by permission, *N Engl J Med* **304**:930, 1981.

change. Dietary fat and fiber, for instance, might be altered in a weight reduction program. Nevertheless, the consistency of cross-sectional and intervention study data makes it highly likely that there is a cause–effect relationship between obesity and blood pressure. Interestingly, even in primitive tribal communities, the relationship between weight and blood pressure can be found (Page, 1980).

The mechanism by which obesity affects blood pressure is not well understood, although recent findings of Reisin and co-workers (1983) suggest some explanations. They found that as compared to hypertensives who did not lose weight, those that did experienced a significant fall in total blood volume, venous return, cardiac output, and plasma norepinephrine at rest. As blood pressure is determined by cardiac output and arteriolar resistance, the reduction in cardiac output and norepinephrine (one determinant of arteriolar resistance) may be important.

The Effect of Diet on Blood Pressure

Diet is well known to effect serum cholesterol, and there is also increasing evidence that hypertension has important dietary determinants. Sodium, potassium, calcium, fat, complex carbohydrate, and alcohol have all been implicated as possible determinants of blood pressure levels, although the evidence is of variable quality.

Two of the earliest and most vigorous protagonists of the idea that increased sodium consumption is associated with increased blood pressure levels were Kempner (1948) and Dahl (1958). Kempner treated hypertension with his famous rice-fruit diet (less than 1 gm salt per day) with excellent results, but the diet was usually described as unpalatable. Dahl experimented with dietary sodium in rats and also compared human sodium consumption and blood pressures in different cultures. For an international comparison of salt consumption/blood pressure data, we return to the examples from Joossens' review of the literature (Tables 10–2 and 10–3), where obvious differences in salt consumption are shown between the countries with higher and lower blood pressures. Gleiberman (1973) reports a similar set of data showing similar relationships. There are a few reports of primitive communities that consume large quantities of salt, and the findings are interesting. Page et al (1974) studied several tribal groups in the Solomon Islands (Table 10–4). The Lau stand out in respect to hypertension, and they were the only tribe studied that boil their food in seawater and presumably have a relatively high salt consumption. Page et al (1978) also studied the Qash'qai, a large tribal confederation of Turkish-speaking nomads in Iran. Evidence of "acculturation' was slight but sodium excretion was high—averaging 186 mEq/day in males and 141 mEq/day in females. Both systolic and diastolic blood pressures showed sharp increases with age in both sexes. Thus, there seems to be a relationship between salt consumption and blood pressure levels, but, as usual with international comparisons, there is much potential for confounding with other variables that differ between these cultural settings.

It has proved difficult to demonstrate a consistent relationship between salt consumption and blood pressure *within* homogeneous Western populations. A few results are positive, but many are nonsignificant. Much of the discussion of similar difficulties in relating diet to serum cholesterol (chapter 5) can be applied to this issue. As Liu et al (1979) have pointed out, blood pressure may be related to some average of an individual's sodium intake. The variation in one individual's daily sodium intake may easily span the extremes of average consump-

Table 10–4 Number (*n*) of subjects aged 20 and over with blood pressure exceeding 140 mm Hg systolic and 90 mm Hg diastolic in six Solomon Island tribes

Tribe	Males			Females		
	n	*n* > 140/90	%	*n*	*n* > 140/90	%
Nasioi	59	2	3.4	63	0	0
Nagovisi	109	3	2.7	101	0	0
Lau	77	6	7.8	101	10	9.9
Baegu	126	1	0.8	109	0	0
Aita	81	0	0	88	0	0
Kwaio	128	1	0.8	114	1	0.9

Source: From LB Page et al: Antecedents of cardiovascular disease in six Solomon Islands societies. *Circulation* **49**:1132, 1974, by permission of the American Heart Association, Inc.

tions within the population. Consequently, it is impossible to rank an individual in the population using one estimation of sodium consumption (or excretion). The theoretical solution is to average several 24-hour urinary sodium values and so stabilize the estimates for different individuals. It seems that 5–10 estimations may be necessary. Few have done this, but relationships are more likely to be found when repeated measures are taken or the population considered is rather heterogeneous with regard to salt consumption, so allowing more accurate ranking (R Cooper et al, 1980; Watson et al, 1980).

Recently, several controlled intervention studies have demonstrated that in *hypertensives*, changing salt consumption will usually change blood pressure (Beard et al, 1982; Holly et al, 1981; McGregor et al, 1982a; T Morgan et al, 1978; T Morgan and JB Myers, 1981; Parijs et al, 1973). All of these studies either had a control group or used the study participants as their own controls in a crossover design. Salt restriction was usually moderate, falling from an average of about 190 mEq/day to between 37 and 157 mEq/day in different studies. In each study there was a significant drop in the subject's blood pressure during the salt-restricted dietary period. The drop was often in the range of 10 mm Hg for both systolic and diastolic pressures. Gillum and colleagues (1983) have demonstrated that the effect of sodium restriction and weight reduction are independent and additive in overweight borderline hypertensives. While it is true that these studies vary in the severity of the subjects' hypertension, the length of intervention, the presence of a preliminary phase, and the magnitude of change in electrolyte intake, the fact that the majority report significant lowering of blood pressure argues for the effectiveness of this type of therapy.

One of the best of these studies was conducted by McGregor et al (1982a). Nineteen hypertensives adopted a sodium-restricted diet. Their sodium intake dropped from 191 to 83 mEq with no significant change in potassium excretion. After 2 weeks of sodium restriction they entered a double-blind, randomized crossover trial. Patients were given either placebo or sodium tablets (estimated to restore sodium intake to the patient's normal intake) for a period of 4 weeks. As can be seen in Fig. 10–7, during the salt restriction and placebo phases, 24-hour urinary sodium levels fell markedly, as did both systolic and diastolic blood pressures. During the 4 weeks of supplementation with sodium, both sodium excretion and blood pressures were restored nearly to the baseline values.

A common finding in primitive tribal communities is that potassium consumption is higher than in Western societies. This is partly explained by a diet including more vegetables and fruits. There are several indications that dietary potassium may also affect blood pressure in an inverse sense to that of sodium. Three experimental studies give support to this (Iimura et al, 1981; Khaw and Thom, 1982; McGregor et al, 1982b). McGregor and co-workers found, in a placebo-controlled, randomized crossover study of hypertensives, that potassium supplementation raising urinary 24-hour excretion from 62 to 118 mmol significantly decreased resting systolic and diastolic blood pressures by 7 and 4 mm Hg, respectively.

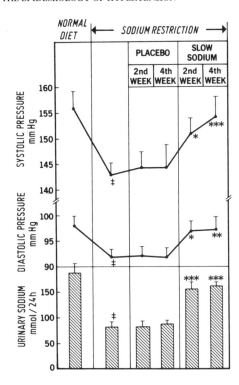

Figure 10–7 Average systolic and diastolic blood pressure and urinary sodium excretion on normal diet, 2 weeks after dietary sodium restriction, and at twice-weekly intervals during the randomized crossover trial of slow sodium versus placebo. (***P <0.001; **P <0.01; *P <0.05 comparing equivalent measurement on slow sodium to placebo. ‡*P* <0.001 comparing measurement on normal diet to 2 weeks of dietary sodium restriction.) From GA McGregor et al, 1982a, with permission.

It has been asked whether the much greater frequency of hypertension in U.S. blacks than whites could be due to different intakes of sodium and potassium. The few studies comparing dietary and excretory patterns of sodium and potassium in blacks and whites do show a higher sodium/potassium excretory ratio in the blacks (Grim, 1980; Watson et al, 1980). Grim and colleagues found that the difference resided mainly in potassium excretion, but Watson and colleagues found differences in both sodium and potassium when they compared 506 black females to 181 white females (Table 10–5).

As with the effect of diet on serum cholesterol, there is a suspicion that everyone in the population is not equally responsive to the influence of sodium on blood pressure. There may be two subpopulations, one responsive and the other less responsive to such changes. Fortunately, it is probably those who most need the responsiveness (hypertensives or potential hypertensives) who get the most effect from sodium reductions. Holly et al (1981) compared the responsiveness of mild hypertensives to nonhypertensives, and of university students with one or two hypertensive parents to students with no family history of hypertension. Statistical significance was often achieved in an experimental protocol that involved progression through several diets with differing combinations of sodium and potassium. The mild hypertensives and the students with hypertensive parents tended to respond more dramatically to the changes in sodium and potassium than the other groups. Luft et al (1982) studied sodium excretion in

Table 10–5   Mean blood pressure, weight, and urinary solute excretion rates per hour for black females and white females

Measurement	1968 and 1969 Black females			1970 White females			
	n	Mean	SD	n	Mean	SD	t
Home measurement							
Weight (lb)	506	125.9	26.4	181	125.6	21.3	0.152
Systolic BP (mm Hg)	506	116.0	11.7	181	109.1	9.0	8.14[b]
Diastolic BP (mm Hg)	506	70.7	11.6	181	69.3	13.0	1.28
24-hr urine[a]							
Cr	355	46.3	12.6	104	43.0	9.7	2.84[b]
Ur	107	248.9	77.4	104	277.3	98.5	2.32[b]
Na	356	4.7	2.0	104	4.1	1.2	3.79[b]
K	356	1.2	0.4	104	1.5	0.5	5.32[b]
Na/K	356	4.1	1.7	104	2.9	1.0	8.54[b]

Source: Adapted from RL Watson et al. Urinary electrolytes, body weight, and blood pressure. *Hypertension* **2**(suppl 1):93, 1980, by permission of the American Heart Association, Inc.

[a] Na and K reported in mEq/hr; units for urea and creatinine in mg/hr; Ur = urea.

[b] $P \leqslant 0.05$.

three groups of individuals at elevated risk of developing hypertension: blacks, persons over age 40, and first-degree relatives of hypertensives. These groups were unable to excrete a sodium load as rapidly as normal. It is not clear whether this inability stems from an intrinsic renal lesion, an abnormality in hormonal regulation of renal electrolyte function, or other factors affecting renal function. Mark et al (1975) demonstrated that increasing sodium consumption while keeping potassium intake constant leads to increased vascular resistance in borderline hypertensives, but not in nonhypertensives. There is recent evidence that sodium–potassium membrane transport in red cells and leukocytes of hypertensives is abnormal, although it is not clear whether this abnormality is involved in the blood pressure elevation or simply a marker for persons at increased risk (Canessa et al, 1980; Forrester and Alleyner, 1981; Garay and Meyer, 1979). Moreover, it has been shown that plasma from hypertensives decreases sodium transport in leukocytes of normotensives (Postan et al, 1980).

One unifying theory is that in hypertensives and potential hypertensives, a humoral substance is produced that affects sodium transport in the kidneys and elsewhere. This could in turn affect the closely linked transmembrane calcium transport system leading to increased intracellular calcium. The effect on calcium on smooth muscle may lead to increased tension of vascular smooth muscle and so heightened peripheral vascular resistance (Blaustein, 1977). A high sodium intake would then expand intravascular volume in the face of increased vascular resistance, thus raising blood pressure. It is possible that the humoral substance is a natriuretic hormone that in itself is stimulated by an excess of sodium consumption (De Wardener, 1982). It is also speculated that potassium supplementation may stimulate the inhibited sodium–potassium pump mechanism of hypertensives, thus tending to reverse these effects (McGregor et al, 1982b). Whatever the exact mechanisms, evidence suggests that a segment of the population cannot tolerate more than about 70 mEq/day of sodium (4 gm of salt) without a deleterious effect on blood pressure (Tables 10–2 and 10–3).

When giving nutritional advice to patients, it is important to realize that the same foods in processed and unprocessed form will often differ dramatically in both sodium and potassium content (Table 10–6). Most canned foods, milk shakes, burgers, pickles, soy sauce, and vegetarian protein foods are very salty— and often this is not apparent to the taste sense. Salt is incorporated into the diet in four main ways: naturally present in the food, added in the factory during processing, added during the cooking process by the cook, or added at the table by salt shaker. It is unfortunate that foods prepared commercially as "low salt" are usually more expensive, when blacks and people of lower socioeconomic status need them most.

The "salt-loving palate" is a learned attribute. It is common clinical experience that modest sodium restriction, while initially unpleasant, becomes entirely acceptable after a period of 1 to 2 months. There is now objective evidence that the preferred level of salt in food is related to the level of salt consumed and that this preferred level is usually lowered after a reduction in sodium intake (Bertino et al, 1982). Because so much salt is added during the commercial preparation of foods, food choice is obviously important for persons on a low-salt diet. The American Medical Association has made recommendations on sodium labeling of foods and the reduction of sodium in processed foods (Council on Scientific Affairs, 1983).

The possible role of calcium metabolism in the genesis of hypertension is of current research interest. As mentioned above, the transport of calcium across membranes is linked to that of sodium and potassium, and calcium is involved in vascular reactivity. McCarron (1982) found that ionized extracellular concentrations of calcium are significantly depressed in hypertensive animals and

Table 10–6 Sodium and potassium contents of some natural and equivalent processed foods

Natural food	Na	K	Processed food	Na	K
Flour, wheat	2.2	94.9	White bread	496.3	122
Rice, raw brown	9.4	214.1	Rice, instant fluffed	272.7	trace
Uncooked peas	2.1	315.9	Canned peas (drained)	236.3	96.2
Ham, fresh lean	72.6	332.5	Ham, light cured	995.4	311.2
Beef, lean flank	53.3	244.1	Corned beef	942.1	59.9

Source: Values derived from Adams, 1975.

humans. This might represent increased binding of ionized calcium to cell membranes and other proteins. Earlier, Langford and Watson (1973) had reported that lower dietary calcium correlated with higher pressures, but a Belgian epidemiologic study revealed a significant association in the reverse direction (Kesteloot and Geboers, 1982). In rats dietary calcium supplements correct low ionized calcium levels and attenuate hypertension (Ayachi, 1979). Preliminary evidence suggests the same may be true for humans. Belizan and colleagues (1983), in a randomized controlled trial, supplemented the diets of an experimental group with 1 gm of calcium per day for a period of 22 weeks. Significantly lower diastolic blood pressures were found in both men (9 percent lower) and women (5.6 percent lower) in the experimental group. Nutritional data from the Health and Nutrition Examination Survey (HANES) Study showed that the most consistent difference between hypertensives and normotensives was a lower intake of calcium in the hypertensives (McCarron, 1983). Other studies reveal similar differences (McCarron, 1982; McCarron et al, 1982). Although the details have not all been worked out, it appears that calcium may represent another link in our understanding of essential hypertension, again implicating the possibility of membrane transport abnormalities in a predisposed segment of the population.

Three randomized studies of normal healthy subjects each suggest the possibility that fat consumption may raise blood pressure levels in humans (Iacono et al, 1975; Puska et al, 1983a; Rouse et al, 1983). Each study was carefully conducted using 6-week dietary periods involving low-fat, high P/S ratio, or lacto-ovo vegetarian diets. In no case was there significant weight change, and in the two studies where they were estimated urinary electrolytes showed no systematic changes; yet there were significant changes in blood pressure. Which component of these diets is the active principle is open to speculation, but possibilities include total fat, saturated fat, polyunsaturated fat, and dietary fiber.

It is well known that persons who drink more alcohol have higher blood pressure levels (Criqui et al, 1981; Harburg et al, 1980; Klatsky et al, 1979). A representative set of results is shown for white males and females in Table 10–7. Findings for blacks were very similar. A small intervention study has shown the effect of stopping and starting alcohol consumption on the blood pressures of 16 men (Potter and Beevers, 1984). The mechanism is uncertain, but the relationship does not seem to be confounded by adiposity, socioeconomic status, cigarette smoking, or coffee consumption (Klatsky et al, 1977).

Exercise and Blood Pressure

The relationship between exercise and blood pressure is controversial, with many but not all observational studies finding that the more physically active have lower blood pressures (KH Cooper et al, 1976; Criqui et al, 1982; Gibbons et al, 1983). One study—that of Harvard University alumni—was longitudinal in design, demonstrating that the exercise habits preceded the different blood

Table 10–7 Number of age-adjusted percentages of white men and women with hypertension according to alcohol use

Alcohol habit (number of drinks/day)	White men		White women	
	n	≥ 160/95 mm Hg (%)	*n*	≥ 160/95 mm Hg (%)
None	5,393	4.6	10,353	6.3
≤ 2	21,366	4.8	31,165	5.3[b]
3–5	4,270	8.2[a]	2,074	8.6[a]
≥ 6	1,430	11.2[a]	346	11.3[b]

Source: Adapted from AL Klatsky et al: Alcohol use, myocardial infarction, sudden cardiac death, and hypertension. *Alcoholism: Clin Exp Res* 3:33, 1979, by permission.

[a] *P* < 0.001 (vs. nondrinkers).

[b] *P* < 0.01 (vs. nondrinkers).

pressure levels on follow-up (Paffenbarger et al, 1983). Most of these studies found that the relationship persisted even after adjustment for, or within categories of body mass. The implication is that weight reduction does not fully explain any relationship between exercise and blood pressure.

Several small experimental studies of hypertensives have sought to answer the same questions (Boyer and Kasch, 1970; Choquette and Ferguson, 1973; Hartung and Vlasek, 1980; Roman et al, 1981). Of nine such studies reviewed, all showed decreases in both systolic and diastolic blood pressures, and in seven of them, changes in systolic, diastolic, or both were statistically significant. A problem in some was the lack of a control group, allowing the possibility that changes ascribed to exercise may have been due to regression to the mean or to increased familiarity with personnel and procedures. However, results were similar in the studies that did have a control group, or else employed a switch-back design with participants stopping exercise and the blood pressure consequently rising. Again, the effect was sometimes seen without there being any mean change in body weight, suggesting an effect independent of weight loss. The evidence for some effect is thus quite strong, although its magnitude is probably modest. The mechanism is unknown, but effects on resting cardiac output or peripheral vascular resistance, or both, are postulated.

Socioeconomic Status and Blood Pressure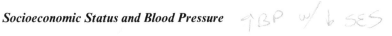

An inverse relationship has frequently been documented between blood pressure and the socioeconomic status (HDFP Cooperative Group, 1977a; JF Kraus et al, 1980; GA Rose and MG Marmot, 1981). Kraus found that for northern Californian whites, over six socioeconomic classes from highest to lowest, the percentage with diastolic blood pressure greater than 95 mm Hg

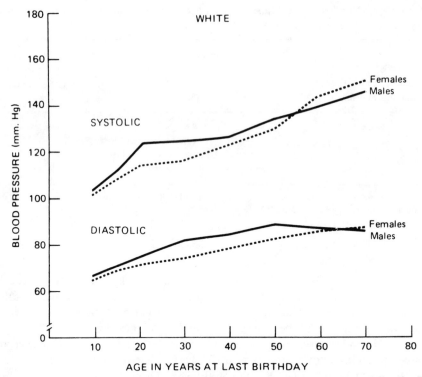

Figure 10–8   Mean systolic and diastolic blood pressure of white males and females 7–74 years, by age: United States, 1971–1974. From National Health Survey. US Dept of Housing, Education and Welfare, 1978.

increased as follows: 9.0, 10.8, 12.0, 13.1, 14.7, 16.1. Kotchen's study of Washington, D.C., schoolchildren (Kotchen et al, 1974) allowed a similar conclusion. He compared two schools, one in a middle-class area having white and black children (school A) and the other from a ghetto area with mainly black students (school B). Within each category of relative weight, blood pressures in blacks at school B were usually higher than those at school A. It is possible, of course, that the apparent effect of the socioeconomic variable may simply reflect differences in other determinants of blood pressure between socioeconomic classes.

Blood Pressure Levels in the United States

There are several sources of information on patterns of blood pressure within the United States. The National Health Survey (1978) collected data from a probability sample of the U.S. population. The response rate was 74 percent, and 20,749 persons were examined. Blood pressure measurements were made in carefully standardized ways, usually with a regular mercury sphygmo-

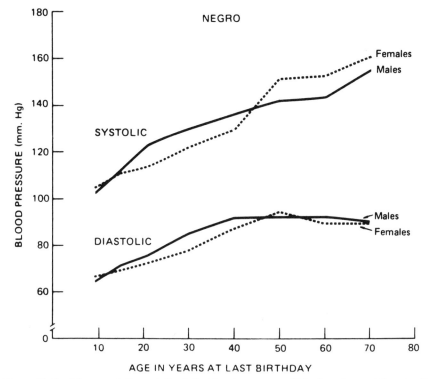

Figure 10–9   Mean systolic and diastolic blood pressure of black males and females 7–74 years, by age: United States, 1971–1974. From National Health Survey. US Dept of Housing, Education and Welfare, 1978.

manometer, although a few centers used an aneroid machine. Diastolic blood pressure was measured as the fifth Korotkoff sound. The results (Figs. 10–8 to 10–11) show the expected rise in blood pressure with age in all race–sex groups. The values shown in these figures are means, and there is of course considerable scatter about these means. A range of ±20 mm Hg at younger ages, and ±40 mm Hg at older ages, would encompass about 95 percent of the population. The Lipid Research Clinics Prevalence Study provided similar findings, notably higher blood pressures in males under age 50 than females and in post-adolescent blacks than whites (Lipid Research Clinics Study Group, 1980). A brief discussion of time trends in prevalence and adequacy of treatment of hypertension is found in chapter 20 (p. 306).

Summary

1. Blood pressure distributions are a continuum. Hypertension can be defined according to statistical criteria (especially in children) or according to

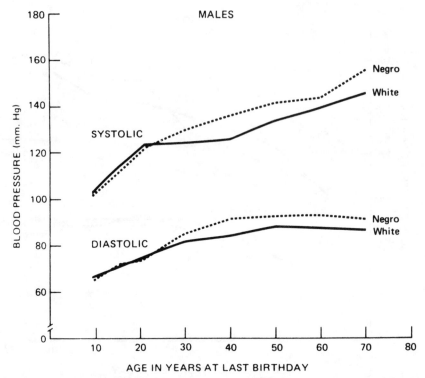

Figure 10–10 Mean systolic and diastolic blood pressure of white and black males 7–74 years, by age: United States, 1971–1974. From National Health Survey. US Dept of Housing, Education and Welfare, 1978.

levels shown to have increased risk of subsequent clinical disease (especially in adults).

2. Practical problems of measurements and interpretation include digit preference, lower value on repeated measurement, and also regression to the mean if a population of "hypertensives" is selected at a screening session and subsequently reexamined.

3. Blood pressure tracks over time, with increases over time being more prominent in those with initially elevated pressures.

4. Primitive tribal communities show little rise in blood pressure with age in contrast with Western society. Migration studies show that environmental influences are important determinants of blood pressure, although this does not deny the importance of heredity also.

5. Various indices relate body size consistently and positively to blood pressure, but it appears that body fat (in adults at least) is the important variable. The relationship is dynamic and probably independent of sodium consumption.

6. International comparisons suggest that salt consumption relates importantly to blood pressure levels. Intranational comparisons show variable results,

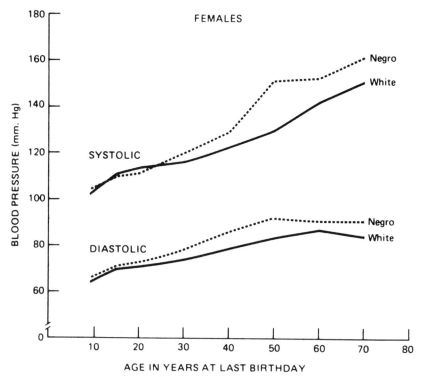

Figure 10–11   Mean systolic and diastolic blood pressure of white and black females 7–74 years, by age: United States, 1971–1974. From National Health Survey. US Dept of Housing, Education and Welfare, 1978.

probably due to measurement errors and variations in day-to-day salt consumption, making it difficult to characterize an individual's intake.

7. Intervention studies in hypertensives show the benefit of moderate salt restriction. There are probably salt sensitive and salt resistant segments of society. Hypertensives are more likely to be salt sensitive. Mild calcium deficiency may be an additional risk factor for hypertension.

8. There is evidence suggesting that a diet with a higher P/S ratio and more vegetables is associated with lower blood pressure. The active components of such a diet have not been clearly defined.

9. Alcohol consumption has a positive relationship to blood pressure levels.

10. The lower socioeconomic classes have a tendency to higher blood pressure levels, but it is not clear whether this is independent of other factors.

11. In the United States, blood pressure increases with age. Blacks have higher blood pressures than whites, and females below age 50 have lower blood pressures than males.

11

Psychosocial, Socioeconomic Variables, and Ischemic Heart Disease

Psychosocial Factors

The effect of our emotions on the force and speed of cardiac contractions is common knowledge to all. However, the role of psychologic factors in the development of chronic heart disease is still a matter of debate. Since traditional risk factors together account for only a proportion of coronary heart disease, there would seem to be room for the influence of other factors. This point was made when a risk equation developed from U.S. data, based on age, systolic blood pressure, serum cholesterol, smoking habits, and body mass index, was applied to a European population (Keys et al, 1972). The Europeans were properly ranked from high to low risk (correlation coefficients 0.93–0.98 in different subgroup analyses), but the U.S. equation consistently and markedly overpredicted risk, as compared to observed cases. The most likely explanation is that there are other risk factors in the United States or protective factors in Europe that have not yet been defined. Psychosocial factors have received considerable attention as potentially helping to fill such a gap. They can be divided into categories of stress, personality, and behavior.

Stress has to do with the environment, but it also involves perception. A stressful environment to one person may not be perceived as such by another. Stress measurement may involve a subjective element, asking the individual his or her perception of an environmental stress. Alternatively, a questionnaire may try to measure the environment in a more objective fashion, as by enumerating deaths or serious illness in the family, changes in marital relationship, changes in employment or salary in the recent past. With *personality type* the focus shifts from the environment to the individual's psychologic "makeup." Personality may be measured by behavior or by the person's feelings about self. Various aspects of neuroticism such as anxiety, depression, and hypochondriasis have been most commonly used. *Behavior patterns* are closly related to both of the above and are often an outgrowth of the interaction between environmental stress and personality type. Behavior can be assessed by observation or by questionnaire.

Most of the studies discussed in this chapter are prospective. This is because the difficulties of retrospective and prevalence studies are especially prominent in the psychosocial sphere. With these study designs there are two main problems. First, did the psychosocial variable cause the disease or the disease produce the value of the psychosocial variable? Often this cannot be answered except by a prospective study. When a serious disorder such as ischemic heart disease is diagnosed, this clearly has the potential for changing the person's psychologic state. A prospective study measures the psychologic state before the cardiac disorder was manifest. The second problem is that prevalence and retrospective studies usually deal only with surviving cases. Rapidly fatal cases cannot be interviewed, although in some situations where the variable in question is relatively objective, information from next of kin may be satisfactory. The practical importance of these two problems was recently demonstrated when the correlations of psychosocial variables to prevalence and incidence portions of the same study led to different conclusions (Reed et al, 1982).

Stress and Ischemic Heart Disease

Many different stressors have been investigated, but the results are not easy to interpret. Stress can take many different forms and these probably do not have the same significance for a particular disease. In addition, different coronary syndromes may have different associations with the same stress. The stressors considered in the literature include the recent life changes of Holmes and Rahe's summary scale (Holmes and Rahe, 1967), social status incongruity, social, occupational, and geographic mobility, workload, tensions, or frustrations with superiors at work, and family problems.

The Holmes and Rahe scale of recent life events includes a spectrum of both pleasant and unpleasant experiences that may be seen as stressful (e.g., marriage, fired from work, recent illness, pay raise). The literature on recent life changes and their relationship with IHD has been summarized by CD Jenkins (1976b). He found that the results were conflicting and that generally the better designed studies were less likely to show positive results.

Social status incongruity refers to inconsistencies between the components of a person's or couple's socioeconomic status such as income, education, and occupation. The idea is that a lack of consistency places an individual at variance with peers, and this may lead to social tension. Social and occupational mobility may be intergenerational or intragenerational. The information relating to these variables is not easy to summarize, and it is also difficult to know whether conclusions in one cultural–geographic–socioeconomic setting can be translated to other situations. Results from three large longitudinal studies are presented below. These relate mainly to social, occupational, and geographic mobility, social status incongruity, family tensions, and frustrations with superiors at work.

In a prospective evaluation of employees from the Chicago Western Electric Company Study, the incidence of IHD was analyzed in 1472 men over 5 years (Shekelle et al, 1969, 1976a). Incidence differences were noted for several types

Table 11–1 Results of a multivariate logistic regression relating social status incongruity, social status, serum cholesterol, diastolic blood pressure, and smoking to risk of myocardial infarction and IHD death

Variable	t score[a]	P value
Social status incongruity[b]	2.33	<0.05
Social status	0.86	0.61
Serum cholesterol	1.93	0.06
Diastolic BP	3.79	<0.001
Smoking[c]	3.41	<0.001

Source: Adapted from RB Shekelle: *J Health Soc Behav* **17**:83, 1976, with permission.

[a] Tests the probability that the regression coefficient equals zero.
[b] Status inconsistency scored as follows: 0, range of status ratings <3; 1, otherwise.
[c] Cigarette smoking scored as follows: 0, currently none; 1, 1–9 cigarettes/day; 2, 10–19 cigarettes/day; 3, 20–29 cigarettes/day; 4, ≥30 cigarettes/day.

of social incongruity. Each of seven variables was first scaled 1–7 (education, occupation, income, neighborhood, dwelling, religion, and membership in voluntary associations). If the difference in scores between the highest and lowest of the seven variables was more than 3, this was considered a positive response for a summary incongruity score. This was significantly correlated with both myocardial infarction and IHD death, independently of socioeconomic status and the traditional risk factors (Table 11–1). Additional scores were given for discrepancies between the subject's class of origin and present socioeconomic class, wife's class of origin and present socioeconomic class, the subject's educational status below the wife's, and the subject's socioeconomic class of origin below the wife's. The first three of these four variables, which reflect both social mobility and social status incongruity, significantly predicted an increased risk of IHD.

Haynes and colleagues (SG Haynes and M Feinleib, 1980; SG Haynes et al, 1980) followed 725 men and 949 women from the Framingham Study, aged 45–77 years at entry, over a period of 8 years. Several variables reflecting situational stress (e.g., marital dissatisfaction, work overload, nonsupportive boss) and sociocultural mobility (e.g., job changes, promotions, social class mobility) were included. The end point was all new ischemic heart disease, and significant associations were sparse. For men aged 55–64 years, work overload and frequency of promotion was associated positively with IHD incidence. Among clerical working women, Haynes reports that IHD rates were higher if the women had a nonsupportive boss, did not express any anger, and showed decreased job mobility.

Another prospective study was of 10,000 Israeli citizens (Medalie and Goldbourt, 1976a,b; Medalie et al, 1973a,b). This study considered angina and myocardial infarction as distinct end points but may have suffered by trying to integrate several groups from diverse cultural backgrounds (although all Jewish) into the one study population. The participants represented a stratified sample of Israeli male civil service and municipal employees aged over 40 years in 1963. The strata corresponded to different geographic locations of birth (e.g., Eastern Europe, Israel, North Africa). In addition to measuring the traditional risk factors, the investigators incorporated a large battery of psychosocial questions. These included an anxiety index, a sociologic questionnaire, and a psychosocial questionnaire that focused on problems relating to past and present work, financial and family life situations. The relationships found differed for angina pectoris and myocardial infarction. When the end point was new angina, univariate results (Table 11–2) showed positive relationships with family prob-

Table 11–2   Angina pectoris incidence in Israeli men (1963–1968) and its relation to psychosocial factors in 1963

Psychosocial area	Severity score[a]	Number of subjects	Number of cases	Age–area adjusted (rate/1000)
1. Family problems	0 (least)	1636	50	31
	1	3972	125	33
	2	1836	68	38
	3	865	41	49
	4 (most)	219	16	88
2. Co-worker problems	0	6482	203	32
	1	1578	74	47
	2	399	18	47
	3	69	5	79
3. "Superior" problems	0	5520	173	32
	1	2116	76	36
	2	635	37	57
	3	257	14	57
4. Financial problems	0	3884	113	29
	1	2421	104	43
	2	1147	38	36
	3	1076	45	46
5. Work problems	0	4264	119	29
	1	3010	124	41
	2	1254	57	45

Source: From JH Medalie et al: *Am J Med* **55**: 583, 1973a, with permission.

[a] Severity score: a score indicating the number of times a subject reported serious or very serious problems in respect to questions within the psychosocial area (e.g., 0 = no serious problems; 3 = a serious problem in each of the three questions related to the relevant problem area).

lems, co-worker problems, boss problems, and financial problems (Medalie et al, 1973a). When the answers from each of these five variables were amalgamated to give a combined "severity score," this was significantly positively associated with risk of angina for the age groups 40–49 and 50–59 years, but not over 60 years (numbers here were small).

A multivariate analysis showed that the total "problem" score was a significant predictor of angina independent of several other traditional risk variables (Table 11–3; Medalie and Goldbourt, 1976a). The components of this score were very similar to those of the "severity score" of the previous publication, and of these, family problems stood out as most important. When myocardial infarction was the end point, one or two such variables showed some univariate significance (Medalie et al, 1973b), but on multivariate analysis, no significant relationships were found (Goldbourt et al, 1975).

Syme and colleagues (1964) conducted a retrospective study of 228 new cases of ischemic heart disease developing over a 1-year period in six counties of North Dakota. For each case, two age-matched controls free of IHD were randomly selected from the same population. It was possible to interview either the patients or their next of kin in 203 of these cases. Thus, this study overcomes the disadvantages of retrospective studies in that all new cases were ascertained (including fatal ones), and the pre-diagnosis values of the variables of interest were objectively identified, since they included such measures as geographic

Table 11–3 Standardized β-coefficients of the age-specific multivariate logistic risk functions, and incidence of angina pectoris (excluding myocardial infarction incidence cases) in Israeli men[a]

	Age group			
	40–44	45–54	$\geqslant 55$	Total
Variable	Multi-variate	Multi-variate	Multi-variate	Multi-variate
Age	(0.16)	0.19	(−0.19)	0.18
Systolic BP	0.26	0.19	(0.18)	0.20
Anxiety	(0.18)	0.26	0.43	0.29
Problems (total score)	0.43	0.26	(0.06)	0.25
Cholesterol	0.21	0.24	(0.20)	0.24
Diabetes	(0.09)	(0.11)	(0.10)	0.10
Electrocardiographic abnormality	0.22	(0.04)	0.23	0.14
Number with all measurements known { At risk	2710	3326	1551	7857
Angina pectoris	55	104	65	224

Source: Adapted from JH Medalie and U Goldbourt: Am J Med **60**:910, 1976a, with permission.

[a] Coefficients underlined are significant at the 0.01 simple-comparison level (B/SE(B) > 2.327). Coefficients in parentheses are not significant at levels below 0.05 (B/SE(B) < 1.645). All others are significant at the 0.05 level.

location of the subjects and their parents, number of occupational changes, and socioeconomic status of the subjects and their parents. Compared to controls, the cases showed more upward intergenerational mobility (Table 11–4, sections A and B), major job changes (Table 11–5), and more changes in geographic location. A similar study in California by Syme et al (1966) produced similar results, and so did a large prevalence study from Evans County in Georgia (Kaplan et al, 1971). However, these two studies involved only prevalent cases and were therefore biased toward survivors.

From a different perspective on stress, there is evidence of increased age-specific risk of IHD mortality following the death of a spouse (Koskenvuo et al, 1980; AS Kraus and AM Lilienfeld, 1959; Parkes et al, 1969). However, agreement is not complete on this point (Helsing et al, 1982).

In summary, the evidence relating chronic social stressors to the risk of IHD needs further support and may differ for angina and myocardial infarction, but for some variables the evidence is impressive. This is so for social status incongruity for social, occupational, and geographic mobility, and perhaps for family and work problems.

That *acute* stress may be related to sudden death has recently attracted some attention (Lown, 1979). Here stress is viewed as a precipitating cause of arrhyth-

Table 11–4 Number of cases and controls and ratio of observed to expected cases by subject's sociocultural background and occupation[a]

Subject's socio-cultural background[b]	Subject's occupation	Number of cases	Number of controls	Ratio of observed to expected cases
A. Rural European	Agricultural	50	138	0.72
	Blue-collar	11	41	0.54
	White-collar	11	12	1.83
B. Rural American	Agricultural	34	75	0.91
	Blue-collar	10	16	1.25
	White-collar	11	7	3.14
C. Urban European	Agricultural	8	17	0.94
	Blue-collar	6	22	0.55
	White-collar	7	17	0.82
D. Urban American	Agricultural	4	3	2.67
	Blue-collar	9	7	2.57
	White-collar	20	18	2.22

Source: From SL Syme et al: Some social and cultural factors associated with the occurrence of CHD. Reprinted with permission from *J Chron Dis* **17**:277, 1964. Pergamon Press, Ltd.

[a] Twenty-two cases and 33 controls were unknown as to either respondent's sociocultural background or occupation. $X^2 = 15.511$ (for parts A and B only); $P < 0.01$ (5 degrees of freedom).

[b] Father's occupational classification (agricultural vs. nonagricultural) and father's nativity (European vs. American).

Table 11–5 Number of cases and controls and ratio of observed to expected cases by number of occupation changes[a]

Number of occupation changes	Number of cases	Number of controls	Ratio of observed to expected cases
0–1	105	278	0.75
2–3	43	77	1.12
⩾4	47	39	2.41

Source: SL Syme et al: Some social and cultural factors associated with the occurrence of CHD. Reprinted with permission from *J Chron Dis* **17**:277, 1964. Pergamon Press, Ltd.

[a] Eight cases and 12 controls are unknown as to number of occupation changes. $\chi^2 = 24.031$; $P < 0.001$ (2 degrees of freedom).

mia in predisposed persons. It has been clearly demonstrated in animals that stressful circumstances can lower the threshold for ventricular fibrillation (Lown et al, 1973; Matta et al, 1976). There is evidence that acute stress will also increase the frequency of premature ventricular beats in humans (Lown and De Silva, 1978). Several case studies have shown that in some individuals ventricular fibrillation can be triggered by emotions such as anger or fright (Lown et al, 1980). Preliminary studies of persons successfully resuscitated from ventricular fibrillation suggest that a proportion of such cases may have been precipitated by psychogenic stimuli (Lown et al, 1980). However, in the absence of a control group and because of the probably important effect of the catastrophic event in affecting recall (potentially increasing or decreasing), firm conclusions are difficult to reach. Probably only a small proportion of sudden deaths could be explained in this fashion.

Social Support and Heart Disease

Another group of variables that are usually thought to decrease environmental stress have been called *social support* factors. Berkman and Syme (1979) gave a social support questionnaire to subjects at entrance to a 9-year prospective study of 6928 adults in Alameda County, California. This questionnaire included four variables thought to contribute to social support: marital status, number of contacts with close friends and relatives, church membership, and membership in informal and formal group associations. Over the 9-year follow-up period, church membership and contacts with friends and relatives were significantly associated with death from all causes for both sexes, and marital status and group membership for individual sexes (Table 11–6). Combining them to form a composite scale of social support, Berkman and Syme found that high scores of social support were associated with twofold to fourfold relative risk differences for all-cause mortality as compared to low scores (Fig. 11–1). Recently this work has been replicated in the Tecumseh Longitudinal Study

Table 11-6   Age- and sex-specific mortality per 100 (all causes) by source of social contact: Human Population Laboratory Study of Alameda County, 1965–1974

Source	Age group						
	30–49		50–59		60–69		
	n	% died	n	% died	n	% died	P^a
Men							
Marital status							
Married	1227	3.0	446	12.1	268	26.9	
Nonmarried	175	8.6	55	25.5	98	33.7	≤0.001
Contacts with friends and relatives							
High	276	2.9	127	11.0	81	22.2	
Medium	865	3.4	303	14.2	173	24.9	≤0.001
Low	236	5.1	62	14.5	59	40.7	
Church member							
Member	391	2.8	168	11.3	88	21.6	
Nonmember	1011	4.1	333	14.7	238	30.3	≤0.05
Group member							
Member	1066	3.6	394	11.9	223	28.2	
Nonmember	336	3.9	107	19.6	103	27.2	n.s.[b]
Women							
Marital status							
Married	1249	3.0	407	7.1	208	14.4	
Nonmarried	286	3.8	167	9.6	179	20.7	n.s.
Contacts with friends and relatives							
High	266	1.9	166	6.6	105	11.4	
Medium	1007	2.9	340	7.6	223	17.0	
Low	239	5.4	57	12.3	42	31.0	≤0.001
Church member							
Member	484	1.4	217	6.9	152	15.8	
Nonmember	1051	3.9	357	8.4	235	18.3	≤0.05
Group member							
Member	1005	2.4	347	7.2	173	15.0	
Nonmember	535	4.5	227	8.8	214	19.2	≤0.05

Source: From L Berkman and SL Syme: Social networks, host resistance, and mortality. *Am J Epidemiol* **109**:186, 1979, with permission.

[a] Chi square values were calculated for differences in age-adjusted mortality rates among categories.
[b] Not significant.

(House et al, 1982) and also in a 30-month follow-up of 331 elderly persons (Blazer, 1982).

These fascinating relationships between social support and all-cause mortality seem consistent for different age groups, for both sexes, and across different studies. It seems probable that social support is protective specifically against

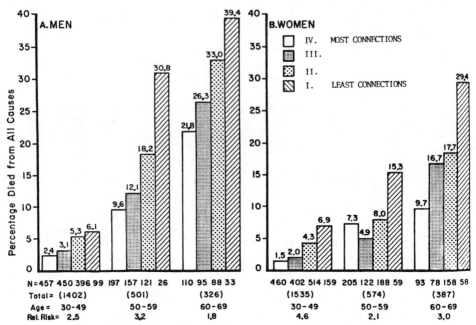

Figure 11–1   Age- and sex-specific mortality rates from all causes by value for the social network index. Population laboratory study of Alameda County, 1965–1974. From L Berkman and SL Syme: Social networks, host resistance, and mortality. *Am J Epidemiol* **109**:186, 1979, with permission.

IHD, but it is uncertain whether it acts independently of the traditional risk factors. Berkman and Breslow (1983) did show that, as their index of social support (see above) increased from I to IV, mortality rates from IHD decreased consistently from 5.1 to 2.4/100 in men and from 3.2 to 1.0/100 in women. The Tecumseh Study found an association with IHD mortality specifically, particularly in women. A longitudinal study of 4653 men of Japanese ancestry living in Hawaii found a significant relationship between social support and lower incidence rates of total IHD and nonfatal myocardial infarction (Reed et al, 1983). On multivariate analysis with the traditional risk factors as covariates, the associations with social support lost statistical significance. Thus, these relationships may be explained by favorable values of traditional risk factors where social support is high, and vice versa. As the authors point out, the effects of social support may be culture dependent, and extrapolation to other societies from the results in Japanese Hawaiians should be cautious.

Personality Factors and Risk of Ischemic Heart Disease

In this section we will consider the evidence relating such variables as general neuroticism, anxiety, depression, and hypochondriasis to risk of ischemic heart disease. Most of the evidence is from retrospective studies, which are very difficult to interpret in that any relationships could represent psychologic results of the disease rather than antecedents. Reviewing this literature, CD Jenkins (1976b) concluded that "this family of variables is associated with coronary heart disease—seemingly more for angina pectoris than for myocardial infarction." We will draw attention here only to results from prospective studies.

In the Western Electric Company Study in Chicago, Ostfeld et al (1964) found over a 4.5-year follow-up that men subsequently developing angina pectoris differed significantly from men subsequently developing myocardial infarction. Before disease developed, the former had a greater tendency to complain about somatic symptoms of all sorts and to be worried about their health even in the absence of objective findings. Men subsequently developing myocardial infarction complained about their health no more than the average citizen. In the study of 10,000 Israeli men, anxiety was also found to have a significant positive association with the incidence of angina pectoris (Medalie et al, 1973a). This variable retained its significance as a risk factor on multivariate analysis, being independent of traditional risk factors (Table 11–3). Some idea of the magnitude of this effect can be gained from Table 11–7. The findings also suggested that a "loving and supportive" wife can ameliorate the adverse effects of anxiety on risk of angina pectoris. Some prospective studies have related depression to risk of IHD, but results are inconsistent (CD Jenkins, 1976a).

Behavior Patterns and Ischemic Heart Disease

In 1910, William Osler observed that "it is not the delicate neurotic person who is prone to angina, but the robust, the vigorous in mind and body, the keen and ambitious man, the indicator of whose engines is always 'full steam ahead.'" Having made similar observations, M Friedman and RH Rosenman (1959) formed their well-known hypothesis about types A and B personalities. The type A behavior pattern has been defined by CD Jenkins et al (1974) as an

overt behavioral syndrome or style of living characterized by excesses of competitiveness, striving for achievement, aggressiveness (sometimes stringently repressed), time urgency, acceleration of common activities, restlessness, hostility, hyperalertness, explosiveness of speech amplitude, tenseness of facial musculature and feelings of struggle against the limitations of time, and the insensitivity of the environment.

In 1960, M Friedman, RH Rosenman, and associates initiated the Western Collaborative Group Study, a prospective investigation of 3154 men free of IHD, aged between 39 and 59 years, who were employed in 10 different companies in California and represented a white, middle-aged working population rather than the general population. The investigators developed a Structured Interview to measure types A and B patterns. This mildly challenging interview

Table 11–7   Association of 5-yr incidence of angina pectoris (cases of myocardial infarction excluded) with anxiety and wife's love/support, Israeli men

Anxiety score	Wife's love and support	Number at risk	Number angina pectoris cases	Rate/1000	
0–1	3+	4110	88	21	
	2+	1090	31	28	
	±	460	11	24	
	–	714	18	25	n.s.
2–3	3+	637	33	52	
	2+	242	11	45	
	±	150	11	73	
	–	183	17	93	$0.01 < P < 0.05$[a]

Source: From JH Medalie and U Goldbourt: *Am J Med* **60**:910, 1976a, with permission.

[a] *P* values are for significance of the incidence slope with rising scores for "wife's love."

Note: The "Anxiety score" (column 1) is based on answers to the following questions:

(a) Do you consider yourself a tense person?

(b) Do you generally or frequently suffer from anxiety (when there is no obvious reason for it)?

(c) Do you generally have sleep problems?

The scores under "Wife's love and support" (column 2) are based on the question:

"Does your wife show you her love?

(a) Does not love me.

(b) Loves me but never shows it.

(c) Loves me and shows it often.

(d) Loves me and shows it occasionally.

takes 10–20 minutes and is tape-recorded. It is assessed by the content of the subject's answers and also by voice and motor characteristics.

Table 11–8 depicts some of the results of this study for 50- to 59-year-old men (Rosenman et al, 1975). There were similar findings for the 30- to 49-year-old men. Within various strata representing other traditional risk factors, the rate of IHD for type A persons is always greater than that for type B persons, so that the predictive ability of the type A–B behavior patterns is independent of these risk factors. A multivariate analysis confirmed this. The relative risk for IHD (type A compared to type B), after adjustment for other factors was 1.87 and 1.98 for the 39–49 and 50–59 age groups, respectively.

The influence of types A and B behavior patterns was also investigated in the Framingham Study, using a questionnaire validated by noting moderate agreement with the Structured Interview (SG Haynes et al, 1980). A psychosocial interview was administered to a subsample of 1674 IHD-free persons, and

Table 11-8 Incidence of IHD according to behavior pattern, within strata of other risk factors: men aged 50–59 in the Western Collaborative Group Study

	Subjects at risk		Subjects with IHD		Rate of IHD[a]	
	Type A	Type B	Type A	Type B	Type A	Type B
Number of subjects	522	383	83	29	18.7	8.9
Parental history of CHD						
Yes	103	64	20	7	22.8	12.9
No	419	319	63	22	17.7	8.1
Smoking habits						
Never smoked	90	89	10	5	13.1	6.6
Pipe or cigar	81	78	17	2	24.7	3.0
Former cigarette	91	41	10	2	12.9	5.7
Current cigarette	260	175	46	20	20.8	13.4
Current cigarette usage						
None	262	208	37	9	16.6	5.1
1–15 per day	65	43	8	1	14.5	2.7
⩾ 16 per day	195	132	38	19	22.9	16.9
Systolic blood pressure (mm Hg)						
< 120	95	80	7	4	8.7	5.9
120–159	381	283	64	21	19.9	8.7
⩾ 160	46	20	12	4	30.7	23.5
Diastolic blood pressure (mm Hg)						
< 95	448	344	64	25	16.3	8.5
⩾ 95	74	39	19	4	30.2	12.1
Serum cholesterol (mg/dl)						
< 220	211	148	20	6	11.2	4.8
220–259	179	142	36	10	23.7	8.3
⩾ 260	130	90	27	13	24.4	17.0
Fasting serum triglycerides (mg/dl)						
< 100	151	99	16	5	12.5	5.9
100–176	238	170	37	11	18.3	7.6
⩾ 177	114	98	26	9	26.8	10.8
Serum β-/α-lipoprotein ratio						
< 2.35	323	263	43	18	15.7	8.1
⩾ 2.36	196	117	39	11	23.4	11.1

Source: Adapted from RH Rosenman et al: *JAMA* **233**:872. Copyright 1975, American Medical Association.

[a] Average annual rate/1000 subjects at risk. Difference of rates between type A and type B subjects are tested for significance by Mantel–Haenszel χ^2, with adjustment for factors indicated. For each factor the adjusted association between behavior and pattern and IHD incidence is significant at $P < 0.001$.

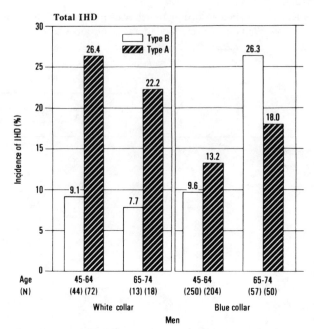

Figure 11–2 Eight-year incidence of ischemic heart disease among men stratified by occupation and Framingham type A and type B behavior. From SG Haynes et al: The relationship of psychosocial factors to coronary heart disease in the Framingham Study. *Am J Epidemiol* **111**:37, 1980, by permission.

results were presented after an 8-year follow-up. Among men, there was an overall excess of ischemic heart disease for type A persons, but further analysis revealed that the type A behavior was predictive only for men in white-collar occupations (Fig. 11–2). It is of interest to recall that 80 percent of the Western Collaborative Group Study participants were "white-collar" workers. In the Framingham Study also, the IHD–type A relationship persisted after adjustment for other risk factors in a multivariate logistic regression.

There was an excess of ischemic heart disease in type A Framingham women (Fig. 11–3). These relationships appeared for both housewives and working women, although they were statistically significant only in the latter after adjustment for other factors. In both sexes the clearest association was between angina and type A behavior. Another report from SG Haynes et al (1982) sheds further light on the complexity of some of these relationships. On a 10-year follow-up of a Framingham sample, she found that the type A status of a husband was an important predictor of his IHD risk only if he were married to a wife who either worked outside of the home or was highly educated.

Despite the above results, there remains some controversy over the validity of

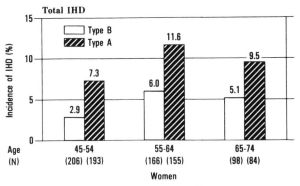

Figure 11–3 Eight-year incidence of ischemic heart disease among women by the Framingham type A and type B behavior patterns. From SG Haynes et al: The relationship of psychosocial factors to coronary heart disease in the Framingham Study. *Am J Epidemiol* **111**:37, 1980, by permission.

type A behavior as a risk factor for IHD. This was recently highlighted by a report from the MRFIT Study of men at high risk for IHD events. Type A behavior was assessed by the Structured Interview, and after a 6-year follow-up there was no hint of any relationship with subsequent IHD death (Shekelle et al, 1983). Of course, this group of high-risk men was not representative of the total population.

The other common method of assessing type A–B behavior is the Jenkins Activity Survey (JAS). This questionnaire contains 72 questions and can be scored by computer. Agreement between the Structured Interview and JAS averages about 67 percent in different situations (CD Jenkins, 1978). Type A–B behavior as measured by this questionnaire was shown to predict ischemic heart disease events (angina pectoris and Q-wave infarctions combined) in the Western Collaborative Group Study (CD Jenkins et al, 1974). However, it is clear that the Structured Interview and the Jenkins Activity Survey type A patterns are not identical. Matthews and colleagues (KA Matthews et al, 1982) found that the common components of the two methods appeared to be in measures of self-reported pressured drive, hostility, competitiveness and energy level. The unique components of the Structured Interview include the subject's speech behaviors, and for the Jenkins Activity Survey, self-reported time pressure. This has furthered the idea that some of the various questions and subscales comprising each measure may be predictors of IHD while others are not.

KA Matthews et al (1977) performed a factor analysis of the Structured Interview, again using the Western Collaborative Group Study population. They identified five main factors—which they called competitive drive, past achievements, impatience, nonjob achievement, and speed—and tried to identify which of these factors and their component questions discriminated significantly between cases of IHD and controls. "Competitive drive" and "impatience" proved the most important. The components of competitive drive that discriminated significantly were "explosive voice modulation," "potential for hostility," and "vigorous answers to questions." The single significant component of the impatience factor was "irritation at waiting in lines."

The Type A Behavior Pattern and Coronary Atherosclerosis

Several autopsy and coronary angiography studies have dealt with the association between type A behavior and coronary atherosclerosis (Bass and Wade, 1982; Blumenthal et al, 1978; Dimsdale et al, 1979; K Frank et al, 1978; M. Friedman et al, 1968; RB Williams et al, 1980; Zyzanski et al, 1976). In the studies of persons undergoing coronary angiography, those who show significant coronary disease are compared to those with little disease for type A behavior. Some studies showed significant differences, but results are conflicting. Of course, in these studies, subjects showing little disease were still symptomatic enough to warrant angiography, so that they probably do not adequately represent the general population as control cases.

M Friedman and colleagues (1968) reported the only prospective study relating type A behavior pattern to coronary disease. This was an autopsy study attempting to follow all deaths occurring in the Western Collaborative Group Study. Thus, it was population based, although the population was a little atypical, representing middle-class employed white males. The degree of coronary obstruction was measured by 21 microscopic sections of right and left coronary arteries. The average obstruction score was significantly higher in type A subjects as compared to type B subjects, and type A subjects were six times more likely to have severe coronary obstruction (more than 50 percent cross-sectional narrowing).

The Prevalence of Type A Behavior

Good population data on the prevalence of type A behavior are difficult to find, but some information is available. In the Western Collaborative Group Study, about 50 percent of the men were rated as type A when assessed by the Structured Interview. As mentioned above, this study group consisted of middle-aged, middle-class white business and professional men (Rosenman et al, 1975). In the Framingham Study population, which was more of a cross section of society, about half the subjects were classified as type A, using the Framingham questionnaire. About 51 percent of the Framingham women were also classified as type A when assessed by the Structured Interview (SG Haynes and M Feinleib, 1980). In the United States, employed men are more prone to type A behavior than employed women, according to one Chicago study that used the Jenkins Activity Survey (Waldron et al, 1977). This study and others indicated that type A behavior is more prevalent in more highly educated persons. KA

Matthews and colleagues (1982) commented that more recent studies using the Structured Interview appear to be classifying much higher proportions of the male population as type A than the older studies. It is unclear whether this is a real change or represents a shift in the interview technique.

The whole issue is complicated by the likelihood that type A behavior may well be a culture-dependent attribute. In Belgium, type A behavior was less common (38 percent) as assessed by the Structured Interview (Kittel et al, 1978). In New Zealand, Spicer et al (1981) found the prevalence of type A behavior in men aged 30–55 to be 27 percent, as assessed by the Structured Interview. In Japanese residents of Honolulu, the prevalence of type A behavior was rated as 15 percent using the JAS (JB Cohen et al, 1978). Note that the JAS scale has been standardized so that approximately half of U.S. white males are scored type A.

Furthermore, there is evidence that the concept of type A may not be relevant in some cultures. Factor analysis of the JAS items produced three new factors, when applied to Honolulu Japanese. This indicates that the component questions mix differently in this population, and that traditional type A behavior reflects a frequent combination of certain items in Europeans, whereas other combinations not clearly type A or type B are more common in Japanese (JB Cohen et al, 1975).

Possible Mechanisms for the Influence of Psychosocial Factors on Risk of Ischemic Heart Disease

There are several potential mechanisms whereby psychosocial factors may influence risk of ischemic heart disease. It is possible that these factors affect values of the traditional risk factors or they act through other physiologic responses that have implications for atherogenesis or the development of arrhythmias. Many of these postulated mechanisms seek to explain the effects of stress on IHD. Presumably social support, by limiting stress, could prevent their activation.

Stress may result in changes in serum lipids. This is not well documented, but M Friedman et al (1958) demonstrated a cyclic rise in serum cholesterol levels in a group of accountants during periods of time pressure and work overload. The relationship between psychosocial factors and blood pressure has been examined by several investigators with mixed results. There is a little evidence that type A individuals have higher blood pressures (Harrel, 1980). The Loma Linda Children's Blood Pressure Study indicates that "type A" and other family environments may be positively related to blood pressure in children (Insel et al, 1981). In a study of factory workers in Belgium, however, De Backer et al (1979) was unable to find any evidence that type A men differed from type B men in any risk factors, or in urinary catecholamine excretion. Shekelle (1976b) came to similar conclusions, using the Jenkins Activity Survey. Thus, it seems that any effects of stress or behavior pattern on traditional risk factors are small and probably do not have substantial influence on IHD risk.

Yet there is firm evidence of interactions between stress, type A behavior, and physiologic responses. Several studies have demonstrated a heightened cardiovascular reactivity to stress in type A individuals. Dembroski et al (1977) investigated reactivity of pulse rate and blood pressure in 10 type A and 14 type B men. The type A men's pulse rates and blood pressures rose significantly more in association with controlled stress. M Friedman et al (1975) compared 15 type A and 15 type B men who had similar plasma catecholamine levels under resting conditions. Under the stress of a competitive situation, the plasma norepinephrine concentration in type A persons rose 30 percent while that of the type B men remained unchanged. It has also been shown that platelet aggregation after stressful exercise is increased in type A as compared to type B subjects (MT Simpson et al, 1974). This may be related to catecholamine release, well known to be a platelet-aggregating stimulus. Thus, we have a hint that type A persons might be susceptible to developing IHD because of a supersensitivity to the metabolic effects of stress.

As mentioned above, there is some evidence that acute stress can precipitate sudden death. It is not difficult to suggest possible mechanisms for such a pathogenic sequence. The electrical activity of the heart is under substantial neuronal and hormonal control. Stimulation of the stellate ganglia and hypothalamus in animals can significantly alter cardiac electrophysiology (Schwartz et al, 1978). Such effects as prolongation of Q–T interval, increased arrhythmias, lowered threshold for ventricular fibrillation, and abnormalities of the T wave have been observed. Consequently, it is quite plausible that the known effects of acute stress on the autonomic nervous system could precipitate ventricular fibrillation in a diseased heart. It has been established that β-adrenergic blocking drugs decrease long-term mortality after a myocardial infarction (chapter 20), and they may act through suppression of abnormal neurohormonal activity. In addition, the possibility of emotionally induced coronary artery spasm has been raised by the data of Schiffer and colleagues (1980). This provides another possible mechanism of emotionally induced sudden death—acute myocardial ischemia.

Socioeconomic Status and Ischemic Heart Disease Events

Lower socioeconomic status is associated with increased incidence of coronary events (Hinkle et al, 1968), and this is particularly evident for IHD death (Comstock, 1971; Fraser, 1978a; Koskenvuo et al, 1980; GA Rose and MG Marmot, 1981; Salonen, 1982a; Weinblatt et al, 1978). In the British Whitehall Study, GA Rose and MG Marmot (1981) followed 17,530 London male civil servants over 7.5 years. They documented dramatically different IHD prevalence by occupation at the beginning of the study, and differences in IHD mortality on follow-up (Fig. 11–4). Social class was defined by occupation and

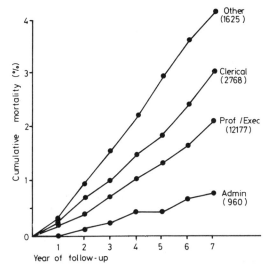

Figure 11–4 Cumulative age-adjusted mortality from ischemic heart disease according to employment grade and year of follow-up (numbers of subjects in parentheses): British civil servants. From GA Rose and MG Marmot: *Br Heart J* **45**:13, 1981, with permission.

classified as administrative, professional/executive, clerical, and "other." These are the five ranked occupational status groups to which British civil servants are commonly classified. The "other" category consists mainly of unskilled manual workers.

These observations are unexplained, but they may involve stress. Persons of lower socioeconomic status probably do experience more stressful circumstances in their lives, whether because of poverty, lack of opportunity for advancement due to poor education, or other conditions. Persons of lower socioeconomic status also have a worse profile for the traditional IHD risk factors. For whites in the Californian study by JF Kraus et al (1980), this result was true for blood pressure, serum cholesterol, and smoking habits. Using the Framingham risk score to convert values of subjects' risk factors to a predicted risk of IHD events over 6 years, a clear trend was seen of higher risk in persons of lower socioeconomic status and vice versa (Fig. 11–5). The relationship was consistent among whites, Asians, and Spanish Americans, but not for blacks. In the Whitehall Study the upper social classes smoked less, had lower systolic blood pressures, got more leisure-time physical activity, but had higher blood cholesterol levels. Despite this last item, overall risk was judged to be considerably lower. Further support for this idea comes from the Lipid Research Clinics Study in which persons of higher socioeconomic status had higher levels of HDL cholesterol (Heiss et al, 1980b).

This inverse relationship between IHD risk and socioeconomic status may not always have been apparent. In fact, older data suggest that in the past men in upper socioeconomic classes were at increased risk. GA Rose and MG Marmot (1981) reported evidence from Britain that while nonvalvular heart disease mortality of upper social class men may have remained rather stable, that of lower social class men has risen steeply, crossing over the rates for the

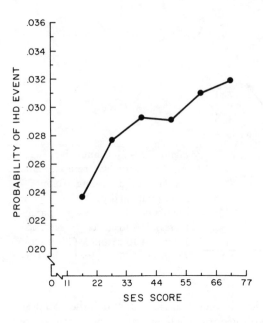

Figure 11–5 Predicted probability of future IHD according to socioeconomic status (SES) for Sacramento, California men 1975–1976. From JF Kraus et al: Socioeconomic status, ethnicity and risk of coronary heart disease. *Am J Epidemiol* **111**:407, 1980, with permission.

upper social class males. The data suggested that lower social class women may always have had higher rates. Cassel and colleagues (1971) traced a similar transition for IHD during the period 1960–1969 in Evans County, Georgia.

One can speculate on the causes of this interesting reversal. Thirty years ago the life-styles and foods now recognized as detrimental for cardiovascular health were most readily available to and affordable by upper socioeconomic class persons. Today, however, such persons tend to be more concerned with physique, better educated about the new-found connections between life-style, diet, and cardiovascular health. Conversely, 30 years ago lower socioeconomic class individuals probably had relatively simple dietary habits and were often involved in manual labor, whereas the same classes can now exist on cheap "junk foods" containing much solid fat, calories, and salt and may work in production-line, automated jobs requiring little physical activity.

Summary

1. The relationship between stress and IHD, although much suspected by laypersons, has been difficult to document consistently. Some consistent relationships appear to exist for social status incongruity, for social, occupational, and geographic mobility, and perhaps for interpersonal problems with family or at the work site. Different relationships may be present for different IHD syndromes. The probable increased risk of the recently bereaved is in keeping with this.

2. Recent interest has centered on beneficial effects of social support on total

(and perhaps IHD) mortality. It is not clear whether this influence is independent of the traditional risk factors.

3. Anxiety is probably a risk factor for angina pectoris at least, as may be a tendency to a hypochondriacal personality.

4. The type A behavior pattern is probably an independent risk factor for IHD. There is some controversial evidence that this may be so also for coronary disease. The effects on IHD disease rates seem most prominent for white-collar men and for working women.

5. The two best-validated instruments for assessing type A behavior are the Structured Interview and the Jenkins Activity Survey (JAS). It is now recognized that these composite scores may contain highly predictive components as well as components not predicting IHD. Future efforts will probably include attempts to separate these.

6. Several mechanisms whereby psychosocial factors can affect IHD are proposed. These include increased cardiovascular reactivity to stress in type A persons and increased platelet aggregability. Stress may provoke coronary artery spasm in susceptible individuals, as well as cardiac arrhythmias. Effects on traditional risk factors are controversial.

7. Persons of lower socioeconomic status are at increased risk of IHD events. This is probably partly because they are likely to have a worse coronary risk profile. They probably also have less social support and thus more stress.

12

Physical Inactivity and Ischemic Heart Disease

Many laypersons view lack of physical activity as one of the important causes of heart disease. Exercise has also received much attention as a key part of cardiac rehabilitation programs (chapter 19). The epidemiologic basis for the value of exercise with regard to ischemic heart disease (IHD) is fairly secure, though it is not an easy variable to measure.

Little thought is needed to appreciate the difficulties involved in trying to summarize a person's daily activities as a single score. Physical activity of some sort is almost continuous for most persons. Various measures have been used to try to quantify either occupational or leisure time physical activity. Some are as simple as obtaining the job title or use questionnaires or interviews. Few methods have been formally validated against caloric expenditure or physiological measures of fitness. One of the best techniques available at present is the Minnesota Leisure Time Physical Activity Questionnaire (Taylor et al, 1978). It was developed through experiments to estimate energy expenditure for a variety of activities. The subject is asked which activities he or she has undertaken, in which month of the year, the number of times each month, and the average duration. From this, a calculation of time spent on the leisure time activity and thus caloric expenditure is obtained.

Physical *fitness* can be quantified rather more precisely than physical *activity* by measuring oxygen consumption at maximum effort. However, this is difficult to measure in the field, and less precise measures, such as pulse rate at a given work load on either a bicycle ergometer or treadmill or the time to run a fixed distance, have also been used. It is important to distinguish between physical activity and physical fitness. These two variables are both of interest in relation to IHD but are not necessarily interchangeable. Persons who are very physically active are not always very physically fit. This may be due to adverse hereditary factors (Klissouras, 1971; 1973). Females also are often less physically fit than males (Matthews and Fox, 1976; Fraser et al, 1983b).

Many studies relating exercise or physical fitness to IHD risk are difficult to interpret because of potential confounding between obesity and physical activity. Physically active people are usually slim. Indeed, there is evidence that regular activity may affect some intrinsic "set-point" regulating energy storage, metabolic rate, and thus body weight (Bennett and Gurin, 1982; Brownell, 1982a). As we will see later, evidence suggests that physical activity and fitness

168

influence risk independent of other major risk factors for IHD. The evidence for obesity as an independent risk factor is less clear (chapter 15).

Epidemiologic Studies of Physical Activity and Ischemic Heart Disease

Information is available from studies with a variety of designs, populations, and measures of physical activity or fitness. The Seven Countries Study compared men aged 40 to 59 years at intake in seven different countries (chapter 4). IHD incidence has been reported over both 5- (Keys, 1970) and 10- (Keys, 1980b) year follow-up. Physical activity was estimated at baseline by occupational category plus two or three extra questions relating to leisure time activities. The relationship between physical activity and IHD incidence in the 5-year follow-up was not very convincing (Fig. 12–1). The striking data against the hypothesis came from Finland, where the percentage off sedentary persons was only 10 percent, but IHD incidence was greatest of all. The 10-year results were similar. This suggests either that physical activity is not protective for IHD or else that excellent habits of physical activity cannot override the effects of other suboptimal health habits of Finns prevalent at the time of this study. The latter seems most likely in view of evidence presented later.

Leon and Blackburn (1977) reviewed many studies that sought to link physical activity with IHD. Nearly as many showed no relationship between lack of exercise and IHD risk as found one. However, all studies are not equal. We are

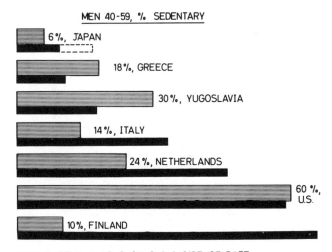

NARROW, SOLID BARS SHOW CHD INCIDENCE RATE

Figure 12–1   Percentage of men sedentary or engaged only in very light physical activity related to IHD incidence in seven countries. From A Keys et al: Coronary heart disease in seven countries. *Circulation* **41**(suppl 1): 1, 1970, by permission of the American Heart Association, Inc.

faced with serious measurement problems and ambiguity over the predictor variable to be measured—physical activity or physical fitness. Ideally, adjustment should be made for the effects of covariates of physical fitness or physical activity on the IHD risk since persons who exercise obviously differ from those who do not in other ways.

Retrospective and cross-sectional studies are often difficult to interpret. Retrospective studies rely on memory or on records not designed for the purpose of the study whereas cross-sectional studies cannot exclude the possibility that either manifest or subclinical IHD may have caused the decrease in physical activity. A special group of retrospective studies deal with the current status of former athletes (Table 12–1). Again, roughly equal numbers of studies are positive as nonsignificant. Such studies usually look back over many years because people tend to be more athletic while young whereas IHD most often strikes the middle-aged or elderly. However, exercise habits of 20 to 40 years ago may have little bearing on present clinical status.

Prospective studies have clear advantages in interpretation and should be given the greatest credibility. Results of older prospective studies are mixed when physical *activity* as variably assessed, is the predictor (Table 12–2). Notice, however, that all five longitudinal studies in which physiologic data are used to measure physical *fitness* show a positive relationship with IHD. The reason for the clearer relationship when fitness rather than activity is investigated may be physiological since fitness has determinants other than exercise. Or it may be related to the greater precision in measuring physical fitness.

A nonsignificant result should be considered a neutral result in most circumstances where difficult-to-measure variables such as diet or exercise or involved. The fact that 7 out of 21 retrospective and prevalence studies, 4 of 9 studies of athletes, 7 of 14 longitudinal studies of physical activity, and all 5 longitudinal studies of physical fitness are positive is highly suggestive of an underlying relationship between physical activity, fitness and IHD. In the absence of such a

Table 12–1 Retrospective studies of former athletes and nonathletes—Longevity and IHD status

	Reduced IHD		Increased Longevity	
	Positive	Nonsignificant	Positive	Nonsignificant
Former athletic status assessed by questionnaire, letters to relatives, and college records. IHD mortality assessed by death certificate.	4	5	6	4

Source: Adapted from AS Leon and H Blackburn: *Ann NY Acad Sci* **301**:561, 1977, with permission.

Table 12–2 Prospective (longitudinal) studies involving initially IHD-free men

Sources of data	Relationship of physical inactivity or exercise test result to subsequent IHD	
	Positive	Nonsignificant
Activity from job title and/or job evaluation; IHD from medical records	2	5
Questionnaire for job and leisure-time activity; IHD by medical evaluation or death certificate	4	2
Leisure-time activity by questionnaire; IHD by medical evaluation	1	—
Physical fitness by physiological data; IHD by medical evaluation	5	—

Source: Adapted from AS Leon and H Blackburn: *Ann NY Acad Sci* **301**:561, 1977, with permission.

relationship, presumably only 1 study in 20 should be statistically significant at the $p = 0.05$ level, representing a random event.

Four specific prospective studies will now be described in more detail as examples. The first is an older study that nicely illustrates the potential problem of confounding between obesity and physical activity. The other three are a representative selection of the six recently reported longitudinal studies with large numbers of subjects and methodological excellence. All six find significant relationships between physical activity and IHD risk. The three not reported in detail are the Framingham Study, in which the relationship was not presented independent of obesity (Kannel and Sorlie, 1979); a 4-to-8-year follow-up of male Los Angeles firemen and law enforcement officers (Peters et al, 1983); and the Puerto Rico Heart Program, which followed urban and rural men for over eight years (Garcia-Palmieri et al, 1982). The Los Angeles study used physical fitness as assessed by treadmill performance as the independent variable, and results indicated that the association of increased fitness with lower risk of IHD was most evident for smokers or where blood pressure or serum cholesterol were relatively elevated.

The London Busmen Study is one of the earliest and most famous of these studies (Morris et al, 1953). Morris and his colleagues compared London bus drivers with bus conductors. Many of the buses were double-deckers, so that while the drivers sat all day, the conductors were very active. On follow-up, clear differences in IHD mortality between the drivers and conductors, favoring the latter, were found (Table 12–3). Most of the excess mortality came from deaths occurring within 90 days of the first clinical manifestation of IHD. However, in a later article entitled "The Epidemiology of Uniforms," Morris and his colleagues (1956) pointed out that the waist size of the drivers' uniforms was substantially greater than that of the conductors so that differences in obesity

Table 12–3 First clinical episodes of coronary heart-disease in drivers and male conductors (aged 35–64 inclusive) of central buses, trams, and trolleybuses of London Transport Executive, 1949–50: Average annual rates per 1000

Ages (years)	Person-years observed	Angina pectoris	"Coronary thrombosis"		Total incidence	
			Coronary occlusion— myocardial infarction	Immediate mortality (first 3 days)	No. of cases	Rate per 1000 p.a.
			Drivers			
35–44	12,360	—	0.4	—	8	0.7
45–54	11,698	—	1.5	0.9	29	2.5
55–64	6,668	1.2	3.3	2.0	43	6.5
Standardized rate at ages 35–64 incl.		0.4	1.5	0.9		2.7
			Conductors			
35–44	9,622	—	—	—	0	—
45–54	5,522	0.5	0.9	0.5	11	2.0
55–64	4,022	2.2	2.0	0.8	20	5.0
Standardized rate at ages 35–64 incl.		0.8	0.8	0.4		1.9

Source: JN Morris et al: 1953, with permission.

may have been important in their subsequent disease experience. We have the same problem mentioned earlier—is it physical activity or obesity?

Morris and his colleagues (1980) have done extensive work on another population of 17,000 British male civil servants. Each man was asked to record meticulously his *leisure-time* activities on the previous Friday and Saturday, having been contacted without warning on the following Monday. They were categorized according to several levels of activity. Almost always, the more active groups—whether it was sports or other "strenuous" activities—had the better IHD experience over the subsequent 8½ years (Fig. 12–2). This was so even when analyses were conducted within strata of obesity and cigarette smoking and across all ages (Tables 12–4, 12–5). These findings indicate that the effect of physical activity is independent of obesity and cigarette smoking. Even in prospective studies like this one, it is possible that some inactive men are that way because the early preclinical phase of IHD has unrecognized manifestations that restrict activity. This could produce a spurious increase in IHD events in the inactive group. Ideally, one should examine and possibly stress-test all men at entry to such a study, but this degree of rigor is usually not feasible in a large

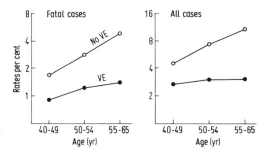

Figure 12–2 Rising incidence of IHD with age in relation to vigorous exercise (VE). British civil servants. From JN Morris et al, 1980, with permission.

population study. This problem seems an unlikely explanation for the findings of the last study (Morris, 1981).

Another methodologically excellent study was the 22-year follow-up of 3975 San Francisco longshoremen conducted by Paffenbarger and his colleagues (Brand et al, 1979). The various job categories of the longshoremen were assessed for energy expenditure by kcal/min of activity required to perform the work. Each year the work status of each man was reassessed. A careful analysis showed that there was a statistically significant decrease in the relative risk of

Table 12–4 Relationship of physique and vigorous exercise to incidence of IHD in British male civil servants[a]

	First attacks CHD 1968–78			
	All men		Reporting VE sports	Reporting no VE
Physique	Cases	Rate (%)	(rate, %)	(rate, %)
Stature (at 40–65 yr)				
<5 ft 5 in.	136	9.7	6.3	10.4
5 ft 6 in.–5 ft 8 in.	474	7.2	3.3	7.8
5 ft 9 in.–5 ft 10 in.	297	6.2	3.1	6.8
5 ft 11 in. +	225[d]	5.3	2.5	6.0
Body mass (at 40–59 yr)[b]				
<23.0	163	4.9	2.4	5.2
23.1–25.0	276	6.2	3.3	6.9
25.1–28.0	375	6.5	4.4	6.9
28.1 +	163	7.5	0.7[c]	8.8

Source: JN Morris et al: 1980, with permission.

[a] Height, weight, and exercise as self-reported at survey, 1968–70. Rates standardized for age.

[b] Quetelet's index of weight in kg/height in inches.^{2}

[c] Fewer than 5 cases.

[d] Totals incomplete because of inadequate information.

Table 12–5 Relationship of smoking and vigorous exercise to incidence of IHD in British male civil servants[a]

| | First attacks CHD 1968–78 | | | |
| | All men | | Reporting VE sports (rate, %) | Reporting no VE (rate, %) |
Smoking	Cases	Rate (%)		
Never smoked	108	3.4	1.5	3.8
Ex-smokers	229	4.6	2.1	5.1
Pipe-cigars only	148	5.7	3.1	6.2
All non-cigarette smokers	485	4.5	2.1	5.0
Cigarette smokers:				
1–10 per day	158	7.7	5.3	8.3
11–20 per day	343	9.0	4.6	9.6
21 + per day	152	10.8 ⎫		11.6
All cigarette smokers	653	9.0 ⎭	4.9	9.7

Source: JN Morris et al: 1980, with permission.

[a] Men aged 40–65 at survey, 1968–70. Smoking and exercise as reported at survey. Rates standardized for age.

fatal heart attack according to the level of energy requirement assigned to an individual's job title (Fig. 12–3). Although IHD status was not assessed initially in this longitudinal study, the investigators were able to show, through the annual job reclassification, that the observed relationship was probably not due to transfer of persons developing IHD to less physically demanding jobs. The

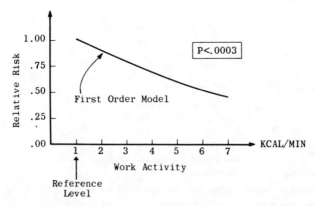

Figure 12–3 Estimated relative risk of fatal heart attack vs. work activity immediately prior to risk period for a population of San Francisco longshoremen studied over a 22-year period. From RJ Brand et al. Work activity and fatal heart attack studied by multiple logistic risk analysis. *Amer J Epidemiol* **110**:52, 1979, with permission.

relationship of relative risk of IHD to work activity was not much altered by adjusting for the potential effects of several other factors (age, race, systolic blood pressure, smoking, obesity, glucose tolerance, and ECG status). Thus, as in the 1980 Morris study, the association between physical activity and IHD proved to be independent of obesity.

Paffenbarger and colleagues (1978) also conducted a 6 to 10 year follow-up study of 16,936 Harvard University male alumni less than 75 years of age and self-reportedly free of IHD at baseline. The responses to baseline and follow-up questionnaires represented 117,680 person-years of observation. The baseline questionnaire asked how many flights of stairs were climbed daily (10 stairs = 1 flight), how many city blocks or equivalents were walked each day, and how many hours per week were engaged in active sports. This activity was then converted to an approximate composite index of kilocalorie expenditure. The dividing line between low and high expenditure was drawn at 2000 kcals/week. Results showed that the age-adjusted risk of a first heart attack apparently decreased up to the range 2000–2999 kcals/day; thereafter no additional benefit was gained (Fig. 12–4). This effect was consistent across all age decades from 35 to 75 years. Bivariate analyses adjusting for other potential risk factors one at a time continued to show clear benefit for the exercisers (Fig. 12–5). It should be remembered that this information is all self-reported, but, where appropriate, presumably doctor diagnosed. An additional observation from this study is that it was physical activity in adulthood (that is, at study baseline) rather than student athleticism that exerted a strong influence (Table 12–6).

The amount of exercise required for benefit is controversial. Some studies suggest that vigorous exercise is more protective for IHD than moderate exercise (Brand et al, 1979; Morris et al, 1980). Others find that the bulk of the benefit is already achieved by a change from sedentary habits to moderate activity levels (Garcia-Palmieri et al, 1982; Kannel and Sorlie, 1979; Magnus et al, 1979; Paffenbarger et al, 1978). Either way, it is clear that moderate activity levels are relatively easy to achieve and will almost certainly give substantial benefit. Easily implemented suggestions include the following: (a) Take one to two

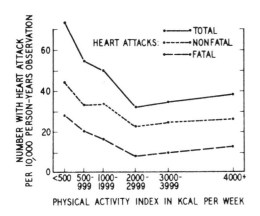

Figure 12–4 Age-adjusted first heart attack rates, by physical activity index in a 6 to 10-year follow-up of Harvard male alumni. From RS Paffenbarger et al: Physical activity as an index of heart attack risk in college alumni. *Amer J Epidemiol* **108**:161, 1978, with permission.

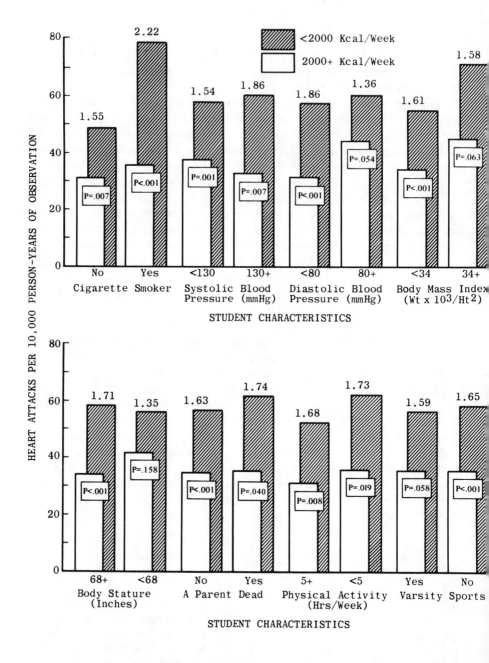

Figure 12–5 Age-adjusted rates and relative risks of first heart attack, by paired combinations of physical activity index and other characteristics of Harvard male alumni in a 6 to 10 year follow-up. From RS Paffenbarger et al: Physical activity as an index of heart attack risk in college alumni. *Amer J Epidemiol* **108**:161, 1978, with permission.

Table 12–6 Age-adjusted first heart attack rates among Harvard male alumni in a 6 to 10-year follow-up, by student and alumni physical activity patterns

Student activity	Alumni physical activity index in kcal/week					
	< 500		500–1999		2000	
	Number[a]	Rate[b]	Number	Rate	Number	Rate
Varsity athlete						
No	92	70.7	183	53.3	98	35.3
Yes	12	92.7	20	45.2	24	35.2

Source: Adapted from RS Paffenbarger et al: Physical activity as an index of heart attack risk in college alumni. *Amer J Epidemiol*, 1978, with permission.

[a] Number with heart attack.

[b] Number with heart attack per 10,000 person-years of observation.

flights of stairs rather than the elevator. (b) Park the car one to two blocks from work. (c) Take a brisk walk during the lunch hour. (d) Develop a regular program exercising at least three times per week for 20 to 60 minutes per occasion. Beneficial forms of exercise include walking, jogging, cycling, swimming. Chapter 21 includes further practical suggestions.

Some consideration of the risks of exercise is appropriate at this point. Generally, the risk of any complication is negligible for moderate intensity exercise such as walking. However exercise such as jogging does have associated hazards. Cardiac complications are rare, but well described (Thompson et al, 1982; Waller and Roberts, 1980). Most sudden deaths occur in persons with clinically silent IHD. Persons over 35 years, at least, should have a preliminary medical examination (see chapter 21). Of greater importance are the orthopedic inuries that are clearly related to mileage run (Koplan et al, 1982). When the weekly mileage was less than 20 miles per week, about 10 percent of persons consulted their doctor for injuries, and 20 to 30 percent reported some injury within one year.

Physical Activity and Cardiovascular Pathology

Several hypotheses have been proposed relating exercise to cardiovascular pathology. We shall consider three of these although more evidence is needed before definitive statements can be made.

The first composite hypothesis is that more active persons have less ischemic myocardial damage, coronary thrombosis, and coronary atheroma. Morris and colleagues (1958) tested this hypothesis in a study of about 3800 autopsies of noncoronary deaths. The state of the myocardium and the coronary arteries was compared with the deceased's last occupation and thus with an estimate of physical activity by occupation. The results showed negative correlations between occupational physical activity and frequency of total occlusion of a coronary artery, large healed infarcts, and ischemic myocardial fibrosis (Fig. 12–6). However, no relationship could be found between occupational activity and indices of severity of atherosclerosis. Others have also reached the latter conclusion (Spain and Bradess, 1960). There is some indication that physically active persons have an increased fibrinolytic response to venous occlusion (Williams RS et al, 1980), and this may be relevant to Morris' observations.

The second hypothesis is that persons who are more active have larger coronary arteries, making obstruction by atheroma or thrombus less likely. There are isolated reports that athletes have rather large coronary arteries, but no consistent picture emerges. Even if it did, the origin could be genetic, allowing superior physical performance rather than vice versa. A study by Rose et al (1967) provides limited information on this question. In 46 autopsies of males with no myocardial scars, the age-adjusted right coronary artery diameter (in areas free of plaque) did not clearly relate to activity by occupation.

The third hypothesis is that active persons with coronary artery disease are more likely to have significant collateral coronary circulation. There is good evidence for such a relationship in certain animals, but very little in humans. The suggestion is that regular exercise in persons with moderate but asymptomatic coronary obstruction may produce mild ischemia and so provoke collateral development. However, there is very little support for this in human studies. Most studies have addressed the effects of exercise training in cardiac patients, and while several beneficial physiological effects have been observed, maximal coronary blood flow is not consistently changed (Ferguson et al, 1978; Sim and Neil, 1974; Verani et al, 1981). No studies of collateral development and physical activity in asymptomatic humans are known to the author.

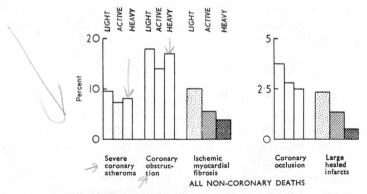

Figure 12–6   The relationship between cardiac pathology at autopsy and antemortem occupational activity. From JN Morris et al: 1958. *Br Med J 2*: 1485, 1958, p. 1485, with permission.

The Effect of Physical Activity on Other Risk Factors

Physical activity probably increases HDL cholesterol and may decrease LDL cholesterol. It is not yet entirely clear whether these are direct causal relationships or whether they could be due to the low body mass indices of physically fit persons. The results of a cross-sectional study comparing HDL cholesterols of runners and control subjects are shown in Table 12–7 (Wood et al, 1976). The runners clearly have higher HDL cholesterols, lower LDL cholesterols, and lower serum triglycerides; but other differences, for example, in obesity and interest in health practices, may exist between runners and controls that could account for this. In a longitudinal study where each subject acted as his own control, before and after an exercise program, Lopez (1974) found significant changes in virtually all lipid fractions by 7 weeks after the exercise started (Table 12–8). There was no significant change in body weight. Although not all longitudinal studies have produced the same results with regard to HDL and LDL cholesterol (Allison et al, 1981), most show an association between increased physical activity and increased HDL cholesterol (or alpha lipoprotein), decreased triglycerides, and decreased LDL cholesterol (or beta lipoprotein).

Table 12–7 Mean plasma lipid and lipoprotein cholesterol concentrations (mg/100 ml) for runners and control subjects

Age group	Triglycerides	Total cholesterol	LDL cholesterol	HDL cholesterol	VLDL cholesterol[a]
35–39					
Runners	71 ± 33^d $(9)^b$	183 ± 23^c	115 ± 19^c	59 ± 10^c	9 ± 7
Controls	120 ± 78 (138)	202 ± 36	135 ± 23 (29)	43 ± 9	24
40–49					
Runners	68 ± 19^c (22)	207 ± 19	133 ± 19	64 ± 11^c	11 ± 41
Controls	151 ± 99 (310)	212 ± 37	145 ± 37 (55)	41 ± 9	30
50–59					
Runners	74 ± 30^c (10)	198 ± 23	116 ± 20	70 ± 19^c	10 ± 12
Controls	152 ± 126 (295)	212 ± 33	136 ± 28 (63)	44 ± 11	30
35–59					
Runners	70 ± 25^c (41)	200 ± 23^c	125 ± 21^d	64 ± 13^c	11 ± 6
Controls	146 ± 108 (743)	210 ± 35	139 ± 31 (147)	43 ± 10	29

Source: PD Wood et al: The distribution of plasma lipoproteins in middle-aged male runners, *Metabolism* **25**: 1249, 1976. Reprinted by permission of Grune & Stratton, Inc., and the author.

Values are means ± SD.

[a] Control group values estimated as triglyceride divided by five.

[b] Figures in parentheses are numbers of subjects included for runners, control group A (triglycerides and total cholesterol), and control group B (lipoprotein cholesterol).

[c] $0.01 < p < 0.05$ for runners versus control subjects.

[d] $0.001 < p < 0.01$ for runners versus control subjects.

[e] $p < 0.001$ for runners versus control subjects.

PREVENTIVE CARDIOLOGY

Table 12–8 Serum lipid changes (mg/100 ml) induced by 7 weeks of exercise in young individuals, $N = 13$

	Before	During[a]		After[b]	
	Mean ± S.D.	Mean ± S.D.	p^c	Mean ± S.D.	P
Cholesterol	169 ± 22	159 ± 22	0.01	162 ± 25	0.03
Triglycerides	110 ± 36	97 ± 36	0.01	83 ± 38	<0.01
β-Cholesterol	104 ± 30	100 ± 25	0.5	86 ± 22	<0.01
β-Lipoprotein	185 ± 57	180 ± 75	0.6	158 ± 39	0.02
Pre-β-Lipoprotein	93 ± 57	75 ± 57	0.01	54 ± 41	<0.01
α-Lipoprotein	286 ± 86	273 ± 72	0.7	332 ± 75	0.01

Source: SA Lopez et al: *Arterosclerosis* **20**:1, 1974, with permission.

[a] Three weeks after initiation of exercise.

[b] Seven weeks after initiation of exercise.

[c] Paired $+/-$ t-test.

One longitudinal study that has been analyzed in detail randomly assigned 81 initially sedentary men to a running program or continued sedentary habits. As expected, differences in fitness and obesity developed. Overall there were no significant changes in HDL cholesterol for either group after 1 year of the study. However, when the analysis was restricted to those exercisers who ran at least 8 miles per week, a significant difference emerged (Wood et al, 1983). An important observation was that persons with initially higher HDL levels were easier to persuade to run, so that nonlongitudinal studies are probably biased (Williams PT et al, 1982). In this study most of the change in HDL could be attributed to weight loss rather than exercise per se (Williams PT et al, 1983). From a clinical perspective, whether it is the exercise itself or the exercise-induced weight loss or both, this will not usually alter recommendations. There is some doubt as to whether the changes in HDL with exercise occur in women (Brownell et al, 1982b).

Many investigators have looked for a relationship between physical activity and blood pressure levels, and this probably does exist (chapter 10). Recently, we accumulated physical fitness and blood pressure data on 218 children at Loma Linda University (Fraser, 1983b). On univariate analysis, both systolic and diastolic blood pressures were lower in children who were fitter than average (Fig. 12–7). A multivariate analysis, adjusting for various anthropometric measures, showed a clear association between fitness and systolic blood pressure in adolescents of both sexes and also in preadolescent boys. The effect was independent of obesity and was such as to predict a difference of 16 mm Hg in systolic blood pressure between very unfit (2.5th percentile) and very fit (97.5th percentile) individuals. This study dealt with fitness, not physical activity, and

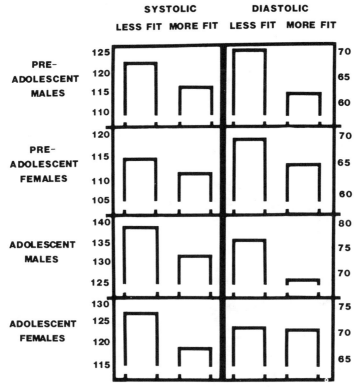

Figure 12–7 The univariate relationship between physical fitness and blood pressure in children. Loma Linda Children's Blood Pressure Study. From GE Fraser et al: Physical fitness and blood pressure in children. *Circulation* **67**:405, 1983, by permission of the American Heart Association, Inc.

an individual's fitness can probably be improved by only about 20 percent. Thus, if this is a dynamic relationship, resting systolic blood pressure could be changed by about 4 mm Hg.

It would not be unexpected to find that increased physical activity is associated with reduced cigarette consumption since the acute and chronic effects of cigarette smoke on the respiratory system do not favor good exercise performance. Results from various studies, however, have been conflicting (Heinzelman et al, 1970; Morgan et al, 1976).

Prevalence of Physical Activity in the United States

Casual observations over the last few years would suggest a decided trend to regular physical activity, such as jogging. Sales of exercise equipment and footwear tend to support this conclusion. Several years ago, exercise habits were

Table 12–9 Reported exercise by Americans in the 1977 Gallup Poll

Stratum	Who Exercises? (%)	Who Jogs? (%)
All	47	11
Men	50	16
Women	45	7
Age		
18–29	60	22
30–49	47	10
50+	38	4
College educated	59	17
High school	47	11
Grade school	30	3
Professional and business	56	13
Clerical and sales	57	16
Manual	45	12

Source: Working Group on Arteriosclerosis of the National Heart, Lung and Blood Institute: 1981b, with permission.

assessed in the Framingham Study population (Dawber, 1980). A scale was used in which a score of 24 was equivalent to sleep. The results suggested that a sizable proportion of the population was barely awake! More recent, but less rigorous data come from the 1977 Gallup Poll (Table 12–9). This suggests that men exercise more than women and that highly educated persons exercise more than others. A recent survey sample of adult Massachusetts residents with a 61.1 percent response rate revealed that 28.3 percent exercised daily and another 29.1 percent two to five times per week. Walking, jogging, and running were most popular (Lambert et al, 1982).

Summary

1. As is true for most complex and frequent activities, physical activity is difficult to measure with precision. The inverse association between exercise and obesity has often hampered interpretation. It is also important to clarify whether a study deals with physical *activity* or physical *fitness*.

2. International comparisons, retrospective, and cross-sectional studies suggest the possibility of a relationship but do not clearly answer the major question of this chapter.

3. The methodologically best studies—prospective with large numbers—strongly suggest that both increased physical activity and physical fitness pre-

dict a reduced risk of IHD. Probably it is relatively recent, rather than remote (e.g., activity in college) physical activity that is important.

4. The relationship between exercise and coronary/cardiac pathology needs more study. There is evidence that physically active persons have less myocardial fibrosis and less likelihood of completely occluded coronary arteries at autopsy. There is little support for reduced severity of coronary atherosclerosis, larger caliber coronary arteries, or increased collateral formation in the more physically active.

5. Persons more physically active have higher serum HDL cholesterol levels, lower levels of triglycerides and LDL cholesterol, and body weight and also probably slightly lower blood pressures.

13

The Relationship Between Alcoholic Beverage Consumption and Risk of Ischemic Heart Disease

The relationship between the consumption of alcohol and the risk of clinical syndromes commonly ascribed to ischemic heart disease has been controversial for decades. Over the last 10 years, many new findings have shown that the relationship is complex. Moreover, it seems quite possible that the effects of alcoholic beverages on the heart may at times mimic the effects of IHD and be ascribed to it, yet in fact be due to other mechanisms.

The epidemiologic data on this question appear conflicting. Approximately equal numbers of studies show a beneficial or detrimental influence of alcohol. A few show no effect (Greig et al, 1980). It is important, however, to specify the effects of alcohol on different "IHD" syndromes (e.g., MI or coronary death) and also to allow for the possibility of a nonlinear relationship between alcohol and IHD events. The apparent conflicts may be resolved by distinguishing between different clinical endpoints and by determining whether alcohol consumption is at the upper or lower end of the range.

Studies Suggesting That Consumption of Alcoholic Beverages Is a Risk Factor for Ischemic Heart Disease

The studies showing a detrimental effect of alcohol all have IHD death as the endpoint and tend to find the relationship at the upper range of alcohol consumption. Several longitudinal studies have related alcohol consumption to an increased incidence of IHD death by comparing the IHD mortality rates in alcoholics and nonalcoholics. Although results have not been unanimous, several of these studies have demonstrated a significant excess of deaths from cardiovascular causes in the alcoholics.

Pell and D'Alonzo (1973) matched Du Pont Company employees who abused alcohol with nonabusers by age, sex, payroll class, and geographic location. They found roughly twice as much cardiovascular mortality in the alcoholics. Schmidt and de Lint (1972) followed 6478 alcoholic men and women who were involved in a treatment program in Toronto for up to 14 years. Again, a highly significant excess mortality from arteriosclerotic and degenerative heart disease as compared to the national age/sex expectation was found in both men and women. It should be pointed out that there is a possibility that persons

Table 13–1   Estimated coefficients of the linear logistic model predicting IHD death in a Swedish longitudinal study

Variable	Nine variables		
	b	s_b	$t = \dfrac{b}{s_b}$
Cholesterol	0.566	0.168	3.4
Smoking	0.503	0.175	2.8
Systolic blood pressure	0.381	0.140	2.7
Dyspnea	0.361	0.140	2.5
Record of intemperance	0.356	0.144	2.5
Physical activity during work	−0.359	−0.173	−2.1
Hematocrit	0.126	0.161	0.8
Triglycerides	−0.055	0.153	−0.4
Place of birth	−0.031	0.173	−0.2
The constant	−3.427	0.224	

Source: L Wilhelmsen et al: Multivariate analysis of risk factors for coronary heart disease. *Circulation* **48**:950, 1973, by permission of the American Heart Association, Inc.

Abbreviations: b = the coefficient estimated by maximum likelihood method; s_b = standard deviation of b.

volunteering for a treatment program may differ from other alcoholics in other IHD risk factors.

Wilhelmsen et al (1973) conducted a longitudinal study in Sweden to find the power of several variables to predict IHD mortality. One variable that had an independent positive association with IHD death was membership in a temperance society for reformed and reforming alcoholics (see the significant logistic coefficient ($t > 1.96$) in Table 13–1). Note the significance, as expected, for the other traditional risk factors. Wilhelmsen et al followed up this study by a population-based, case-control study of young men, using Swedish social registry data. They found that significantly more cases of IHD death than controls had a record of alcoholic problems (Wilhelmsen et al, 1983). A Finnish longitudinal study found that those in the upper social classes who became inebriated or experienced a hangover once weekly had a twofold risk of IHD death over a 12 year follow-up (Poikolainen, 1983). Two Chicago longitudinal studies (Dyer et al, 1977; 1980) showed that heavier drinkers have higher mortality from IHD (also from cancer). After adjustment for the traditional risk factors, this excess risk no longer quite reached the traditional level of statistical significance. In these last studies, the possible effect of alcohol on IHD mortality could not be discerned until the highest consumption category (see Table 13–2). In 1968, Kramer and colleagues studied mortality from cirrhosis of the liver in Baltimore. They found that a surprising proportion of these deaths (51 percent)

Table 13-2 Age-adjusted, 17-year mortality rates by level of alcohol intake—1832 white males age 40–55 from the Chicago Western Electric Company Study, 1957–1975

Average daily consumption	Number of men	All causes		CHD death	
		Number	Rate	Number	Rate
All	1832	296	152	149	79
0–<1	632	96	141	53	80
0	77	13	153	4	49
<1	555	83	139	49	84
1	542	77	134	43	77
2–3	428	66	147	32	73
4–5	152	25	146	9	55
6+	78	32	404	12	155
χ^2 Test of age-adjusted rates		33.10		11.27	
		$P<0.001$		$P<0.05$	
χ^2 Test of rates adjusted for age and cigarettes		20.76		7.99	
		$P<0.001$		$P<0.10$	
χ^2 Test of rates adjusted for all variables[a]		15.35		7.80	
		$P<0.01$		$P<0.10$	

Source: Adapted from AR Dyer et al: *Prev Med* **9**:78, 1980, with permission.

[a] *Adjusting variables:* All causes: age, diastolic blood pressure, cigarettes/day, pulse; CV death: age, diastolic pressure, cigarettes/day, pulse, serum cholesterol; CHD death: age, diastolic blood pressure, cigarettes/day, serum cholesterol; cancer death: age, systolic blood pressure, cigarettes/day; other death: age, diastolic blood pressure, cigarettes/day, serum cholesterol.

were sudden and unexpected. It is not clear whether these sudden deaths were attributable to the cirrhosis or whether alcohol consumption had also affected other body organs, including the myocardium.

A study from Auckland, New Zealand, (Fraser and Upsdell, 1981) found that among cases of acute IHD events, those who suffered sudden death consumed significantly more alcohol than cases of myocardial infarction (194 compared to 118 grams of alcohol per week). This implies that when a coronary event occurs in a high alcohol consumer, it is more likely to be a sudden death than a myocardial infarction (Table 13.3). The data also showed that patients suffering acute myocardial infarction who drank heavily were more likely to die suddenly with that infarction.

Evidence Suggesting That Alcohol Beverage Consumption Is Protective Against Ischemic Heart Disease

The epidemiologic studies supporting a protective hypothesis have largely used myocardial infarction or the combination of myocardial infarction and IHD

Table 13–3 Observed proportion of IHD events[a] as sudden deaths, for different values of alcohol consumption

	Alcohol (grams per week)				
	0–100	101–300	301–500	501–750	>750
Number of cases	212	59	20	11	9
Percent as sudden deaths[a]	34	40	47	70	93

Source: GE Fraser and M Upsdell: Alcohol and other discriminants between cases of sudden death and myocardial infarction. *Amer J Epidemiol* **114**:462, 1981, with permission.

[a] Observed proportions, adjusted for the effects of other significant covariates, using a logistic discriminant analysis. Events include all sudden deaths and myocardial infarctions (fatal or not).

death as an endpoint. The supportive evidence was often found within the low to moderate alcohol consumption range.

In the Honolulu Heart Study (Yano et al, 1977), there is a clear and statistically significant gradient between alcohol consumption and rates of IHD death and myocardial infarction combined (Fig. 13–1). No such evidence was found for the combination of angina pectoris and coronary insufficiency. The alcohol consumption reported even at the highest level was relatively low.

In a population-based study from Yugoslavia (Kozarevic et al, 1980), a statistically significant trend was found between alcohol consumption and the rates of nonfatal MI and IHD death combined. The alcohol data were rescored combining recent intoxication and daily consumption. There was then no significant relationship with total IHD, but a significant negative relationship was found with nonsudden IHD death (Kozarevic et al, 1983).

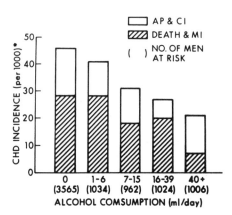

Figure 13–1 Six-year incidence of coronary heart disease according to alcohol consumption. The Honolulu Heart Study. From K Yano et al: Reprinted, by permission of the *N Eng J Med* **297**: 405, 1977.

The Framingham Study also showed a significant negative relationship between alcohol consumption and all IHD (Gordon and Kannel, 1983). As the authors point out, the relationship was significant for only some of the smoking and sex subgroups analyzed. The Puerto Rico Heart Health Program measured alcohol by 24 hour recall in 9150 Puerto Rican males aged 35–79 years and followed them for 12 years (Kittner et al, 1983). In a simple analysis comparing drinkers to nondrinkers, there were apparent overall advantages for drinkers for angina pectoris, nonfatal myocardial infarction and nonsudden IHD death. However, inclusion of more detailed alcohol consumption values suggested "J-shaped" relationships between alcohol and incidence of these same endpoints, indicating a slight decline in risk with low intake as compared to teetotalers, but a striking increase in risk with heavy consumption. Presumably the results for the simpler comparison of drinkers and nondrinkers can be explained by most of the drinking population having intakes close to the lowest portion of the "J." There was no relationship found with sudden death (defined as death within 1 hour of onset of symptoms). Further analyses found a lack of consistency of results by age and social class subgroups.

A case-control study was reported in 1978 (Hennekens et al, 1978) showing an apparently protective effect of alcohol consumption over the preceding 3 months before sudden death. Problems include the possibility that patients may reduce intake in response to prodromal symptoms during this 3 months. Also the participant response rate was only 56 percent, raising the possibility of biases. In addition, there was an unexpected dose-response effect with the protection apparently being only in the lower consumption ranges. The Kaiser-Permanente Study (Klatsky et al, 1979) was another case control study which found a significant negative association between alcohol consumption and myocardial infarction (see Table 13–4).

In addition, ecological evidence has recently been presented in favor of the

Table 13–4 Comparison of drinking habits of myocardial infarction (MI) patients and risk-factor-matched controls[a]

Drinking habit	MI patients (%)	Risk controls (%)
No alcohol	32.4[b]	24.7[b]
≤2 Drinks daily	48.1	53.5
3–5 Drinks daily	10.0	10.3
6+ Drinks daily	2.6[c]	5.4[c]

Source: AL Klatsky et al: Alcohol use, myocardial infarction, sudden cardiac death, and hypertension. *Alcoholism: Clin Exp* **3**:33, 1979, by permission.

[a] Among the 405 matched pairs, of which both members supplied adequate alcohol habit information.

[b] $p < 0.01$.

[c] $p < 0.05$.

protective hypothesis. In ecological studies, each data point represents a whole community or even country. Such evidence is very liable to confounding by other factors and cannot provide strong support, only rather untrustworthy clues. St. Leger et al (1979) found that national alcohol consumption data from several European countries revealed a statistical association between high alcohol consumption and low IHD rates on a whole-country basis. As others pointed out later, however, milk, milk products, garlic, and total sugar consumption also correlate with IHD. Which, if any, of these variables represent causal influences is open to debate. LaPorte et al (1980) reported that national beer consumption in the United States correlated inversely with the age-adjusted IHD death rates over time. The problem is that a lag period is presumably required between the alcohol consumption and the clinical manifestation. The author chose 5 years, but, depending on how long the period is defined, the correlation coefficient can fluctuate widely. Also, the people responsible for most of the alcohol consumption (young and middle-aged) are not the people experiencing most of the IHD events (older persons).

Little is known of these relationships for women. The Framingham Study found a significant negative association for the endpoint of all IHD events (Gordon and Kannel, 1983). Petitti, in a longitudinal study, divided women as drinkers and nondrinkers and found evidence of lower rates in drinkers (Petitti et al, 1979).

Before trying to resolve this conflict in the epidemiological evidence, I will review the effect of alcoholic beverage consumption on the traditional risk factors, pathology, and physiology.

Mechanisms Whereby Alcoholic Beverage Consumption May Affect Risk of Ischemic Heart Disease

The relationship between alcoholic beverage consumption and high-density lipoprotein particles is well established. In cross-sectional epidemiologic investigations of free-living people, a positive relationship between alcohol consumption and HDL cholesterol has been repeatedly demonstrated (Castelli et al, 1977). Experiments using small numbers of subjects have also been conducted. The advantage of these is that many potentially confounding variables can be controlled. Figure 13–2 shows the results from one such study (Belfrage, 1973) of eight subjects who consumed 441 grams of alcohol per week as light beer. During the experimental period alpha-lipoprotein cholesterol rose significantly. In a feeding experiment controlled or adjusted for the effects of diet, body weight, exercise, and cigarette smoking, we found that alcoholic beverage consumption raised the levels of apolipoprotein A1 (Fraser et al, 1983a). Suggestive evidence was also found for an effect of apolipoprotein A2. Thus, alcoholic beverages seem also to affect the protein portion of the HDL particle. Although alcohol is the prime contender for causing these effects, other substances contained in alcoholic beverages could yet turn out to be responsible.

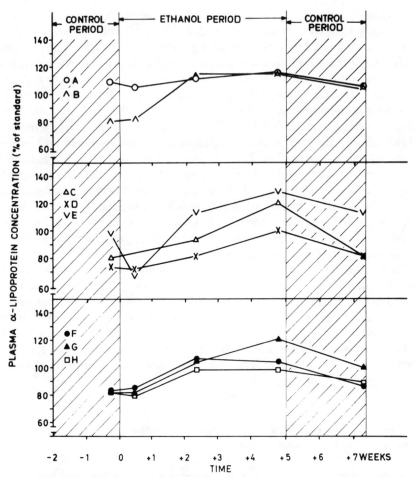

Figure 13–2 Plasma alpha-lipoprotein levels in fasting plasma during the control and ethanol periods. The values are arbitrarily expressed in percent of the normal mean for adult men (range 65–135%). From P Belfrage et al: *Acta Med Scand*, suppl: 552, 1973, with permission.

Alcohol induced thrombocytopenia is well described, and it has been shown that platelet function is acutely impaired by alcohol ingestion (Haut and Cowan, 1974). An association of increased fibrinolytic activity with increased alcohol consumption (Meade et al, 1979), along with the platelet effects, could be additional mechanisms of any postulated protective effect of alcohol.

There is clear evidence of an association between blood pressure levels and the consumption of alcoholic beverages (Klatsky et al, 1977; Mathews, 1976). Heavy consumers of alcohol have higher blood pressures than other age/sex/race matched individuals (see chapter 10).

Alcohol-induced myocardial damage, which frequently remains subclinical, is well known. This is not the relatively rare alcoholic cardiomyopathy known to clinicians but rather a more common phenomenon. Chronic excessive alcohol consumption is known to induce a variety of abnormalities in both skeletal and cardiac muscle. These include dilatation of the sarcoplasmic reticulum, abnormal mitochondria, interstitial fibrosis, and accumulation of an abnormal glycoprotein in the myocardial interstitium (Hognestad and Teisberg, 1973; Portal, 1981; Regan et al, 1975; 1981; Rubin et al, 1976; Steinberg and Hayden, 1981). Heavy drinkers often have cardiac hypertrophy, as seen by echocardiography (Askanas et al, 1980) and at autopsy (Steinberg et al, 1981). These effects on the myocardium appear to result in a rather subtle but definite deterioration in cardiac function in alcoholics, even in the majority of alcoholics with no *manifest* cardiac disease. This deterioration has been documented by systolic time intervals (Levi et al, 1977; Spodick et al, 1972) and also by in invasive measurement of cardiac contractility. Abnormal rises in left ventricular end diastolic pressures in response to increased afterload were demonstrated (Regan et al, 1969). Animal work shows similar results (Thomas et al, 1980). Furthermore, there is evidence that high alcohol consumption can be associated with myocardial infarction in the presence of normal coronary arteries (Regan et al, 1975; Moreyra et al, 1982). Limited information from humans and animals raises the possibility of some association between alcohol consumption and coronary artery spasm (Fernandez et al, 1973; Friedman, 1981; Sato et al, 1981; Webb and Degerli, 1965).

That alcoholics are subject to excessive cardiac arrhythmias is without question, and it is perhaps to be expected given the pathologic changes descibed earlier. It has been shown that alcohol consumption delays atrioventricular conduction and allows easier stimulation of atrial and ventricular tachycardias during electrophysiologic studies (Greenspon and Schaal, 1983). The clinical significance of this is unknown. Most reports have emphasized that the majority of arrhythmias in alcoholics are supraventricular and generally not life-threatening. However, ventricular arrhythmias apparently induced by alcohol have been described (Ettinger et al, 1978; Singer and Lundberg, 1972). They may not account for the majority of alcohol associated cardiac deaths as in the Auckland Suburbs Coronary Study; we found that high alcohol consumers who died suddenly (within 24 hours of the onset of acute symptoms) actually died significantly later than low alcohol consumers within this 24-hour period (Fraser and Upsdell, 1981). This would not be expected if these deaths were due to primary arrhythmias.

The Relationship Between Alcoholic Beverage Consumption and Coronary Atheroma

Many have attempted to relate alcohol consumption to coronary artery pathology by angiography or by autopsy. Although it is commonly held that high alcohol consumers are relatively protected from coronary atherosclerosis, the evidence does not clearly support this viewpoint. In several autopsy series cirrhotics have had less myocardial infarction and coronary atheroma than noncirrhotic controls (Hall et al, 1953; Howell and Manion, 1960). In an autopsy study of both cirrhotic and noncirrhotic high alcohol consumers, Hirst et al (1965) found decreased atherosclerosis in the cirrhotic but not in the noncirrhotic group. There are several problems inherent in the interpretation of such studies. Persons dying of cirrhosis have often been chronically undernourished and many may also have been chronically ill. Metabolic changes associated with chronic disease alone have been associated with reduced coronary atheroma (Wilens, 1947a). Wilens (1947b) demonstrated that apparent protection explained by several older studies could be well explained by differences in age and other risk factors between the alcohol abusers and others, not necessarily by the alcohol itself.

Control groups based on all autopsies will be heavily biased towards IHD, as a high proportion of deaths are attributable to this disorder. A more appropriate control group would consist of deaths due to accidental or violent causes, as often used in the International Atherosclerosis Project (see chapter 3). A recent autopsy study that paid close attention to methodology compared coronary pathology between four autopsy groups chosen according to a retrospective assessment of alcohol consumption (Lifsic, 1976). No clear differences were seen between groups, except that coronary calcification was less common in high consumers. Another autopsy study showed that although fatty streaks were less common in alcoholics, the amount of plaques and stenotic coronary lesions was similar to that in controls (Rissanen et al, 1974).

Autopsy results of deaths in the follow-up period of the Puerto Rico Health Program were used to associate baseline alcohol consumption with coronary atheroma, but no significant relationship emerged (Sorlie et al, 1981). However, only 14 percent of all deaths had acceptable autopsies. A similar study of deaths from the Honolulu Heart Study population found that myocardial infarction at autopsy was associated with lower baseline alcohol consumption, but there was no relationship with coronary atheroma (Rhoads et al, 1978). Coronary arteries were examined in 28 percent of deaths in this study.

Barboriak et al (1977) studied 909 male, nondiabetic patients who were referred for coronary angiography. Those consuming no alcohol or less than 180 mls absolute alcohol per week had higher occlusion scores at angiography than those consuming higher quantities of alcohol. Barboriak (1977) suggested that this finding might be interpreted as indicating that high alcohol consumers develop chest pain and/or myocardial infarction at a lesser severity of coronary obstruction than lower alcohol consumers; as a prerequisite for entry to the study was chest pain or a previous myocardial infarction.

An Attempt to Explain the Apparently Contradictory Epidemiologic Evidence

Several points should be stressed. First, chronic alcohol use has a toxic effect on the myocardium resulting in microscopic damage and decreased ventricular performance. This is probably unrelated to coronary disease, and it probably becomes important only at relatively high intakes. These myocardial changes, as well as the frequent cardiac hypertrophy in heavy alcohol consumers, probably promote cardiac death.

Secondly, chronic alcohol consumption at low to moderate levels may reduce the incidence of myocardial infarction and nonsudden cardiac death. This could be a consequence of reduced coronary atheroma although the evidence is not very convincing. The existence of a possible mechanism—increase in HDL levels—gives this notion some credibility. Changes in platelet function and fibrinolysis may also be important.

Thirdly, there is a possibility that the apparent increased risk in teetotalers may be partially artifactual. Several studies have divided teetotalers into lifelong teetotalers and former alcohol consumers. Three found that the *former* consumers had markedly higher mortality whereas two others found no differences (Chafetz, 1974; Day, 1979; Dyer et al, 1977; Klatsky et al, 1981; Yano et al, 1977). This raises the possibility that the apparent disadvantage of the teetotal status could be due to the mortality experience of former drinkers. More evidence is needed.

Fourthly, IHD is not a homogeneous disorder. Although certain basic similarities probably underlie all of the syndromes, alcohol may be important for some syndromes but not others.

Fifthly, it is possible that the effects of alcohol directly on the myocardium may interact with ischemic pathophysiology already present rather than being the only causal factor.

The negative relationship between alcohol and IHD at lower to moderate intakes involves different syndromes of IHD in different studies and sometimes showed quite different trends with different subgroups of the population. As also stated by others (Ashley, 1982; Gordon and Kannel, 1983; Kittner et al, 1983), this negative relationship at low and moderate intakes, cannot yet be considered proved as causal. Potential problems include different methods of measuring alcohol consumption, the possibility that binge drinking is important, and the inability to exclude confounding by social and psychosocial correlates of alcohol intake.

There seems little doubt that very heavy drinking is associated with an excess of cardiac deaths. The evidence is quite consistent in studies containing substantial numbers of participants consuming sufficient alcohol. Moreover, plausible mechanisms exist. While some of these deaths may be arrhythmic, another possibility is as follows. Alcohol consumption is often associated with an increased frequency of elevated coronary risk factors such as cigarette smoking and hypertension. As hypercholesterolemia is present in at least 50 percent of many Western populations, this will also be a frequent association on a chance basis. Thus, it would not be unexpected to find a modest frequency of myocardial infarction in heavy alcohol consumers. The acute reduction in pumping capacity due to a fresh myocardial infarction, aggravated by the preexistent reduced myocardial functional reserve ascribed to the chronic effects of heavy alcohol consumption, may result in a greatly increased fatality of such acute infarctions.

Thus, advising patients to drink a little alcohol for their heart either for primary or secondary prevention cannot be clearly supported by the evidence at present. Alcohol has well documented detrimental social and physical effects apart from its controversial effects on IHD. The effects of alcohol on traditional IHD risk factors show some apparently beneficial and other detrimental influences. The epidemiologic evidence is complicated; also there is no clear evidence of pathologic benefit—perhaps the opposite. A randomized trial of alcohol dosing would probably be the only way to assess the ratio of long-term risks to benefits. Until this type of information is available, there are too many unanswered questions to make any positive public health recommendations.

Summary

1. Epidemiologic studies are about equally split between those showing benefit or detrimental effect of alcohol on risk of IHD.

2. Those suggesting alcohol to be harmful tend to show this at moderate-to-high doses and to have IHD death as the endpoint.

3. The evidence that alcohol is protective for IHD at low doses is still controversial with the evidence being inconsistent.

4. Alcohol modestly raises HDL cholesterol but also is associated with hypertension.

5. Alcohol-induced myocardial damage is well described at moderate-to-high doses and may occur in the absence of symptoms or signs of heart disease.

6. There is no good evidence that alcohol consumption is associated with less atherosclerosis of the coronary arteries despite long held views to the contrary.

cxcessive Alcohol → arrhythmia

14

The Epidemiology of Sudden Death

Sudden death is a major clinical and public health problem. It is the first indication of ischemic heart disease in 25 percent of all persons who develop that condition and accounts for about 50 percent of all IHD deaths. Doctors in hospital practice are never exposed to 90 percent of the cases, and even in office practice the physician's role usually amounts to signing the death certificate. Investigating the circumstances of death, even prodromal symptoms, is often hampered by a lack of data. Most information must be collected from the dead person's spouse, friends, and doctor.

The definition of sudden death is also a problem, affecting the interpretation and comparability of results from different studies (Goldstein, 1982). One definition that is fairly representative is given in Chapter 2, but uncertainties remain. What time lapse between onset of symptoms and death is equated with "sudden"? Different studies use criteria of death within 1 hour, 6 hours, or 24 hours of the onset of symptomatic change. The next problem is what constitutes a meaningful symptomatic change from which to measure the time lapse. In practice this is usually quite clear, but on rare occasions it is not (e.g., when there is a "stuttering" onset), There is no simple answer. No standardized definitions are available, and probably the most important need is for criteria to be clearly documented and applied within a particular study. Should sudden death include patients who die after a slow deterioration, perhaps from chronic heart failure? After all, death is "sudden" (usually instantaneous) for most. It is necessary to exclude noncardiac sudden deaths, such as massive pulmonary emboli and ruptured aortic aneurysm and also to decide how to handle cardiac sudden deaths that may not be attributable to ischemic heart disease.

The Descriptive Epidemiology of Sudden Death

Rates of sudden death are available from several locations and appear to be remarkably similar in such sites as Edinburgh, Scotland (Armstrong et al, 1972), Tecumseh, Michigan (Chiang et al, 1970), Nashville, Tennessee (Hagstrom et al, 1971), Helsinki, Finland (Romo, 1972), and Auckland, New Zealand (Fraser, 1978b). Preliminary indications are that much of the decline in IHD mortality over recent years is a decline in rates of sudden death. Folstrom et al (1981)

195

Table 14–1   Socioeconomic class and sudden death[a]

	Socioeconomic class[b]		
	I	II	III
Number of cases	48	64	64
(Expected number)	(51.7)	(75.6)	(48.7)

Source: From GE Fraser, 1978b, with permission.

[a] $\chi_2^2 = 6.85$ ($P < 0.05$) Calculated according to the null hypothesis of no differences across socioeconomic class.
[b] Social class was defined according to area of residence, based on a previous factorial analysis.

found that the decline in Minnesota was largely in "out of hospital deaths." Most of these were undoubtedly sudden deaths. In the Chicago Peoples' Gas Company Study population, the marked decline in mortality occurred in the rate of sudden death, particularly where it was the first evidence of IHD rather than a secondary event (Anastasiou-Nana et al, 1982). Beaglehole and colleagues (1984) repeated the study of ischemic heart disease I conducted seven years earlier in Auckland, New Zealand. We found virtually no change in the attack rate for myocardial infarction, but there was a significant 16 percent decline in the rate of sudden death.

The relationship of the sudden death rate to age is similar to that for myocardial infarction, changing from 1.0 to 2.0 to 5.8 per thousand population per year in the fourth, fifth, and sixth decades of life (both sexes combined) in Tecumseh, Michigan. The average age tends to be two to three years older than for myocardial infarction and the usual 3:1 or 4:1 ratio between males and females is also seen (Armstrong et al, 1972; Chiang et al, 1970; Fraser, 1978a; Fraser, 1978b; Hagstrom et al, 1971; Romo, 1972). As with total IHD mortality, an excess of sudden deaths in the lower socioeconomic classes has often been found (Fraser, 1978b; Romo, 1972). Table 14–1 shows the relevant data from New Zealand.

The place of the fatal event shows remarkable consistency between different studies (Armstrong et al, 1972; Fraser, 1978b; Simon et al, 1973). In New Zealand these were largely "out-of-hospital" deaths; 73 percent died at home, 6 percent at work, and only 9 percent in hospital and 12 percent elsewhere. There is a seasonal variation in IHD deaths, with a significant excess in the cooler half of the year (Dunnigan and Harland, 1970; Fraser, 1978a; Rose, 1966). In New Zealand, 59 percent of the sudden deaths occurred in the cooler six months ($p \sim 0.005$). The reasons for this excess are not well understood but may include coronary artery spasm in cooler weather (Mudge et al, 1976), and seasonal increases in blood pressure (Rose, 1966) and serum cholesterol (Warnick and Albers, 1976).

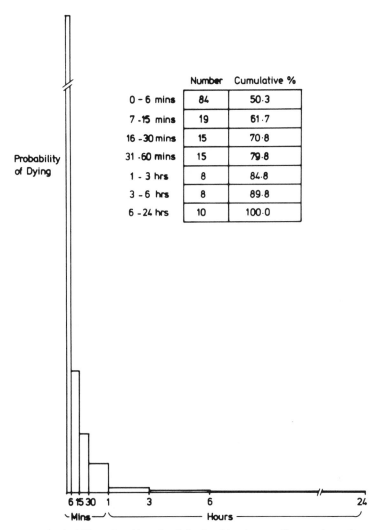

	Number	Cumulative %
0 - 6 mins	84	50·3
7 -15 mins	19	61·7
16 -30 mins	15	70·8
31 -60 mins	15	79·8
1 - 3 hrs	8	84·8
3 - 6 hrs	8	89·8
6 -24 hrs	10	100·0

Figure 14–1   Probability of sudden death in Auckland according to time after onset of symptoms. From GE Fraser, 1978b, with permission.

The Medical Care Problem

The difficulty of the therapeutic approach to sudden death is illustrated in Figure 14–1, which shows a pattern typical of many studies (Armstrong et al, 1972; Kuller et al, 1972; McNeilly and Pemberton, 1968; Simon et al, 1973). Fifty percent of sudden deaths in the 24 hours after onset occurred within 6 minutes, and 71 percent, within 30 minutes. The majority occurred before any medical aid could be summoned, let alone arrive. Indeed 30 to 40 percent of sud-

Table 14–2   Comparison of sudden death and living controls by history of symptoms in preceding 2 weeks and history of heart disease[a]

Race and sex	History of heart disease		n	Symptoms (number of people)			
				Chest pain	SOB[b]	Palpita- tions	Fatigue
White males	Yes	Case	119	40	66	13	79
		Control	119	19	22	8	20
	No	Case	83	22	23	5	35
		Control	83	11	16	5	13
White females	Yes	Case	24	7	14	8	12
		Control	24	7	8	8	8
	No	Case	39	10	15	3	19
		Control	39	8	18	10	15

Source: From LH Kuller, 1978, with permission.

[a] History of heart disease in case only.

[b] Shortness of breath.

den deaths are unwitnessed during the first critical five minutes after the cardiac arrest (Fraser, 1978b; Simon et al, 1973). In Auckland, of those who survived till the arrival of medical aid, two thirds died before hospitalization. This dramatically underlines the obstacles to treatment after the event and highlights the need for a preventive approach. As most people have not used appropriate preventive measures during most of their lives, coronary disease is usually well advanced by middle age. When considering prevention of sudden death in such a population, it would be important to identify those persons for whom sudden death is a probability. If this could be done, specific monitoring and preventive steps could be undertaken. Different studies indicate that about two-thirds of sudden death victims have warning symptoms of some kind in the preceding 30 days (Alonzo et al, 1975; Fraser, 1978b; Kuller et al, 1972; Kuller, 1978). Unfortunately, many of these are very nonspecific, such as lethargy or breathlessness, and are frequently ignored by patients or ascribed to "flu or overwork." Kuller (1978) compared the frequency of some of these prodromal symptoms in sudden death victims to that in healthy controls and found that they were not uncommon in the latter (Table 14–2). Think what a nightmare it would be trying to monitor everyone in the population who complained of fatigue!

The Pathology and Pathophysiology of Sudden Death

About 50 percent of deaths ascribed to ischemic heart disease are sudden, as stated earlier, but about 50 percent of sudden cardiac deaths occur in persons with no previous diagnosis of ischemic heart disease. What is the relationship of sudden death to the pathology usually associated with ischemic heart disease? Several investigators have described the coronary artery pathology of sudden death victims (Reichenbach et al, 1977; Roberts and Jones, 1979). Roberts et al compared 31 sudden death cases to matched control autopsies. All the sudden death victims had significant obstructions (>75 percent narrowing of cross-sectional area) of at least one coronary artery. In two thirds of the cases, narrowings involved all three main coronary arteries. The control subjects showed much less pathology. This is a typical finding demonstrating that severe coronary artery disease is almost invariably present when sudden death occurs. However, the percentage of cases with a fresh identifiable infarction at autopsy or a fresh coronary artery lesion, such as thrombosis or a ruptured plaque, is much more variable from study to study (Baba et al, 1975; Fraser, 1978b; Kuller et al, 1973; Liberthson et al, 1974; Lie and Titus, 1975; Spain and Bradess, 1970). In the New Zealand study (Fraser, 1978b) only 26 percent of cases had a fresh identifiable infarction at autopsy, and only 29 percent had a fresh coronary artery lesion. However, 73 percent of the cases showed old myocardial scarring (Table 14–3). The high prevalence of myocardial scars has been well documented by others (Bashe et al, 1975; Spikerman et al, 1962). These pathological findings are at some variance with those in fatal myocardial infarction, where a much higher proportion will show acute coronary artery lesions (Buja and Willerson, 1981; Horie et al, 1978). These and other findings led Baroldi et al (1979) to question whether acute infarction always precedes sudden death. Further clinical evidence (see below) has made it clear that indeed this is not always the pathogenic sequence.

The frequency of old myocardial infarction is striking and is implied by the fact that many sudden death victims have a history of IHD symptoms. In addition, a pattern of fine, focal myocardial fibrosis is commonly described. Baroldi (1975) found that the only *acute* myocardial lesion in 67 percent of sudden deaths was what he called *coagulative myocytolysis*. This appeared to be the result of highly focal damage to myofibrils or small numbers of myocardial cells, which often heal to form discrete scars. There is some evidence that this lesion is

Table 14–3 Autopsy results of 98 sudden deaths[a]

	MMI and no ACAL	No MMI and ACAL	MMI and ACAL	LVH	Myocardial fibrosis (fine discrete lesions and/or old MI)
Number of cases	12	16	12	40	72
Percentage of total	13	16	13	41	73

Source: From GE Fraser, 1978b, with permission.

[a] Abbreviations: MMI, macroscopic myocardial infarction; ACAL, acute coronary artery lesions; LVH, left ventricular hypertrophy.

identical to that produced by catecholamine excess, and Baroldi speculated that such an excess might be present and could even provoke sudden death in some cases. Another possible precipitating mechanism is microthrombi or micro-emboli to small vessels of the coronary circulation. This could produce patho-physiological conditions for lethal arrhythmias. Frink et al (1978) found evidence of nonobstructive thrombi along the walls of the coronary arteries of all six sudden death cases they investigated. They also found distal micro-thrombi, perhaps of embolic origin from the large lesions, in four of the six hearts. Finally, disturbances of the sympathetic nervous system arising from acute stress can apparently alter the ventricular fibrillation threshold (see Chapter 11) and might play a role in some sudden deaths. Thus, sudden death victims usually have extensive coronary atheroma—myocardiums previously damaged either by an old infarction or a fine fibrotic process.

The terminal electrical event admits several possibilities, including ventricular fibrillation, asystole, ineffective ventricular tachycardia, and bradyarrhythmia. Cardiac rupture or severe pump failure during sinus rhythm may also occur. Nevertheless, it is clear that ventricular fibrillation is by far the most common cause (Liberthson et al, 1974; Cobb et al, 1980a). Liberthson and colleagues found that 72 percent of the cases encountered by a rapid mobile coronary care unit were in ventricular fibrillation when the ambulance arrived.

Out-of-Hospital Resuscitation for Cardiac Arrest

Since the advent of mobile coronary care units, several studies of resuscitated "would-be sudden deaths" have demonstrated that in only 19–44 percent of cases is there an evolution of the typical ECG pattern of a transmural myocardial infarction during their subsequent hospital stay (Cobb et al, 1980a; S Goldstein et al, 1981; Liberthson et al, 1974; CR Webb et al, 1981). Another 30–40 percent show cardiac enzyme elevations without new Q waves on the electrocardiogram, though often in association with ST–T wave changes. Although these latter changes may relate to resuscitation efforts, it is possible that some also represent an acute ischemic etiology for the cardiac arrest. Figures may be different for the 40 percent who could not be resuscitated. The results from Liberthson's group are shown in Table 14–4 where infarction was diagnosed by new Q waves and ischemia by ST–T wave changes on the ECG.

A proportion of sudden deaths result from ventricular fibrillation that is *not* secondary to an acute myocardial infarction but appears to be the result of an electrically unstable myocardium. This is reinforced by the observation that patients resuscitated from such *primary* ventricular fibrillation are at increased risk of subsequent sudden death: 22 percent in the first year compared to 2 percent in those whose initial episode of ventricular fibrillation is associated with a transmural myocardial infarction (Cobb et al, 1980b).

The most extensive reports of "out-of-hospital resuscitation" come from Seattle (Cobb et al, 1980a,b). About 60 percent of persons found in ventricular

Table 14-4 Characterization of defibrillated survivors of out-of-hospital cardiac arrest

	Patients (%)	Patients (%)
Acute myocardial infarction	31 (39%)	
Anterior wall		16 (52%)
Anterior wall and inferior wall		4 (13%)
Inferior wall		11 (35%)
Ischemia without infarction	27 (34%)	
Anterior wall		19 (70%)
Anterior and inferior wall		5 (19%)
Inferior wall		3 (11%)
No acute ECG change	15 (19%)	
Complete left bundle branch block[a]	7 (8%)	

Source: From RR Liberthson et al: Pathophysiologic observations in prehospital ventricular fibrillation and sudden cardiac death. *Circulation* **49**:790, 1974, by permission of the American Heart Association, Inc.

[a] Possibly masking an acute myocardial change.

fibrillation are resuscitated and about 30 percent live long enough to be discharged from hospital, representing considerable improvement since the program was begun (Fig. 14–2). Patients discharged home following a successful resuscitation had a 26 percent mortality in the first year, and 36 percent over 2 years. Of these deaths, 75 percent were "recurrent sudden deaths." Several patients have had three or four such episodes (Cobb et al, 1980b; Schaffer and

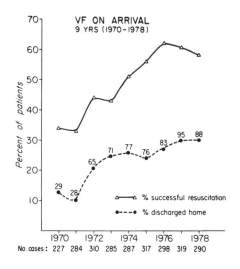

Figure 14–2 Outcomes in patients found in ventricular fibrillation (VF) outside the hospital during 9 years' experience. From LA Cobb et al: Sudden cardiac death. I. *Mod Concepts Cardiovasc Dis* **49**:31, 1980a, by permission of the American Heart Association, Inc.

Table 14–5 Percentage of IHD sudden deaths with prior history of heart disease by race and sex and comparison with Baltimore population sample

	Male	Female
White		
Sudden death	55	46
Population sample	11	6
Black		
Sudden death	45	71
Population sample	10	11

Source: Adapted from L Kuller et al: Epidemiology of sudden death. *Arch Intern Med* **129**:714, 1972. Copyright 1972, American Medical Association. Reprinted by permission.

Cobb, 1975). About 40 percent of survivors have some neurologic deficit (Cobb et al, 1975; Liberthson et al, 1976). Thus, after 1 year only 23 percent of those originally found in ventricular fibrillation survive, many with some neurologic deficit. The 30–40 percent of sudden deaths unwitnessed within the first few minutes at present are not salvageable. Despite these problems, there is much interest in the use of such mobile coronary care units, and techniques continue to improve (Eisenberg et al, 1979a, 1982; Pozen, 1979; Siltanen et al, 1979). The group at very high risk for further cardiac arrest are those with no evidence of infarction with the first arrest. Electrophysiologic testing may provide a guide to drug therapy in reducing their subsequent risk.

Risk Factors for Sudden Death

Most studies of antecedent characteristics predicting sudden death have included all cases of sudden cardiac death as valid end points, disregarding the fact that about 50 percent of these carried a previous diagnosis of heart disease (Table 14–5). As a result, it would seem likely that there would be some considerable overlap between predictors of sudden death and predictors of mortality for persons with established ischemic heart disease (chapter 18). Strictly speaking, sudden deaths with a previous history of IHD should not be included in a study of disease incidence, as the antecedent disease may result in changes in health habits and risk factors.

It is not surprising that electrocardiographic abnormalities predict sudden death in view of pathologic evidence of previous myocardial damage. The Tecumseh Study indicated that certain ECG abnormalities increased sudden-death risk by more than 100-fold as compared to persons with a normal electrocardiogram (Table 14–6). Although the data are not adjusted for age and

Table 14–6   Relationship of selected antecedent ECG abnormalities to incidence of sudden death in the Tecumseh population (age 30 or older)

ECG findings	Number of sudden deaths		Number observed in total population		Six-year incidence of sudden death per 1000 population
Bilateral BBB[b] syndrome	3	(68.6)[a]	4	(69.3)	750
Left BBB	5	(59.6)	18	(63.2)	277
Old myocardial infarction	5	(62.6)	26	(60.5)	192
Ventricular premature beats	10	(65.1)	165	(57.6)	61
Left ventricular hypertrophy	6	(74.1)	124	(58.1)	48
First degree A–V block	3	(57.6)	100	(53.4)	30
Normal ECG (no codable items)	7	(49.8)	2700	(45.3)	2.6

Source: Adapted from BN Chiang et al: Predisposing factors in sudden cardiac death in Tecumseh, Michigan. *Circulation* **41**:31, 1970, by permission of the American Heart Association, Inc.

[a] Mean age in years of the group.

[b] Bundle branch block.

although persons with ECG abnormalities tended to be older than those with normal ECGs, this could not account for the very large relative risks of sudden death found. One of those variables, premature ventricular contractions, predicts overall cardiac death (chapter 18) as well as sudden cardiac death (Chiang et al, 1969; Rengo et al, 1979).

The Framingham Study has reported relationships between risk factors and separate syndromes of IHD, including sudden death within 1 hour of onset of symptoms. A problem is that such subdivisions result often in quite small numbers of cases, making statistical significance difficult to achieve. This is particularly so for females. Despite this, results from the 18-year follow-up of this study show that elevated blood pressure, serum cholesterol, and cigarette smoking are all associated with increased rates of sudden death in men. Non-significant trends are similar in women, but numbers of cases are very small (Tables 14–7 to 14–9). A multivariate analysis showed these relationships in the men to be statistically significant independent of each other (Kannel and Gordon, 1974). Results from a 26-year follow-up in Framingham have recently been published (Schatzkin et al, 1984) and essentially confirm the older findings with somewhat larger numbers of cases being available. These analyses from Framingham are for true incident cases of sudden death who did not have previous indication of IHD. Similar findings have been reported from a longitudinal study in North Karelia, Finland (Salonen, 1982c). This correspondence of risk factors between sudden death and all IHD is further evidence that obstructive coronary artery lesions are an important part of the causal network for sudden death.

Table 14–7 Sudden death according to level of systolic blood pressure: The Framingham Study, 18-year follow-up (men and women aged 45–74)

Systolic BP level at each examination (mmHg)	Number of sudden deaths		Age-adjusted annual incidence of sudden death (per 1000)[b]	
	M	F	M	F
74–119	2	1	10.6	3.0
120–139	21	2	15.1	3.6
140–159	11	6	21.6	4.2
160–179	6	3	30.7	5.0
180–300	8	2	43.8	6.0
Significance of trend			$P < 0.005$	N.S.[a]

Source: From WB Kannel and T Gordon, 1974.

[a] Not significant.

[b] Smoothed rates.

Table 14–8 Sudden death according to serum cholesterol level: the Framingham Study, 18-year follow-up (men and women aged 45–74)

Serum cholesterol level at each examination (mg/dl)	Number of sudden deaths		Age-adjusted annual incidence of sudden death (per 1000)[a]	
	M	F	M	F
96–204	7	0	14.1	2.4
205–234	17	2	16.9	3.0
235–264	11	3	20.5	3.6
265–294	7	3	24.7	4.4
295–1124	6	5	29.7	5.3
Unknown		1		
Significance of trend			$P < 0.05$	$P < 0.10$

Source: Adapted from WB Kannel and T Gordon, 1974.

[a] Smoothed rates.

Summary

1. There are problems with the definition of sudden death potentially affecting comparability between different studies.

2. Sudden death is more common in males (as for total IHD); it occurs more frequently in the cooler months and in the lower socioeconomic classes.

Table 14–9 Cigarette smoking and sudden death: the Framingham Study, 18-year follow-up (men and women aged 45–74)

Daily cigarette smoking at each examination	Number of sudden deaths		Age-adjusted annual incidence of sudden death (per 1000)[b]	
	M	F	M	F
None	12	9	12.1	2.8
<20	12	0	16.6	4.2
20	11	3	22.7	6.2
>20	13	1	31.1	9.3
Unknown		1		
Significance of trend			$P < 0.02$	N.S.[a]

Source: Adapted from WB Kannel and T Gordon, 1974.

[a] Not significant.

[b] Smoothed rates.

3. Prevention is of great importance for sudden death, as therapy after the event is very difficult. Unfortunately, "late prevention" during the prodrome may not be practical, as prodromal symptoms are very non-specific. Most deaths occur away from medical care.

4. Sudden-death victims usually have significant coronary disease and evidence of myocardial fibrosis (focal or confluent). Obstructing thrombus in major coronary arteries is much less common than for myocardial infarction.

5. Rapid coronary care ambulances in selected locations can save a modest proportion of "would-be" sudden deaths. Follow-up indicates that less than half of resuscitated victims develop transmural infarction, and a significant proportion have no ECG change.

6. This introduces the idea of "primary" ventricular fibrillation. The pathogenesis is uncertain, but the arrhythmia may result from ischemia without infarction or be unrelated to acute ischemia.

7. Risk factors for sudden death include electrocardiographic abnormalities, previous heart disease, hypertension, cigarette smoking, and elevated serum cholesterol.

15

Implications of the Multifactorial Etiology
of Ischemic Heart Disease for Clinical Practice

The Possibilities and Problems of Preventive Cardiologic Practice

In some areas of medicine, prevention is the accepted norm. The obvious examples are immunization and other public health measures that have virtually eliminated many infectious diseases. In cardiology, it is now common practice to give antibiotics as a preventive measure to certain persons at high risk of bacterial endocarditis or recurrent rheumatic fever, as it is to prescribe anticoagulants to persons at risk of mural or valvular thrombosis. The treatment of hypertension is another excellent example of preventive medicine. The occurrence of stroke in uncontrolled hypertension is appropriately considered a medical failure. Notice that all of these examples of preventive cardiology involve the administration of drugs. The effort to use life-style change as a preventive measure is given little more than lip-service by most medical practitioners, even though such changes have probably accounted for a substantial portion of the 30 percent drop in IHD mortality over the past 16 years in the United States. Still, the attitude is understandable, as the evidence has not been clear-cut and patient compliance with recommendations for changing their habits is often very poor. This is particularly so for primary prevention when people are healthy, and the possibility of avoiding future difficulties is usually a poor motivation. In secondary prevention, however, many intelligent patients will be sufficiently motivated by their current problems to undertake the recommended measures.

Should Prevention Be Directed Only at the High-Risk Patient?

The traditional medical care model requires the person to go to the physician. As medical consultation is relatively expensive in many countries, this may require considerable motivation. Such motivation is usually generated by symptoms, often resulting from established chronic disease. In these circumstances, the possibility of the physician becoming involved in primary prevention is less likely. Often it is only patients at relatively high risk levels who are treated or counseled, but attitudes are changing. This high-risk philosophy may be appropriate for the individual, since high-risk individuals stand to gain the most from preventive measures, but in terms of the community burden of disease, it is not optimal.

The following discussion is based on the assumption that the standard risk factors are causal and that interventions that change risk factor values do reduce the person's level of IHD risk. "Risk" in this chapter is calculated by using the Risk Slide Rule developed by the Laboratory of Physiological Hygiene at the University of Minnesota (Thorsen et al, 1979). This instrument is one of several available for office use, which allow a prediction of risk over a specified number of years, according to present values of the major risk factors (see also American Heart Association, 1973; *Coronary Risk Calculator*, 1983). Suppose a 50-year-old man who has a diastolic blood pressure of 85 mm Hg and a serum cholesterol of 310 mg/dl, and is a nonsmoker, changes his diet or loses weight so that his blood cholesterol drops to 235 mg/dl. This cuts his calculated risk of developing IHD over the next 20 years by half from 17 percent to 8.5 percent. Suppose another man similar in all respects, except that his serum cholesterol reading is initially 230 mg/dl, undergoes an identical intervention. One would expect that he may not respond so dramatically; however, let us assume that his serum cholesterol also drops by 75 mg/dl. His risk declines from 8.3 percent to 4.8 percent, a much less striking change in absolute terms. The high-risk individual clearly improves his status more.

To assess the potential intervention gains for the community, it is necessary to include in our calculation the *number* of persons at very high risk. For simplicity, let us consider a change in only one variable, serum cholesterol. Take a hypothetical population of 10,000 forty-year-old white American males who do not smoke, who have diastolic blood pressures of 85 mm Hg, and who are currently free of clinical ischemic heart disease. Data from the Lipid Research Clinics Study Group (1980) suggest that this population would have a serum cholesterol distribution similar to that shown in Table 15–1. The risk of IHD over 20 years for this population is calculated for each serum cholesterol category, using the Risk Slide Rule. These risks are probabilities that can be multiplied by the number of persons at risk in each category to arrive at the predicted numbers of new cases as shown in the table. If we intervened only in those with serum cholesterol levels above 285 mg/dl, for instance, this would leave 93 percent of potential coronary victims untouched by the preventive effort (left side of Table 15–1).

Of course, all their risk is not due to serum cholesterol. Some is apparently due to age (or some unknown variable correlated with age) and some slight amount to the diastolic blood pressure level of 85 mm Hg. In assessing the preventive potential of lowering serum cholesterol, it is also unrealistic to assume that dietary or weight intervention will reduce all individuals' serum cholesterol to some ideal level. It is common clinical observation, and in accord with experimental experience (Keys et al, 1965c), that persons with higher initial levels of serum cholesterol will react more dramatically to the intervention. The "achievable" decreases assumed in Table 15–1 are a drop of 10, 30, 50 mg/dl of serum

Table 15-1 Predicted numbers of cases of IHD within 20 years at age 40 for 10,000 white males

Decile of serum cholesterol (mg/dl)	Number at risk	Number of cases	Cumulative (%)	Cases attributable to serum cholesterol >achievable baseline	Cumulative (%)
<160	1000	40	6.0	—	—
160–173	1000	48	13.0	—	—
174–184	1000	55	21.0	3	2.4
185–194	1000	61	29.6	5	6.5
195–203	1000	66	38.6	6	11.3
204–213	1000	72	48.2	6	16.1
214–223	1000	77	58.2	16	29.0
224–234	1000	84	70.0	18	43.5
235–250	1000	97	81.8	24	62.9
251–284	750	89	93.6	31	87.9
>285	250	43	100.0	15	100.0
Totals	10,000	732		124	

cholesterol if initial values are in the respective ranges 174–213, 214–250, and over 250 mg/dl. It is now possible, using the Risk Slide Rule, to calculate within each initial serum cholesterol category the predicted number of cases if there were no intervention, and also the prediction after intervention. The difference is shown in the fifth column of Table 15–1. Notice that an intervention cutpoint of 285 mg/dl still leaves untreated 88 percent of the IHD caused by cholesterol levels above the "achievable" baseline values. This is because of the large numbers at risk in the moderately elevated categories. Similar calculations can be made for hypertension and smoking. Thus it seems to be justifiable to intervene also on those at only modest risk, if not the whole community.

The Potential Gains for an Average Person

It is common knowledge that preventive measures must be applied to many, for the benefit of a few. Immunization or wearing seatbelts involves hundreds of people taking action to prevent one serious or fatal event. Also with chronic diseases, preventive action by many is needed to reach a few. Consider a group of 100 white American men who are 45 years old, smoke 30 cigarettes per day, have serum cholesterol levels of 210 mg/dl, and have diastolic blood pressures of 85 mm Hg. What are the potential IHD gains if they were all to quit smoking? Risk over the next 20 years would drop from 9.6 to 4.3 percent, an excellent result proportionately. But consider that 100 men had to stop smoking so that 5 could avoid IHD. In a higher risk group of men, the gains in IHD prevention would be greater.

By comparison with other preventive measures these figures are quite favorable, yet it is easier to be immunized than to stop smoking. Also, this does not take into account reduced risk of smoking-associated morbidity and mortality from lung cancer, bronchitis, emphysema, and so on. Dietary change toward high fiber, fewer animal products, and less calorie-dense foods will probably decrease risk of diabetes, diverticulosis, and possibly colon cancer, in addition to IHD. It also promotes an optimal body weight and so helps prevent other obesity-related disorders. Reducing elevated blood pressure decreases the risk of stroke, other arterial disease, renal disease, and damage to the ocular fundi, in addition to hypertensive heart disease. Thus, the life-style changes that may help prevent IHD seem to represent "principles of healthy living" that apply to many other chronic diseases common to Western society.

What Is a "Safe" Intervention?

As with any therapeutic prescription, the physician must weigh the risk/benefit ratio. The same intervention may be acceptable in one population, but not in another. In particular, the average risk of the population is an important determinant of this ratio. Consider a group of 100 patients with IHD (such persons are at high risk for subsequent events), who have been prescribed an intervention. It is known that this intervention will reduce the rate of subsequent IHD events by 40 percent per year over 5 years. However, it is associated with a side effect as severe as developing IHD at a rate of 3 percent over 5 years, so that about three persons will develop it during the 5-year period. If we assume that in this population the recurrent IHD event rate is 8 percent per year and that half are fatal, then it would be expected that 37 events would occur. With intervention the predicted number of events is 23, a saving of 14. This yields a risk/benefit ratio of 3:14, which favors the intervention. Consider now the same intervention applied to 100 healthy low-risk individuals over a 5-year period to prevent the first manifestation of IHD. Assume that the risk of this first manifestation is 1 percent per year and that the intervention as before reduces risk by 40 percent. Assume that the serious side effect rate is still 3 percent over the 5 years. Then about five IHD events would be expected to occur, but if the intervention had been applied, this would have been reduced to three, representing a saving of two. Now the risk/benefit ratio is 3:2, which does not favor the intervention.

This illustrates that in a primary preventive situation where the population is at low risk of disease, the preventive measure must be virtually risk free. It is doubtful that any drug therapy could be justified for the population at large as a preventive measure. A controversial example is the use of thiazide diuretics to treat mild hypertension in order to prevent subsequent morbidity and mortality. There is some evidence for the benefit of this over a 5-year period. Yet, some worry about the potential hazards of 35 million Americans taking daily thiazides for decades. This is because all the possible side effects have not been well quantitated, particularly over a long period of time. The effects of thiazides on blood lipids (chapter 20) has only recently been discovered and is a case in point.

It may be prudent to advocate "natural" life-style interventions (such as weight loss and salt restriction) before resorting to drugs. There are two different types of interventions: those that have been used by some cultures for generations with apparent safety, and those that appear to make good physiologic sense—perhaps by restoring an abnormal risk factor toward an optimal value—but have not had the benefit of long-term use by large numbers of people.

Normal Versus Optimal

To assess the risk factor status of a patient, a physician must make decisions concerning the implications of individual risk factor values. When laboratories report values of tests, they usually include a normal range. Patients, and often physicians, are commonly satisfied providing the values fall within this normal range. However, the concept of normality is tied to the population in which the patient lives. Often the normal range cited represents percentile values from this population. How appropriate is this if the population as a whole has *suboptimal* values for the risk factor?

What is normal may not be optimal. The latter can only be decided by comparison with other populations. Clearly, these considerations apply to blood pressure, serum cholesterol, and dietary variables. Physicians should be guided by evidence regarding *optimality* rather than normality in a population that is suffering an epidemic of ischemic heart disease.

The Epidemiologic or the Clinical Approach?

Clinicians deal with individual patients, whereas epidemiologists deal with populations. Clinicians often see this as a conceptual gulf difficult to bridge. However, the differences are largely illusory. A patient across the office desk from the physician shares many qualities with other individuals, but remains unique. No matter how thorough the clinical and laboratory examination, there is no known way to predict that individual's risk or response to therapy precisely. When assessing risk and risk reduction, or when making a therapeutic decision where disease already exists, physicians must rely on their past experience with or on reports in the literature about *groups* of broadly similar persons.

While clinicians may use their intellect and knowledge of their patients to try to compensate for perceived differences between individual patients and the group mean, they are otherwise reliant on experiences with groups. They must extrapolate from these and assume that their patients will respond roughly similarly. Epidemiologists work with groups of patients and often report on mean values from these groups. Clearly, individuals vary around these means, but in most circumstances the variations appear to be random.

The two approaches are in fact complementary. Epidemiologists help define the broad outlines of the therapeutic or diagnostic situation. Physicians use their clinical experience, knowledge of physiology and human behavior, and familiarity with the patient to allow a more precise fit to each individual.

Conceptual Problems Related to the Multivariate Nature of the Disorder

Clinicians often express doubts about the risk factor basis of IHD by recalling several cases in their experience where clinical IHD was manifest, but the patient displayed none of the traditional risk factors. Such cases do occur, of course, as we cannot explain all the causal forces associated with increased risk of IHD. Frequently, however, the lack of risk factors may be more apparent than real, and again the concept of normality is relevant. Risk factor levels represent a continuum, and while clinicians usually react to markedly elevated levels of particular risk factors, they do not always appreciate that modest elevations (often within normal ranges) of several risk factors can produce the same risk status as severe hypertension or hyperlipidemia. Three individuals hypothesized in Table 15–2 have isolated but substantial elevations of individual risk factors; the fourth has levels of these variables that are common and are often considered unremarkable. Yet all four have the same overall risk. The Framingham Study (Gordon et al, 1971) and other sources indicate that traditional risk factors have a synergistic effect (i.e., more than additive). Changes in

Table 15–2 Risk factors of four patients with approximately equal risk of developing IHD

Risk level[a]	Patient	Diastolic BP	Number of cigarettes per day	Serum cholesterol (mg/dl)
Equal	A	110	—	200
	B	80	40	200
	C	80	—	310
	Joe Bloggs	90	10	240

[a] Patients A–C have risk factors that are relatively rare, while Joe Bloggs has levels that are common and often considered unremarkable.

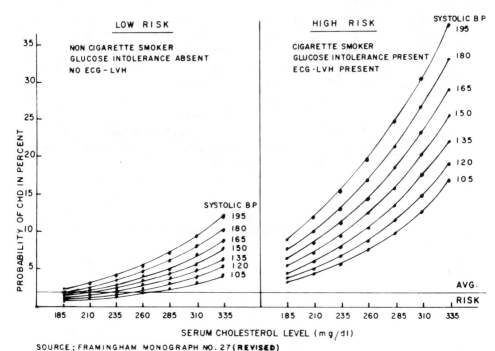

SOURCE : FRAMINGHAM MONOGRAPH NO. 27(**REVISED**)

Figure 15–1   Probability of developing coronary heart disease in 6 years, in 40-year-old men: Framingham Study, 16-year follow-up. From T Gordon et al, 1971.

serum cholesterol or blood pressure or cigarette smoking have decidedly different effects depending on the levels of other risk factors (Fig. 15–1).

Another reason for physicians' doubts is related to measurement of serum cholesterol levels within 4 weeks of myocardial infarction. For unknown reasons, it is usually substantially lower than usual during this period (Fyfe et al, 1971). Yet another finding cited by doubters is that young patients who develop IHD may have only one elevated risk factor. Commonly this will be cigarette smoking or marked hyperlipidemia, and it must be remembered that smoking seems to be a particularly potent risk factor in younger persons, both male and female.

The multifactorial etiologic nature of ischemic heart disease raises another potential complication: Are the main risk factors independently distributed throughout the population, or do persons who are hypertensive, for instance, tend also to have elevations in other risk factors? There are indications that the traditional risk factors are not entirely independent (Criqui et al, 1980b). Individuals showing suboptimality of more than one risk factor occur more frequently than expected. This may imply the presence of a common cause for certain risk factors. If such a cause could be found and proved amenable to intervention, such intervention might be particularly effective, treating several risk factors at once. Obesity may be such a variable.

There is good evidence that obesity is dynamically related to both total and HDL cholesterol levels, tending to increase the total cholesterol/HDL ratio (FW Ashley and WB Kannel, 1974; Blacket et al, 1979; Garrison et al, 1979; Hulley et al, 1979). Obesity is also dynamically related to hypertension and inversely related to physical activity. If the observational results of the Framingham Study have causal implications, it is noteworthy that for men each 10-unit change in Framingham relative weight was associated with an 11.3 mg/dl change in serum cholesterol and 6.6 mm Hg change in systolic blood pressure (FW Ashley and WB Kannel, 1974). Although physical inactivity clearly promotes obesity, it is also possibly true that obesity promotes physical inactivity. Given the prevalence of obesity in American society, one may speculate that an effective treatment for this disorder applied on a mass scale to those who need it, could achieve a great deal in preventing future cardiovascular diseases. Interestingly, although obese people are at higher risk of developing ischemic heart disease than persons of medium body build (Noppa et al, 1980; Schroll, 1981), there is little evidence that it has an independent effect beyond its contribution to hypercholesterolemia and hypertension (Kannel et al, 1967a; Schroll, 1981).

A similar variable is diabetes mellitus. Diabetics have increased ratios of total to HDL cholesterol, more hypertension, and increased platelet reactivity. It seems likely that these factors may largely explain the increased IHD risk of diabetic men at least (Garcia et al, 1974; Kannel and McGee, 1979; Pyorala et al, 1983).

The relationship of serum triglycerides to ischemic heart disease is controversial (Hulley et al, 1980). Persons with higher levels of triglycerides are at higher risk of ischemic heart disease, but generally not independently of other risk factors. In contrast to obesity and diabetes, we have no evidence that hypertriglyceridemia promotes changes in the other traditional risk factors, rather triglyceride levels are statistically linked to some of the traditional risk factors but probably not actually in the causal chain leading to ischemic heart disease. Obesity, physical inactivity, and diabetes are all known to lead to hypertriglyceridemia, and it is probably these relationships that lead to a statistical link with little causal implication.

Different studies have developed equations allowing an individual's risk of developing IHD over some time period to be calculated. Obviously, this has potential for use in patient education and motivation. The usual model is based on a logistic function and so is rather complex. However, as it is increasingly common for physicians and others to own or have access to programmable calculators or microcomputers, some equations and a simple computer program in the BASIC language is shown below. These equations are based on the analysis of Framingham Study data (Kannel and Gordon, 1971) and should only be applied to persons who have not yet developed IHD between the ages of 35 and

70 years. The equations also allow the computation of risk, relative to that of an individual of similar age and sex, but with risk factors close to optimal levels. For illustration, in the computer program, these optimal comparison values are set at nonsmoker; serum cholesterol = 200 mg/dl; systolic blood pressure = 120 mm Hg; no left ventricular hypertrophy; no glucose intolerance.

Risk of developing IHD over the next 8 years $= (1 + e^x)^{-1}$ where

1. For men: $x = 22.41 - 0.49 \times \text{age} + 0.0032 \times \text{age}^2 - 0.027 \times \text{sc} - 0.013 \times$ SBP $- 0.49 \times \text{cigs} - 0.75 \times \text{LVH} - 0.23 \times \text{GI} + 0.0004 \times \text{sc} \times \text{age}$
2. For women: $x = 19.31 - 0.35 \times \text{age} + 0.0021 \times \text{age}^2 - 0.015 \times \text{sc} - 0.013 \times$ SBP $- 0.035 \times \text{cigs} - 0.43 \times \text{LVH} - 0.56 \times \text{GI} + 0.00018 \times \text{sc} \times \text{age}$

    SC = serum cholesterol (mg/dl)
   SBP = systolic blood pressure (mm Hg)
  cigs = cigarettes (enter 1 for a smoker, else 0)
  LVH = left ventricular hypertrophy (enter 1 if diagnosed on ECG, else 0)
    GI = glucose intolerance (enter 1 if diabetic or casual blood sugar
        > 120 mg/dl or trace or more of sugar in the urine, else 0)

10 PRINT "THIS PROGRAM CALCULATES PROBABILITY OF DEVELOPING IHD OVER 8
       YEARS,"
20 PRINT "ALSO THE RELATIVE RISK AS COMPARED TO AN INDIVIDUAL WITH
       OPTIMAL"
30 PRINT "RISK FACTOR VALUES (SERUM CHOLESTEROL = 200, SYSTOLIC BLOOD
       PRESSURE = 120, NONSMOKER,"
40 PRINT "NO LVH OR DIABETES)"
50 INPUT "SEX, ENTER M OR F"; S$
60 INPUT "AGE"; A
70 INPUT "SERUM CHOLESTEROL"; SC
80 INPUT "SYSTOLIC BLOOD PRESSURE"; SBP
90 INPUT "DOES PATIENT SMOKE CIGARETTES, ENTER Y OR N"; K$
100 INPUT "DOES PATIENT HAVE LVH ON THE ECG, ENTER Y OR N"; L$
110 INPUT "DOES PATIENT HAVE GLUCOSE INTOLERANCE, ENTER Y OR N"; M$
120 IF K$ = "Y" THEN K1 = 1 ELSE K1 = 0
130 IF L$ = "Y" THEN L1 = 1 ELSE L1 = 0
140 IF M$ = "Y" THEN M1 = 1 ELSE M1 = 0
150 IF S$ = "M" THEN ODDS = EXP (− 22.41 + .49*A − .0032*A^2 + .027*SC +
    .013*SBP + .49*K1 + .75*L1 + .23*M1 − .0004*SC*A)
160 IF S$ = "F" THEN ODDS = EXP (− 19.31 + .35*A − .0021*A^2 + .015*SC +
    .013*SBP + .035*K1 + .43*L1 + .56*M1 − .00018*SC*A)
170 RISK = ODDS/(1 + ODDS)
180 IF S$ = "M" THEN ODDS1 = EXP (− 22.4 + .49*A − .0032*A^2 + .027*200 +
    .013*120 − .0004*200*A)
190 IF S$ = "F" THEN ODDS1 = EXP (− 19.31 + .35*A − .0021*A^2 + .015*200 +
    .013*120 − .00018*200*A)

200 RR = (ODDS/ODDS1)
210 PRINT "RISK OF IHD IN 8 YEARS = "; RISK
220 PRINT "RISK RELATIVE TO AN INDIVIDUAL WITH OPTIMAL RISK FACTORS = ";
        RR
230 END

The Most Important Risk Factor

Which of the main risk factors is the most important is a question with no simple answer. A variable that is associated with a major change in risk for a comparatively small change in its value would seem to be more important. However, there is no obvious way to decide "equal" magnitudes of change for different risk factors.

The logistic regression coefficients of multivariate analyses describe the slopes of the relationships between the various risk factors and IHD risk. Simply comparing regression coefficients is not appropriate. Their values are markedly dependent on the measurement scales used for the risk factors. For instance, changing measurement of serum cholesterol from milligrams per deciliter to milligrams per liter would reduce the calculated value of the regression coefficient 10-fold, and yet choice of measurement scale is often arbitrary.

This problem is resolved in one sense by using *standardized* regression coefficients, which are independent of measurement scale and can be thought of as describing the relationship between the variable and risk in standard deviation units. If B is a standardized regression coefficient, a change by one standard deviation of the risk factor is associated with a change of B standard deviations of risk. Thus, it is possible to compare the relative changes in risk associated with a 1-SD change in each of the risk factors. Note that these relationships are unique to the particular population being studied, as the values of the standardized coefficients depend on the standard deviations of the various variables in this population. The assumption is that single standard deviation changes in different risk factors are equivalent in some sense. They could be thought of as representing roughly similar changes in rank for each risk factor, within the population. On this basis, using Pooling Project equations, for men, smoking was ranked first for younger men (40–44 years), hypertension for older men (55–59), with serum cholesterol, smoking, and hypertension having about equal importance in middle-aged men (Pooling Project Research Group, 1978).

Another way of looking at this question in a more absolute sense is to compare the relative gains if a population was to change values of each of the risk factors in turn to some optimal level that is found in other cultures. This may seem a less practical perspective, but it estimates the degree of hazard imposed on the community by its culture. The idea is that a risk factor that is markedly suboptimal is very important. For illustration, assume optimal values of risk factors are nonsmoking, serum cholesterol 180 mg/dl, and diastolic blood pressure 75 mm Hg. Obviously, the optimum levels chosen will influence the results.

For serum cholesterol and blood pressure these are based on values from cultures with little IHD. There would seem to be little controversy about the optimal value for smoking. The predicted reduction in risk by change to optimal levels is calculated for men using Pooling Project equations and the more recent Lipid Research Clinics data for average values of risk factors in the United States (Lipid Research Clinics Study Group, 1980). Results show smoking as most important for the 40–44-year age range, but all three of about equal importance during the ages 50–59 years. Using the Framingham Study equation for the age group 60–69 years, hypertension is most important. Thus, the results here are very similar to those using the standardized regression coefficient approach to this question. It should be pointed out that the calculated contribution of lipids cannot be considered definite, as equations are not available containing HDL and LDL cholesterol rather just total cholesterol. Such equations may be available in the future, and would be expected to increase the calculated importance to some degree.

The Unit of Intervention

Physicians and health care providers at different levels of organization have very different views on the unit of intervention. Those involved in government tend to regard the state or even the whole country as the population unit to influence. Those involved in county public health departments view a smaller geographic area as their domain of influence. The physician in office practice is most likely to consider the individual patient as the focus for any particular therapeutic endeavor. However, changes in a patient's living habits may have implications for other family members. When physicians are dealing with risk factors and behavioral problems, a case can be made for considering the whole family as the unit of intervention. There is evidence that to a significant extent elevated risk tends to run in families.

Children of parents with elevated levels of blood lipids often have similar elevations (Godfrey et al, 1972; Tyroler et al, 1980a). The same is true with blood pressure (Annest et al, 1979; Donner and Kavall, 1981; Havlik et al, 1979; Higgins et al, 1980). There is also evidence that relatively hyperlipidemic children are more likely to be found in families with increased premature IHD mortality (Schrott et al, 1979). That there is a familial tendency toward similar smoking habits has been well documented (US Public Health Service, 1976), and so has a familial tendency toward obesity (Garn and Clarke, 1976; Garn et al, 1980; Mayer, 1968). A child with two obese parents has a three times greater chance of being an obese child than a child with two lean parents. There is evidence of some correlations of risk factors between spouses that must be nonhereditary and probably are due to a shared environment (Barrett-Connor et al, 1982; Kannel, 1976). Table 15–3 compares Framingham husbands with low, medium, or high risk status with the values of their wives' risk factor standing. Clearly, risk values for wives tend toward those of their husbands. This under-

Table 15–3 Correspondence of risk factors among spouses: Married couples 30–62 (Framingham Heart Study). Values of risk factors in wives of husbands with low, medium, and high risk factor values

Status of husbands[a]	Level of risk factors in wives							
	Serum cholesterol		Systolic BP		Obesity		Cigarettes	
	No.	Mean	No.	Mean	No.	%	No.	%
Low	402	214	604	120	165	9	151	24
Medium	804	227	242	131	132	17	138	37
High	310	235	110	136	23	22	960	47

[a] Definitions:

	Serum cholesterol	Systolic BP
Low	< 200 mg/dl	< 120 mm Hg
Medium	200–259	120–147
High	> 260	> 148

	Obesity	Cigarettes
Low	< 100 Rel. Wt.	Never smoked
Medium	100–119	Former smoker
High	> 120	Cigarette smoker

lines the logic of considering the family as the unit of therapy when risk factor change is being addressed. A further cogent reason for this is the need for strong family support of the at-risk individual who is trying to change his or her behavior (chapter 21). It is difficult for one member of the family to remain eccentric with respect to eating habits, for instance.

Summary

1. The potential for preventive practice in cardiology is great, but more professional education is necessary.

2. Directing preventive measures at only the high-risk patient gives the best gain/effort ratio for an individual patient but is an inferior approach as far as affecting the community burden of disease.

3. Preventive efforts usually involve changes on the part of many for the benefit of a few. Fortunately, the changes advocated in preventive cardiology have preventive potential outside of IHD alone.

4. Interventions applied to the "well" population (that is, primary prevention) need to be very safe. This may preclude the use of most drugs as *primary* prevention.

5. What is "normal" for a population suffering an epidemic of heart disease is often not "optimal."

6. The multivariate synergistic nature of risk factors for IHD results in minor elevations of several risk factors causing important elevations in IHD risk. Persons with such multiple minor elevations are common.

7. Although obesity may not be associated with IHD independent of its association with other risk factors, it is an antecedent cause of several of these risk factors. In view of this and its high prevalence, it becomes one of the prime targets for intervention.

8. It is suggested that the optimal unit for behavioral intervention in clinical practice should be the family rather than the individual.

16

An Approach to the Child at Risk for Ischemic Heart Disease*

Very few diseases provide health professionals the opportunities that athero-sclerosis does. The potential victims begin life with normal arteries and with the passage of time may develop strokes, gangrene of the extremities, and ischemic heart disease (IHD). The causes of atherosclerosis have not been fully identified, but the environment associated with its development is known. This opens the possibility of preventing or deferring clinical manifestation of the disease by changing life-styles. Such changes probably are maximally effective when initiated in childhood and continued throughout life.

From a chronologic point of view (Fig. 16–1), the first gross atherosclerotic changes are evident in the aorta within a few months of birth, and these are small lipid deposits in the aortic intima. A rapid increase in the number of these fatty streaks occurs after age 8 years, so that by age 15 years, approximately 15

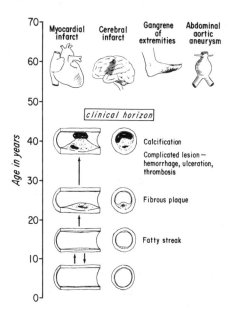

Figure 16–1 Chronologic pro-gression of atherosclerosis.

* I wish to thank Dr. William Strong, Medical College of Georgia, Augusta, Georgia, for supplying much of the original material for this chapter and for also helping with its organization.

percent of the aortic intima is covered by fatty streaks. Between ages 10 and 20 years, fatty streaks become evident in the coronary arteries, and in the cerebral arteries between ages 30 and 40 years (McGill, 1980). Fibrous plaques are first seen in the coronary arteries at about age 20 years, and they increase in number with increasing age. The anatomic distribution of fatty streaks in the coronaries is similar to the distribution of fibrous plaques. This relationship is not observed for these two types of lesion in the aorta (McGill, 1980).

Risk Factors

Epidemiologic studies of adult subjects have identified certain independent factors (hypertension, hypercholesterolemia, low HDL, cigarette smoking, diabetes mellitus, type A behavior) (American Heart Association, 1980) that predispose to atherosclerosis. Whether these characteristics identified in children are the precursors of adult disease has not been substantiated, as longitudinal studies need to be done. Cross-sectional studies strongly suggest that these childhood characteristics are precursors of adult disease.

An important concept in the consideration of risk factors in the pediatric years is that of "tracking." Childhood is a period of growth and change. Do risk factors change in severity as children grow, and if they do, at what ages do the changes occur? The Bogalusa (Frerichs et al, 1979; Webber et al, 1979) and Muscatine (Clarke et al, 1978; Lauer et al, 1975) studies performed on schoolchildren have shown that individual children roughly tend to maintain their positions relative to other children (in terms of risk factors) as they grow. Therefore, a child who when initially evaluated had a cholesterol level above the 80th percentile for age and sex, had a 60 percent chance of being above the 80th percentile if reevaluated after a 6-year interval (Clarke et al, 1978). It seems that childhood values of risk factors are likely to track with time in a manner similar to height and weight.

Lipids and Diet

The ability of genetic or environmental factors to affect neonatal lipid levels was demonstrated in the Bogalusa studies comparing black and white Americans (Frerichs et al, 1976, 1978). At birth, white infants were found to have higher levels of total cholesterol and LDL. White female infants had the highest levels of total cholesterol, HDL, and LDL, when the data were analyzed by race and gender. Another study compared the cord blood HDL levels of infants in Leningrad and Cincinnati (Klimov et al, 1979). While American neonates had higher HDL levels than the Russian neonates, this situation was reversed in adults, with the Russian adults having higher HDL levels.

During the first year of life, remarkable changes are observed in serum lipid and lipoprotein levels. In the Bogalusa studies (Berenson et al, 1982) it was

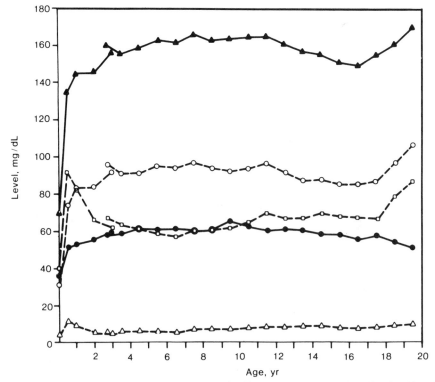

Figure 16–2 Serum lipid values in children of different ages: the Bogalusa Study. Closed triangles, total cholesterol; open circles, β-lipoprotein cholesterol; open squares, triglycerides; closed circles, α-lipoprotein cholesterol; open triangles, pre-β-liproprotein cholesterol. From GS Berenson et al: Cardiovascular risk factors in children. *Am J Dis Child* 136:855, 1982. Copyright 1982, American Medical Association. Reprinted by permission.

found that these levels begin approaching adult levels by age 2–3 years (Fig. 16–2). In relative terms, this means that by age 3 years, total cholesterol has increased by 129 percent, triglycerides by 69 percent, LDL by 212 percent, and HDL by 64 percent. Between the ages of 5 and 14 years, 9 percent of white children were found to have cholesterol levels higher than 200 mg/dl.

Early puberty is another stage in growth at which changes in lipoprotein levels occur. After the significant increases in total cholesterol, LDL cholesterol, and HDL cholesterol during the first 3 years of life, the levels of these lipids and lipoproteins tend to remain stable until early puberty, when their levels decrease slightly (Berenson et al, 1982). Then, between the ages of about 12 and 17 years, changes differ by sex and race (Fig. 16–3). Notice the dramatic rise in the LDL/HDL cholesterol ratio for adolescent white males not seen either in black males or in females of either race. Work done at the Cincinnati Lipid Research Clinic (JA Morrison et al, 1981) demonstrated that adult whites (especially males)

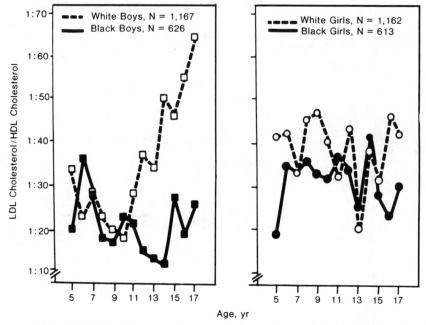

Figure 16–3 Trends in the ratios of LDL to HDL cholesterol in white and black children. From GS Berenson et al: Cardiovascular risk factors in children. *Am J Dis Child* **136**:855, 1982. Copyright 1982, American Medical Association. Reprinted by permission.

have higher LDL levels and lower HDL levels when compared to blacks. There are therefore changes in lipoprotein and lipid patterns with growth. At birth, cholesterol is approximately equally distributed between HDL and LDL, while by adulthood 21 percent of total cholesterol exists as HDL while 66 percent exists as LDL (Frerichs et al, 1978). Percentile values for U.S. children in Bogalusa, Louisiana are shown in Fig. 16–4 (Frerichs et al, 1976).

Many studies of adults have shown that serum cholesterol levels, and probably as a result IHD, are influenced by diet. Similar evidence exists for children but is less complete. International comparisons are generally supportive of the usual diet–cholesterol hypothesis. Mexican schoolchildren have markedly lower serum cholesterol levels than similar-aged Wisconsin schoolchildren (Golubjatnikov et al, 1972). The staple diet of the Mexican children was beans, chile, and tortillas (although chicken, beef, and pork were also consumed), and obesity was rare. In Wisconsin, meat and dairy products are more important dietary components, and obesity in children is much more common. Comparison of serum lipids of Tarahumara Indian boys from northern Mexico and their U.S. counterparts shows a similar picture (Table 16–1).

Natives of New Guinea have markedly different lipid patterns through childhood and adolescence as compared to Australians, although at birth there are

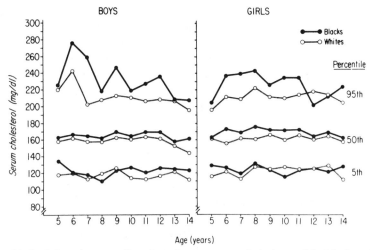

Figure 16–4 Selected percentile values for serum total cholesterol in black and white children in Bogalusa, Louisiana. From RR Frerichs et al: Serum cholesterol and triglyceride levels in 3,446 children from a biracial community. *Circulation* **54**:302, 1976, by permission of the American Heart Association, Inc.

no differences (Whyte and Yee, 1958). The New Guinea children are breast-fed, in part at least, often for 4 years (the maternal breast milk has much less fat than European human milk), and thereafter the diet is virtually devoid of fat. Lipid patterns in children of the various racial groups in South Africa (white, Indian, colored, and Bantu) closely follow expectations based on their respective diets (Du Plessis et al, 1967).

Serum cholesterol levels of samples of 7- to 8-year-old boys have been compared from 16 countries, using standardized techniques and one laboratory to

Table 16–1 Comparison of mean cholesterol and lipoprotein levels in Tarahumara Indian and U.S. boys

	Mean serum cholesterol (mg/dl)		
	Total	HDL	LDL
Tarahumara Indian boys	118	23	75
Muscatine, Iowa boys	163	50	103

Source: Adapted from WE Connor: Cross-cultural studies of diet and plasma lipids and lipoproteins, in Lauer RM, Shekelle RB (eds): *Childhood Prevention of Atherosclerosis and Hypertension*, New York, Raven Press, 1980. Reprinted by permission.

measure cholesterol (Knuiman et al, 1980). Large differences were shown, with African, Asian, and Mediterranean countries tending to have lower levels as compared to the United States and to European countries other than the above. This is consistent with the usual dietary hypothesis and, interestingly, correlates well with the comparative IHD incidence among adults in the same countries. As for the adults, the above intercultural comparisons cannot prove the diet–lipid hypothesis but are only supportive of it. It is interesting that, as for adults, on cross-cultural comparison HDL cholesterol levels are positively associated with total cholesterol, and in countries where disease is more common, HDL levels tend to be *higher*. Comparison of the ratio of total cholesterol to HDL cholesterol shows that this is also often higher in Third World countries, leading one to question its validity as a risk factor outside of westernized cultures.

Several epidemiologic studies have searched for correlations within homogeneous populations. Again, as for adults, the results have been mixed. The Busselton Study in Australia (Hitchcock and Gracey, 1977), and a study of 103 white children aged 6–16 years (Weidman et al, 1978), could find no significant correlations between diet and serum cholesterol. This must be interpreted within the range of nutritional habits encountered within a single community. A study of 1669 children from the Princetown School District (Cincinnati, Ohio) found few significant correlation coefficients treating the data on an individualized basis, but demonstrated significant associations comparing mean lipid values of subgroups representing upper, middle, and lower nutrient intakes (JA Morrison et al, 1980). Low-density lipoprotein levels fell as polyunsaturated fat and carbohydrate increased, and rose as dietary cholesterol increased. Another study (Mendoza et al, 1980) found that Venezuelan schoolchildren attending private schools had marginally higher Quetelet Indices of obesity but substantially higher levels of serum cholesterol than public schoolchildren. The private schoolchildren ingested nearly twice as great a percentage of calories as fat.

The Bogalusa Heart Study (GC Frank et al, 1978) reported results from 185 ten-year-old children (35 percent black and 65 percent white) and found significant associations only when comparing nutrient intakes of groups defined according to high, medium, or low percentiles of serum cholesterol. The expected trends were seen with total fat, animal fat, saturated fatty acids, and carbohydrates, but an unexpected positive relationship between unsaturated fats and serum cholesterol (presumably unsaturated fats here included the inactive *mono*unsaturates). This study also showed associations between several nutrients and serum cholesterols of infants during the first year of life (Berenson et al, 1979; Farris et al, 1982). Other investigators also have found evidence of some relationships between diet and serum cholesterol in observational studies (Rasanen et al, 1978; Ward et al, 1980).

Very few experimental studies of children appear to have been performed in closely controlled "metabolic ward"-type situations. Two studies that come close to this investigated infants (Glueck and Tsang, 1972; Nestel et al, 1979), the study of Nestel et al being of infants with familial type II hyperlipoproteinemia. Another study (McGandy et al, 1972) investigated the effect of diet on 220 boys aged 13–18 years at a boarding school. All found important effects of diet on serum cholesterol in the expected directions.

Consequently, it is probable that the relationships found for adults apply to children in at least a qualitatively similar manner. Similar problems of measurement, individual responsiveness, and homogeneity of dietary habits, make results of cross-sectional population studies difficult to interpret. At this time, longitudinal studies have not been done in children to determine the effect on IHD incidence of modifying diet during childhood to achieve desirable serum cholesterol levels. In childhood, the more important goal of dietary intervention is the establishment of appropriate nutritional patterns that will be maintained into adulthood. Twelve to twenty-four months has been proposed as the age at which intervention should be instituted. It has been suggested but not definitely proven, that a very low dietary cholesterol intake before this age could cause impaired myelinization of the central nervous system, as this process requires fatty acids (Tsang and Glueck, 1975).

When dietary intervention is undertaken, it should be in keeping with recommendations of the American Heart Association Nutrition Committee (AHA, 1982):

1. The intake of saturated fatty acids should be maintained at less than 10 percent of total caloric intake.
2. Replace saturated fatty acids by polyunsaturates up to a maximum of 10 percent of total caloric intake. (The caloric intake from fats would then be limited to 30 percent of total calories ingested.)
3. Increase the intake of carbohydrates so that they constitute approximately 55 percent of total caloric intake.
4. Reduce cholesterol intake. For adults and older children, the recommended cholesterol intake is less than 300 mg/day. For younger children, one recommendation is 100 mg/1000 calories/day, not to exceed 300 mg/day (Weidman et al, 1983).
5. Caloric intake should be adjusted to achieve and maintain a desirable weight (in children this includes an appropriate weight gain with growth).

The recommendations listed above are appropriate for the population as a whole, and if such behavior patterns are adopted at an early age, they will probably be maintained into adulthood. Adolescent white males may particularly benefit from intervention efforts. There are no data as yet on which to support a particular serum cholesterol level as being ideal in children. The data on adults (Stamler, 1979) would suggest an ideal range for children's serum cholesterol of 130 to 190 mg/dl. Maintenance of such low levels from childhood into adulthood would probably decrease the risk of IHD (Fig. 16–5).

Some children will require more intensive intervention—for example, children with known or suspected familial hypercholesterolemia, and children with abnormally high cholesterol levels detected on screening. Screening should be done at the time of entry into school and again in adolescence (Glueck, 1980). Special attention should also be paid to those children with a family history of

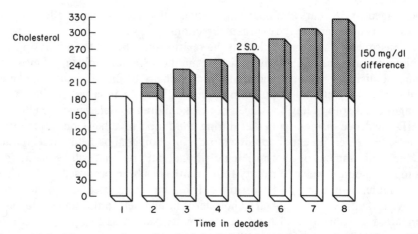

Figure 16–5 The comparison of an initial relatively hypercholesterolemic infant maintaining early childhood levels of serum cholesterol to adult life, with the usual natural history.

early myocardial infarcts, that is, before age 55 years (Boulton, 1980; Glueck et al, 1974), as such children frequently have elevated lipid levels. Similarly, there is increased IHD mortality in young relatives of hyperlipidemic children (Blonde et al, 1981; Schrott et al, 1979). These familial aggregations are probably due to both shared environment and genes. In those children with unacceptably elevated cholesterol levels or familial hypercholesterolemia that do not respond to diet after 1 year of compliance, drug therapy with cholestyramine or other drugs may be indicated.

Hypertension

Data from the Framingham Study (Kannel et al, 1969) demonstrated that there is an increased risk of atherosclerosis in adult hypertensive subjects. The incidence of IHD in men aged 45–62 years with blood pressures greater than 160/95 mm Hg was five times greater than that in normotensive men. Autopsy data and animal studies (Wissler and Vesselinovitch, 1974) have also demonstrated a similar relationship between hypertension and the severity of atherosclerosis. Hypertension is thought to increase the shearing force on the intima of blood vessels and thereby cause damage to the intima. In addition, the increased pressure may lead to increased deposition of lipoproteins.

Blood pressure normally increases with increasing age and growth. Because of the "dynamic" nature of blood pressure in the pediatric years, no single value

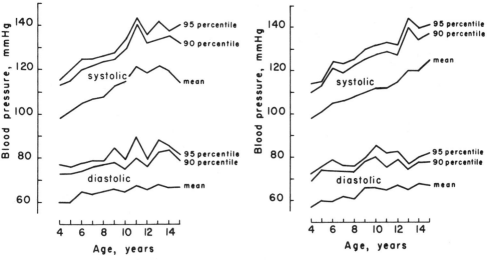

Figure 16–6   Selected blood pressure percentiles by age, from 795 healthy boys and 798 healthy girls seen in the office. Blood pressure was measured in supine position. From S Londe and D Goldring, 1976, with permission.

can be used as a cutoff to separate normals from hypertensive individuals. If the usual adult cutoff points of 140 mm Hg for systolic blood pressure and 90 mm Hg for diastolic pressure were used for all children, mildly hypertensive adolescents could be detected, but younger children would have to be moderately to severely hypertensive to be recognized (Fig. 16–6, Table 16–2). In the evaluation of blood pressure in children, age-related blood pressure percentiles provide a better assessment of significance. Children whose blood pressures are on or above the 95th percentile for age should be considered as being at

Table 16–2   Suspect blood pressure levels in children and adolescents

Age group	Blood pressure (mm Hg)
3–5	≥110/70
6–9	≥120/75
10–13	≥130/80
14–19	≥140/85

Source: Adapted from S Londe and D Goldring: *Am J Cardiol* **37**:650, 1976, with permission.

increased risk of developing hypertension. Blood pressure values in children appear to track, but not to the same extent as serum cholesterol or body weight.

The Evans County Study (Heyden et al, 1969) detected hypertension (>140 mm Hg systolic or >90 mm Hg diastolic, or both) in 11 percent of a group of 435 adolescents. On follow-up examination 7 years later, approximately one-third of the hypertensive group (11 of 30) were found to have sustained hypertension. Factors that predicted the future development of sustained hypertension were (1) high initial blood pressure, (2) a family history of high blood pressure, and (3) excessive weight gain. In the Muscatine Study (Clarke et al, 1978), carried out over 6 years, schoolchildren were seen at 2-year intervals, some children being evaluated on four separate visits over the 6 years. Diastolic blood pressure was found to track poorly, while systolic blood pressure exhibited somewhat better tracking. The probability of an individual's diastolic blood pressure remaining above the 80th percentile on all four visits was 9 percent, while the probability that systolic blood pressure reading would remain above that percentile was 17 percent. These studies underscore the necessity of making several blood pressure readings in children, since one reading may not be predictive of future values. This does not mean that a patient in whom blood pressure readings are found to be only transiently elevated has a completely benign prognosis. Some adolescents—56 percent in one study (Falkner et al, 1981)—who have intermittently elevated blood pressure levels (90th–95th percentile for age) will go on to develop sustained hypertension. Borderline hypertensives should therefore be followed closely. Londe and Goldring (1976) found on serial evaluations (over 3 to 9 years) of a group of children with initially high blood pressure readings that 35 percent of the group subsequently had normal readings. Those children who had elevated readings on three consecutive evaluations exhibited better tracking, as 65 percent of these children remained hypertensive on future evaluations. These data also emphasize the importance of serial determinations in the pediatric years.

Blood pressure should be measured at least yearly in children 3 years of age and older. Before the age of 3 years, the technical difficulty in measuring blood pressure on a small uncooperative patient with a sphygmomanometer makes readings inaccurate. The Doppler method is more suitable for these younger children. The prevalence of *sustained* hypertension in the pediatric years is thought to be between 1 and 3 percent (Londe and Goldring, 1976).

In the pediatric years, intervention on hypertension will be directed toward screening children to identify those who have readings above the 95th percentile, avoidance of excess salt intake to prevent or control hypertension, weight loss when indicated, adequate physical activity, and, finally, drug therapy for those unresponsive to the first two measures or those who are severely hypertensive when first seen. In view of the clear relationship between hypertension and IHD and the putative relationship between salt and hypertension, it is probably beneficial to recommend moderation in salt intake to less than 5 gm/day (Jesse et al, 1981), and less for small children. This can be achieved by eliminating

most highly salted processed food and salt-containing condiments, and by eliminating additional salt at the table.

Smoking

Cigarette smoking by itself is associated with an increased incidence of IHD in
adults, usually about double that of nonsmokers (Gordon et al, 1974). Smoking
is thought to increase platelet adhesiveness and to have an effect on the endothelium of the arteries. High-density lipoprotein levels are lower in smokers,
who therefore lack the protective effect of this lipoprotein. In addition, nicotine
may cause elevations of heart rate and blood presure while carboxyhemoglobin
affects oxygen transport and utilization (AHA, 1980).

Many children begin smoking at an early age. Public awareness of the complications of smoking—lung cancer, chronic respiratory disease, IHD—has led to
a decline in the frequency of smoking in adults. In contrast, smoking in adolescents is increasing. It has been estimated that 41 percent of high school-age children smoke, and the number of new smokers increases with increasing age
(Berenson et al, 1982).

The smoking behaviors of parents and siblings seem to be the strongest
influences on the smoking behavior of the adolescent. Of those teenagers who
come from nonsmoking households, 2 percent smoke. If a parent and a sibling
are smokers, almost 25 percent of teenagers from these households can be
expected to smoke (Committee on Youth, 1976). Since smoking is an acquired
habit, the aim should be to prevent children from acquiring this habit. Prevention of smoking in childhood is even more important, since the incidence of
IHD is highest in individuals who begin smoking before age 20 years, and cessation of the habit becomes more difficult the longer the individual smokes.

Exercise

Surveys suggest that children are not as fit as they should be (President's Council on Physical Fitness and Sports, 1977; *Fitness Profile of American Youth*,
1983; Canada Fitness Survey, 1983). The question is "What is physical fitness in
children, and how should it be measured?" There is no general agreement on
standards. However, what is clear is that few school systems promote or teach
physical fitness as a lifetime goal.

Studies in both Canada (Canada Fitness Survey, 1983) and the United States
(*Fitness Profile of American Youth*, 1983), as well as our own data (BS Alpert et
al, 1982), demonstrate that the aerobic power of adolescent girls decreases significantly while that of boys decreases slightly with body growth as measured by
surface area (Fig. 16–7). The percentage of educated middle-aged Canadians
achieving the recommended level of fitness increases after the trough in late adolescence and during the third decade (Canada Fitness Survey, 1983).

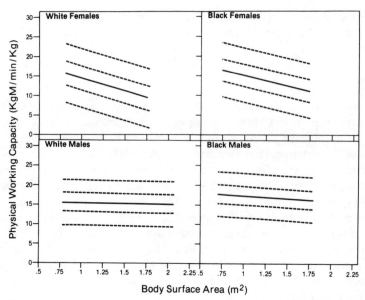

Figure 16–7 Nomogram showing trends in fitness, based on stress tests of 405 healthy children (5th, 25th, 50th, 75th, and 95th percentiles). From BS Alpert et al, 1982, with permission.

Physical activity has been shown to be beneficial in influencing other IHD risk factors also in children. Linder and DuRant (1982), and Nizankowska-Blaz and Abramowicz (1983) have found a positive relationship between exercise and HDL cholesterol in children, similar to that known in adults. Significant lowering of blood pressure by an aerobic exercise program in hypertensive adolescents has also been demonstrated by a carefully controlled experiment (Hagberg et al, 1983). This did not seem to be due to changes in body weight.

Other Risk Factors

Juvenile diabetes mellitus and type A behavior are also considered to be independent risk factors. The increased sense of time urgency, competitiveness, and increased drive to achieve typical of type A behavior are difficult to assess in young children. One method of assessment that has been tried is to ask parents to answer the type A behavior questionnaire for adults relative to their children (Nora, 1980).

Obesity and hypertriglyceridemia have not been definitely established as independent risk factors. However, their presence suggests that other factors likely to increase the risk of IHD will be present. The Bogalusa (Webber et al, 1979) and Muscatine (Lauer et al, 1975) studies have shown a correlation between obesity and hypertension, and between obesity and serum cholesterol levels in children. In the Muscatine study, of those children above the 90th percentile for

Table 16–3   Children with clustering of three risk-factor variables at or above the 75th percentile by race, sex, and year of examination[a]

	1973–1974		1976–1977		1978–1979	
Race and sex	Total number	High-risk number (%)[b]	Total number	High-risk number (%)[b]	Total number	High-risk number (%)[b]
White						
Male	1133	43 (3.8)	1026	40 (3.9)	946	40 (4.2)
Female	1025	29 (2.8)	965	27 (2.8)	909	26 (2.9)
Black						
Male	661	18 (2.7)	543	15 (2.8)	516	12 (2.3)
Female	604	24 (4.0)	540	9 (1.7)	505	18 (3.6)

Source: Adapted from GS Berenson et al: Cardiovascular risk factors in children. *Am J Dis Child* **136**:855, 1982. Copyright 1982, American Medical Association. Reprinted with permission.

[a] Ages ranged from 5 to 14 yrs.

[b] Children in the 75th percentile for diastolic BP, total cholesterol level, and a weight-for-height index (on serial evaluations) were considered high risk. The percentage of high-risk children (1.56% expected) tended to increase with age, particularly for white boys.

weight, 18 percent were above the 90th percentile for serum cholesterol, 29 percent had systolic blood pressures above the 90th percentile, with a similar percentage having elevated diastolic pressures above the 90th percentile. It seems therefore that clustering of risk factors occurs (Table 16–3). Obesity is of particular importance in view of its association with hypertension and adult-onset diabetes mellitus. Obesity may be prevented by appropriate dietary habits and a reasonable amount of exercise.

Intervention

The rationale for instituting preventive measures in pediatric populations is based largely on evidence from epidemiologic data and on studies that must be regarded as incomplete in view of the multifactorial nature of the disease and the prolonged time course of its development. More definitive statements concerning the effects of risk factor intervention in childhood on the eventual development of atherosclerosis and its resultant symptoms cannot be made at present. The longitudinal studies required to confirm beneficial effects on free-living initially pediatric populations are probably not feasible. Such studies in adult populations are in progress. At present, the epidemiologic data on the association of risk factors with disease and the beneficial effects of specific interventions on individual risk factors such as hypertension, cigarette smoking, and elevated serum cholesterol are sufficiently consistent to justify risk factor intervention in childhood.

Three concepts are important when considering intervention for athero-sclerosis in the pediatric years:

1. The risk of developing IHD increases as the number of risk factors present in an individual increases.
2. The risk of developing IHD increases with an increase in the severity of the risk factor.
3. Although one would prefer to eliminate or decrease the severity of a risk fac-tor, a significant decrease in risk may be achieved by preventing an increase in the risk factor with age.

To illustrate the third point, a 10-year-old child with a total serum cholesterol of 212 mg/dl would be on the 95th percentile for his age (Berenson et al, 1982). If by intervention this level could be maintained into adulthood (i.e., further in-crease prevented), by age 30 years, a total cholesterol level of 212 mg/dl would now fall between the 50th and 75th percentiles, resulting in a lower risk than if tracking had occurred. Intervention should therefore be directed at (1) prevent-ing and eliminating risk factors and (2) decreasing the severity of risk factors, which includes the prevention of tracking to higher risk values over time (Fig. 16–5). For the whole pediatric population, intervention should be directed toward adaptation to an appropriate life-style, that is, appropriate diet, exer-cise, and other measures. In addition to these general recommendations, the high-risk group may require pharmacologic intervention to lower their blood pressure or total serum cholesterol. Nora (1980) has developed a questionnaire and scoring system based on analysis of a study of early-onset IHD to identify children at increased risk (Tables 16–4 through 16–6). A child who has a family history of a first-degree relative with IHD before age 55 years would start with a score of 3 points. Should this child also smoke, his score would increase to 4.5 points, and his risk of future IHD would increase to six times that of the general population.

Is Intervention Effective?

Short-term studies have been undertaken to evaluate the efficacy of educational programs directed to children on knowledge of, and behavior toward IHD and probable IHD-producing behaviors. Attempts at modifying attitudes of chil-dren toward IHD are hindered by many problems. One of the more significant problems is the fact that adherence to healthy habits may require the child or adolescent to go against the prevalent behavior patterns of his or her peer group. A second significant problem is that, since the goal is to prevent a disease that may not manifest itself until 30 to 50 years in the future, the risk is not per-ceived by children or adolescents as an immediate one. Perhaps this explains why educational programs for IHD have been less successful than similar pro-grams geared toward problems such as teenage pregnancy and drug use, which are much more immediate consequences of risky behaviors. A third major prob-

Table 16–4 Questionnaire for children and adolescents aged 1–19 years to use in heart attack risk formula

---

The following information can be obtained when a child is as young as 1 to 2 years.

1. Has a first-degree relative (parent or sibling) had a heart attack or coronary disease with onset before age 55?
2. Has a first-degree relative had a heart attack or coronary disease with onset before age 65?
3. Has a second-degree relative had a heart attack or coronary disease with onset before age 65?
4. Is the cholesterol level greater than 220 mg/dl on two tests?
5. Is the cholesterol level greater than 190 mg/dl on two tests?
6. Are the triglycerides higher than 120 mg/dl on two tests?
7. Does the child or a first-degree relative have juvenile-onset diabetes?
8. Is the relative weight greater than 1.20?

The following information will be obtainable as early as 5 years and as late as 19 years.

1. Is the blood pressure tracking at the 95th percentile or 140/90 mm Hg or higher?
2. Does the child show excessive type A behavior?
3. Does the child get daily, vigorous exercise some of which is aerobic?
4. Does the child smoke?

Source: From JJ Nora, 1980, with permission.

lem is that successfully modifying a given child's habits necessitates also modifying the habits of his or her siblings and parents.

Interventions in children have often been successful in increasing knowledge and modifying attitudes, but have not been very successful in changing behavior patterns (Casper et al, 1977). Goldberg et al (1980), in an intervention program in Arizona carried out in school over a 3-year period, demonstrated increased knowledge of atherosclerosis in the intervention group. However, no difference was found between the control and intervention groups when the prevalence and severity of risk factors were compared for both groups. The risk factors studied included cholesterol level, blood pressure, and obesity. Coates and co-workers in the Heart Healthy Program (Coates et al, 1981) were able to change the dietary habits of a group of fourth and fifth graders at their school mealtimes; these changes persisted over the summer vacation of these students. Significantly, changes were detected in the dietary habits of family members, although this was detected by telephone interview and may therefore not have been accurate. This program did, however, involve family members and utilize a reward system, and these aspects probably contributed to its effecting dietary changes. The follow-up period was short (4 months), and it remains to be seen whether the changes will be maintained by the students and families.

Some promising results have recently been reported on the impact of training adolescents to resist social pressure to smoke cigarettes, particularly when student peer leaders were used in the learning process. Three studies have used intervention and control schools in quasi-experimental designs. Hurd et al

Table 16–5   Scoring system for the Risk Index

Risk Index factors	Circle and add points
Family history (take the single highest value, maximum score is 3)	
Coronary disease in first-degree relative before age 55	3.0
Coronary disease in first-degree relative before age 65	2.5
Coronary disease in second-degree relative before age 65	1.0
Stroke in first-degree relative before age 55	1.0
Stroke in second-degree relative before age 65	0.5
Cholesterol and triglycerides (add values to a maximum score of 2)	
Cholesterol greater than 220 mg/dl	2.0
Cholesterol greater than 190 mg/dl	1.0
Triglycerides greater than 220 mg/dl	0.5
Other risks (add all values)	
Smoking regularly	1.5
Diabetes in patient or juvenile diabetes in first-degree relative	1.0
No regular aerobic exercise	1.0
Blood pressure greater than 140/90 mm Hg or systolic or diastolic pressure greater than 95th percentile	0.5
Relative weight greater than 1.20 (>20% overweight)	0.5
Type A behavior	0.5

Source: From JJ Nora, 1980, with permission.

(1980) found that students at school IV who were given all of a social pressures training program, the use of peer leaders, monitoring by questionnaire, and salivary thiocyanate estimation, as well as the opportunity to make a verbal commitment (which was videotaped) had a lesser increase in the frequency of

Table 16–6   Risk scores and increased risks of early-onset coronary heart disease

Risk score	Increased risk
3.0	2×
3.5	3×
4.0	5×
4.5	6×
5.0	15×
5.5	Not calculable by present methods

Source: From JJ Nora, 1980, with permission.

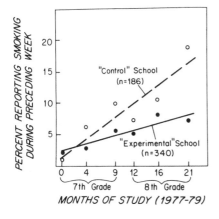

Figure 16–8 Changes in the reported prevalence of weekly smoking from longitudinal observation of seventh- and eighth-grade students of two schools. From A McAlister et al: *Am J Public Health* **70**:719, 1980, with permission.

regular smoking as compared to schools I and II (control schools) or school III (similar to school IV but peer leaders were not used).

A similar study, emphasizing skills in coping with social pressures to seventh- and eighth-grade students, found that students in the experimental school reported a lower prevalence of smoking over the subsequent 21 months (McAlister et al, 1980) (Fig. 16–8). Perry and colleagues (1980) also showed reductions in smoking over 6 months when they emphasized the *immediate* physiologic effects of smoking and educated tenth graders regarding social pressures and how to cope with them.

A communitywide multifactorial intervention effort in North Karelia, Finland, has been under way now for more than a decade. It involved not only adults but also children (Puska et al, 1982). As described in chapter 17, the intervention used not only mass-educational and small-group sessions, but also involved industry and commerce. A special focus on 13- to 15-year-old children involved two schools where more intensive education and behavioral change was attempted with regard to smoking, dietary change, and exercise. This program involved older peer leaders teaching skills to resist social pressures to smoke. School lunches were changed in a more healthful direction with the cooperation of the food industry. Parent gatherings, written recommendations, posters, and a project magazine were also used. Other children in North Karelia were also exposed to a less intensive intervention as part of the countrywide project. Two other schools in North Karelia and two schools in a nearby county were chosen as controls.

The resulting changes in risk factors generally favored the intensive-intervention schools compared with either pair of control schools. However, the results need to be interpreted with caution, as pointed out by the authors. The schools chosen were not necessarily comparable with respect to confounding variables, although a socioeconomic match was attempted. There is no assurance that the schools in either North Karelia or the reference county fairly represented all children in these counties. Nevertheless, the program was judged economically feasible, and the outcome was encouraging.

In spite of the decreasing IHD mortality, atherosclerosis and its complications are still the main cause of death in this country. Intervention has so far been primarily directed at adults, yet because of this high mortality and morbidity from atherosclerosis, our efforts should be directed at intervening at the earliest possible age to attempt to prevent the disease more effectively. At this time there is no conclusive proof that childhood interventions as outlined here will prevent the disease, but the evidence is highly suggestive and there are no obvious risks associated with the interventions. Certainly an appropriate diet, avoidance of smoking, and reasonable exercise will not harm our children, but will make them look and feel better and possibly live better, longer, more productive, and more active lives.

17

Community-Based, Multiple Risk Intervention Studies

The need for intervention studies to support a causal hypothesis has already been discussed. In observational studies there is always the possibility that the true cause is not the variable being measured, but one closely associated with that variable. This could result in a statistical association between the variable measured and the disease outcome that is spurious from a causal viewpoint. An intervention study has the potential to strengthen a causal inference as well as to answer the practical question: "Does the intervention on the measured variable affect risk of ischemic heart disease?" Most of the intervention studies we have discussed so far involved either small groups of persons in "metabolic ward"-type experiments or groups of persons gathered from sources suiting the investigator's expediency (e.g., patients attending a clinic).

Causal factors, as well as the effectiveness of interventions, may differ in different subgroups of a community. This highlights the possibility of drawing false conclusions when extrapolating results from small groups to all individuals at risk in a community. One alternative is to assess the effects of an intervention in a whole population, then search for subgroups that show a greater or lesser responsiveness. But an intervention can be successful only to the degree that the target population chooses to comply. So a second reason for community studies is to evaluate compliance in the entire population and in subgroups. Such subgroups might represent males, females, different age groups, racial groups, and social classes. A third reason for community studies in preventive cardiology has to do with the theory behind behavioral-change endeavors. Social learning theory predicts that social pressures to conform exert a powerful influence on our behavior. Thus, if the attitudes and behavior of large segments of a community could be changed, this would exert pressure on others to change also in the direction recommended.

In this chapter we consider two study designs, the first of which is intervention studies of representative samples from whole communities or large segments of communities. Often the population of interest is all persons in a community with elevated values of the risk factors in question. Individuals are randomly assigned to intervention or control groups. These are true randomized controlled trials. Second, we will consider intervention studies where a *whole* community is the experimental unit being targeted by the mass media or public health agencies, or both. This often limits the study to two or to a few large experimental units, to serve as intervention or control, rather than the minimum 30–50 smaller units (individuals) usually required to make randomization effective in the typical experiment. This design is called quasi-experimental, as the matching of intervention and control units is inevitably only approximate with such small numbers, despite attempts to choose two communities that are as comparable as possible. Any perceived differences could theoretically be adjusted for in the analysis, but the design has the weakness that unthought-of differences between the communities may be present and could influence the frequency of the outcome measures. An additional problem of all large intervention studies is their expense.

Intervention on Diet and Smoking in Oslo, Norway

During 1972–1973, all men in Oslo, Norway, between 40 and 49 years of age were invited for coronary risk factor screening (Hjerman et al, 1981). A total of 65 percent (16,202) responded, and of these, 1232 were selected as fulfilling the criteria of being in the upper quartile of the coronary risk distribution, having serum cholesterol values between 290 and 380 mg/dl, and being relatively normotensive (mean of two systolic pressures less than 150 mm Hg). Another criterion was a normal resting electrocardiogram and no chest pain on exercise. These criteria found a high-risk group whose elevated risk was not due to hypertension or an abnormal electrocardiogram. Thus, they were ideally suited to a dietary and smoking reduction intervention. The men were randomly allocated to either a dietary and smoking intervention group ($n = 604$) or a control group ($n = 628$). The two groups were comparable at baseline with respect to all variables documented, including the traditional risk factors.

A physician spoke to each man in the intervention group individually for 10 to 15 minutes about the risk factor concept and the purpose of the study. A dietitian at baseline obtained a dietary record and gave individualized dietary advice. The recommendations consisted of lowering intake of foods high in saturated fats, slightly increasing foods high in polyunsaturated fats, and increasing dietary fiber. For those also with elevated triglycerides, reducing total calorie consumption was advocated. Individualized advice was given to smokers about quitting smoking; the importance of this was especially emphasized if their lipid levels were very high. Wives of participants were also given dietary and smoking information in group sessions. Every 6 months, the men in the intervention group were reexamined, blood cholesterol was measured, and dietary and cigarette smoking information was obtained. Control subjects were examined each year.

After 5 years the diets of a random half of the intervention group were assessed by estimating the percentage of subjects using various dietary items. As expected, those showing the greatest reductions in serum cholesterol had implemented the larger changes in dietary saturated fats. Over 5 years there was a sustained 25- to 30-mg/dl difference in serum cholesterol levels between the intervention and control groups, and also an average reduction of about five cigarettes per day in the intervention group.

Among the effects of these dietary and smoking interventions was a statistically significant 46 percent reduction in IHD events (Fig. 17–1). Total mortality was 32 percent lower in the intervention group, but this was not statistically significant given the moderate numbers of deaths observed. As there were two interventions involved (diet and smoking cessation), the investigators wished to dissect out the effectiveness of each independently. A multivariate analysis indicated that for the intervention group, both the initial serum cholesterol ($P < 0.05$) and the dietary-induced *changes* in serum cholesterol ($P < 0.01$) were predictive of IHD deaths. The less impressive changes in cigarette smoking could not be shown to have had significant effect on IHD mortality.

This important study demonstrates the following:

1. It is possible to alter dietary habits meaningfully in high-risk middle-aged men with modest effort.

2. These dietary changes are effective at reducing the level of blood cholesterol, which in turn reduces the rate of subsequent IHD events, with no identifiable increase in noncardiovascular mortality.

The Multiple Risk Factor Intervention Trial

The Multiple Risk Factor Intervention Trial (MRFIT) was an enormous effort to test whether simultaneous intervention with regard to diet, blood pressure,

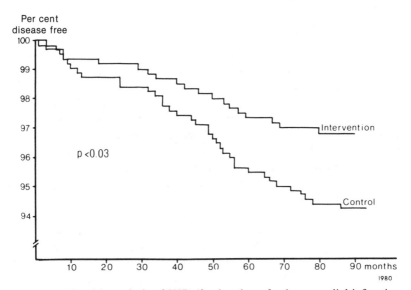

Figure 17–1   Life table analysis of IHD (fatal and nonfatal myocardial infarction and sudden death) in intervention and control groups. From I Hjerman et al, 1981, with permission.

and cigarette smoking protects against IHD mortality in high-risk men (MRFIT Research Group, 1982; Neaton et al, 1981). It was intended not so much to dissect the role of components of the intervention, as to assess the influence of the whole. Serum cholesterol levels were to be decreased by diet; hypertension was treated by drugs and also by weight loss; cigarette smoking was to be reduced. The follow-up period was 6 years. There were 22 clinical centers, a coordinating center, an ECG center, and a laboratory center involved. To find the study population, 366,287 men were screened, and over three sequential visits a group of 12,866 men aged 35–57 years were identified as being at high risk according to the Framingham Risk Equation. These were the men who were randomly assigned to special intervention (SI) or usual care (UC). This number was that calculated as necessary to give sufficient statistical power to detect the predicted effect, under assumptions mentioned below as to the degree of intervention. As in the HDFP Study (chapter 20) the UC group was not a true control group because these participants were sent back to their own physicians to receive care. Thus, it was also possible that subjects in this usual-care group would change both diet and smoking under their own motivation. All participants were told initially that they were at high risk of developing IHD.

The intervention was organized according to a fairly traditional medical model. Specialists in behavioral change, dietitians, nurses, physicians, and administrators were involved in most centers. There were initial group educational and therapeutic sessions, but most of the study follow-up was done through clinic visits. The participants visited a physician at least once each 4 months and saw other therapists such as nutritionists and smoking intervention specialists as required.

It was assumed that the special-intervention group would achieve a 10 percent reduction in serum cholesterol if baseline cholesterol was greater than 220 mg/dl (this was so for most participants), and a 10 percent reduction in diastolic blood pressure if it was 95 mm Hg or higher at baseline, while cholesterol and blood pressure would not change in the usual-care group. It was also assumed that cigarette smoking would decline in both the UC and SI groups, but more so in the former. A problem soon arose. The usual-care group was changing also—always in the same direction as the intervention group, and more than expected. This may be explained by the educational effects of the screening process and the yearly examination, but it was probably also partly a result of changes in dietary and smoking habits in American society as a whole. This dilution of the experimental effect made it more difficult to find statistically significant differences between the two groups.

About 64 percent of the intervention group were identified as hypertensive at some time during the study. Most of them were put on drug therapy, using a stepped-care approach similar to that of the HDFP study (see chapter 20). As for the HDFP study, blood pressure dropped in both the SI and UC groups (Table 17–1). However, in MRFIT the expected difference between the two groups was not achieved, largely because of changes in the UC group.

Table 17–1 Mean diastolic blood pressure change for SI and UC participants by month of follow-up

Follow-up visit (months)	Mean change (mm Hg)		Observed SI–UC difference	Expected SI–UC difference	Observed/ expected ratio
	Special intervention	Usual care			
12	− 6.3	− 2.6	− 3.8	− 7.2	0.53
24	− 8.6	− 4.0	− 4.6	− 6.6	0.69
36	− 9.0	− 4.6	− 4.4	− 6.0	0.74
48	− 9.4	− 5.2	− 4.2	− 5.4	0.77

Source: Adapted from JD Neaton et al: *Prev Med* **10**:519, 1981, with permission.

Dietary intake was reported regularly by the participants, using the 24-hour recall method. The changes in fat intake were all in the anticipated direction. Nutrition goals for the intervention group were saturated fat = 10 percent of calories, polyunsaturated fat = 10 percent of calories, total fat = 35 percent of calories, dietary cholesterol < 300 mg/day. Later in the study, this was changed to saturated fat = 8 percent of calories and dietary cholesterol < 250 mg/day. Consistent differences were soon established between the SI and UC groups for nutrient consumption, and the nutrition goals apparently came close to being achieved (Table 17–2). Notice that the UC group also made some minor changes, always in the more "healthful" direction. The changes in serum cholesterol for the SI group, however, were less than those predicted from the dietary changes, and less than the goal requirements (Table 17–3). The 8.4-mg/dl difference between the two groups at 48 months finally shrank to a 4.8 mg/dl difference at 6 years (MRFIT Research Group, 1982).

The poor serum cholesterol response in the SI group (about 50 percent of that predicted from the dietary change) is due probably to a combination of factors. Possibilities include (1) erroneous dietary reporting, with participants indicating changes more favorable than in truth occurred, (2) changed dietary habits in the 24 hours before appointments, leading to an atypical 24-hour recall result, and finally (3) the concurrent effect of diuretic medications tending to elevate serum cholesterol (chapter 20).

The cigarette smoking quitting rate of 40–45 percent in the SI group is by contrast a success story. Although the self-reported percentage of smokers in the UC group dropped from 64 to 48 percent, the drop in the SI group was a greater 64 to 34 percent, and so the goal difference between the SI and UC groups was achieved (Fig. 17–2). Serum thiocyanate levels were measured and used to adjust the reported smoking rates to what was probably a closer approximation of the truth, and the goal difference persisted (Fig. 17–2). It was noted that the heaviest smokers had more trouble quitting (Neaton et al, 1981).

Table 17-2 Means of selected nutrients for SI and UC participants by month of follow-up

	Special intervention[a]	Usual care[b]
Total calories		
Screen 3	2497.2	2478.7
12 Months	1990.1	2310.2
24 Months	1948.9	2311.1
36 Months	1955.2	2325.3
Total fat (% total calories)		
Screen 3	38.3	38.2
12 Months	33.9	38.1
24 Months	33.9	38.0
36 Months	33.8	38.0
Saturated fatty acids (% total calories)		
Screen 3	14.0	14.0
12 Months	10.1	13.7
24 Months	10.1	13.7
36 Months	10.0	13.5
Polyunsaturated fatty acids (% total calories)		
Screen 3	6.4	6.4
12 Months	8.8	6.5
24 Months	8.6	6.6
36 Months	8.7	6.7
Dietary cholesterol (mg/day)		
Screen 3	454.4	448.2
12 Months	264.6	422.0
24 Months	262.1	423.5
36 Months	264.7	429.3

Source: Adapted from JD Neaton et al: *Prev Med* **10**:519, 1981, with permission.

[a] The entries for screen 3 and 12, 24, and 36 months are based on 6421, 6098, 5967, and 5825 participants, respectively.

[b] The entries for screen 3 and 12, 24, and 36 months are based on 6426, 6070, 5906, and 5766 participants, respectively.

Assuming that the relationship between risk factor levels and risk is a dynamic process, it is possible, using the Framingham Equation, to estimate the relative risk (approximated by relative odds) of the UC compared to the SI group. This ratio did not achieve the design goal (Fig. 17–3), thus resulting in decreased power to find a statistically significant difference in the IHD event rates.

The results of this large study are disappointing in that they did not reject the possibility of no IHD or total mortality difference between the two groups of

Table 17–3 Mean serum cholesterol change for SI and UC participants by month of follow-up

Follow-up visit (months)	Mean change (mg/dl)		Observed SI–UC difference	Expected SI–UC difference	Observed/ expected ratio
	Special intervention	Usual care			
12	−15.5	−7.0	−8.5	−19.0	0.45
24	−15.8	−7.5	−8.3	−17.4	0.47
36	−17.1	−9.6	−7.5	−15.8	0.48
48	−18.6	−10.2	−8.4	−14.2	0.59

Source: Adapted from JD Neaton et al: *Prev Med* **10**:519, 1981, with permission.

high-risk men, despite the multidisiplinary intervention. Although a possible interpretation is that the intervention had no benefit, it is also true that the study design was finally inadequate to test the hypothesis. There were three major problems (MRFIT Research Group, 1982): (1) the unanticipated favorable changes in the usual-care group, (2) the less than anticipated reduction in serum cholesterol, and (3) one major subgroup may have reacted adversely to the intervention: men who were hypertensive and also had an abnormal resting electrocardiogram at baseline. These men showed a 65 percent *greater* IHD mortality than the UC group, and this may account for the apparently poor response in hypertensives overall. In fact, for those hypertensive men with a normal electrocardiogram at baseline there was a 24 percent lower IHD mortality in the SI group. Similarly, nonhypertensive men with an abnormal electrocardiogram showed an 18 percent lower IHD mortality. The abnormalities

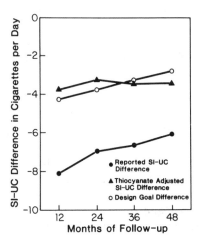

Figure 17–2 SI–UC difference in cigarettes per day compared with design goal. From JD Neaton et al: *Prev Med* **10**:519, 1981, with permission.

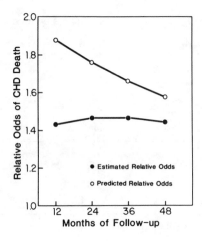

Figure 17–3 Estimated relative odds of IHD death according to actual and predicted risk factor profiles. From JD Neaton et al: *Prev Med* **10**:519, 1981, with permission.

present on the electrocardiograms of the men who apparently reacted adversely, consisted mainly of tall R waves or intraventricular conduction defects not directly indicating ischemia. The mechanism of this possible adverse response is not known although a recent British randomized study of mild hypertensives has demonstrated a significant increase in ventricular ectopy among those allocated to thiazide therapy (Greenberg et al, 1984).

Results in other subgroups were close to or exceeded the 22.2 percent lower IHD mortality for the SI group, predicted by the Framingham Equation: observed SI rates were 21 percent lower for all nonhypertensives and 49 percent lower for hypercholesterolemic nonhypertensives (similar to the population of the Oslo Diet Study—see above). Over 90 percent of the participants performed a standardized submaximal, Bruce Protocol stress test (Multiple Risk Factor Intervention Trial Research Group, 1985). Among the approximately one-eighth of each group showing ischemic ST changes at study baseline, there was highly suggestive evidence of benefit from the intervention with only 17 IHD deaths in this ST group compared to 38 in the UC group. Analysis of such subgroups has dangers in that it involves testing hypotheses that were not previously determined and may have been suggested by the data. Consequently, traditional statistical tests could not be used for these comparisons.

Interventions on Whole Communities

The Stanford Three-Community Study was designed to investigate the feasibility and effectiveness of intervening on risk factors in whole communities (Farquhar et al, 1977). The end points were changes in risk factors rather than disease events. Reasoning that interventions aimed only at high-risk persons miss much preventive potential, the investigators directed their efforts to whole communities. They emphasized health education through mass media and also the application of social learning theory (Bandura, 1977).

Farquhar and colleagues selected three somewhat similar small towns in northern California: Watsonville, Gilroy, and Tracy. Tracy did not share the mass media of the other two communities and acted as a control community in this quasi-experimental design. Health education campaigns were carried out in Watsonville and Gilroy. The hope was that the "ideals" of the whole communities could be shifted so that a citizen's reference group would become supportive of change (Maccoby and Farquhar, 1975; Maccoby et al, 1977). At Watsonville only, some high-risk individuals were offered intensive instruction in small groups (Watsonville Intensive Intervention Group) dealing with cigarette smoking, physical inactivity, poor dietary habits, and methods of making changes. The rest of Watsonville and all of Gilroy were reached only through the mails and mass media intervention (mailing of booklets and cookbooks, publishing of newspaper articles, airing of public services announcements and educational programs on radio and TV). Risk status and health habits were ascertained by surveying random samples of all three communities before the intervention began, and again in two annual follow-up surveys of the same samples. One problem was that only 62–74 percent of these samples participated in both the first and last surveys, so that some bias is possible.

The results (Farquhar et al, 1977; Stern et al, 1976) were reported as changes from the values ascertained at baseline (Fig. 17–4). Changes in knowledge of risk factors, diet, and blood pressure control in Gilroy and Watsonville were greater than in Tracy, the control community. Overall risk status (using the Framingham Risk Equation) was reduced by more than 23 percent. This was accomplished by mass media alone, and even more impressive changes were seen in the Watsonville Intensive Intervention Group.

The somewhat similar study carried out in the county of North Karelia, Finland, had an interesting origin. Epidemiologic evidence had consistently indicated that the highest mortality from ischemic heart disease in the world occurred in east Finland. Faced with this problem, representatives of the 180,000 inhabitants of the county of North Karelia asked the government for assistance. The North Karelia Project was the response. Beginning in 1972, it was a comprehensive 5-year effort to investigate the feasibility of changing health-related behavior, clearly with the hope of reducing disease in the community, although the study was not optimally designed to demonstrate this last result. The investigators deliberately avoided singling out high-risk citizens for intervention; instead, the problem was conceived of as communitywide and the "life-style" of the *community* was the focus.

A baseline survey of risk factors in North Karelia and in a neighboring reference county, Kuopio, was carried out in 1972. Similar surveys were repeated in both counties 5 and 10 years later, to assess risk factor changes. The baseline data confirmed the poor risk profiles of these citizens: 52 percent of North Karelians aged 25–59 years were cigarette smokers; the mean serum cholesterol was about 270 mg/dl, and the mean casual blood pressure about 150/92 mm Hg,

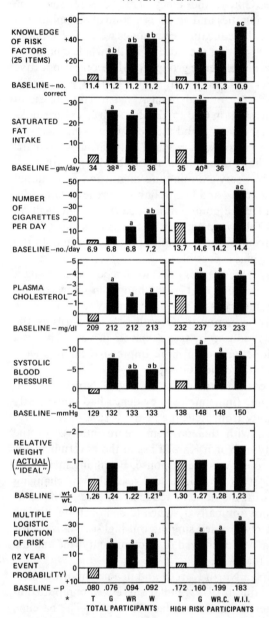

PERCENT CHANGE FROM BASELINE AFTER 2 YEARS

Figure 17–4 Absolute baseline values and percentage change in selected variables after 2 years in control (shaded) or treatment (dark) group. a, $P < 0.05$ for differences in baseline percentage change of control vs. treatment; b, $P < 0.05$ for differences in percentage change within treatment G vs. W (total) or WR; c, $P < 0.05$ for differences in percentage change within treatment WR C vs. W.I.I. T, Tracy; G, Gilroy; WI.I., Watsonville Intensive Intervention group (2/3 of high-risk group); W, total Watsonville participant; WR.C, randomly selected 1/3 of Watsonville high-risk participants not having intensive intervention; WR, A statistical treatment of Watsonville results to estimate the effect of mass media alone in this community. From JW Farquhar et al, 1977, with permission.

246

Table 17–4 Effect of intervention on mean levels of risk factors of IHD in North Karelia[a]

	North Karelia			Reference county			Net reduction (%)[b]	
Risk factor	1972	1977	1982	1972	1977	1982	1972–1977	1972–1982
Men								
Systolic BP (mm Hg)	149	143	145	146	146	147	3	3
Diastolic BP (mm Hg)	92	89	87	93	93	89	3	1
Hypertensives on therapy (%)	13	45	—	14	33	—		
Cigarettes (number per day)	10.0	8.5	6.6	8.5	8.5	7.8	15	28
Serum cholesterol (mg/dl)	274	259	243	266	262	243	4	3
Women								
Systolic BP (mm Hg)	153	142	142	148	144	144	5	5
Diastolic BP (mm Hg)	93	87	85	92	89	85	4	1
Hypertensives on therapy (%)	30	68	—	33	53	—		
Cigarettes (number per day)	1.1	1.1	1.7	1.2	1.3	1.9	9	14
Serum cholesterol (mg/dl)	270	255	239	262	251	232	1	1

Source: Adapted from P Puska et al: *Br Med J* **287**:1840, 1983b, with permission.

[a] Persons aged 30–59 at the time of each survey.

[b] All changes statistically significant except smoking and serum cholesterol in women, this being true for both follow-up periods.

with 34 percent having diastolic pressures greater than 95 mm Hg (Puska et al, 1979; Salonen et al, 1981; Tuomilehto et al, 1980). The intervention was broadly based and used existing public health and medical personnel and facilities, with some reorganization. Information was conveyed to the public by radio, newspapers, leaflets, and posters, as well as at schools and workplaces. Smoking restrictions were enforced, sales of low-fat dairy and meat products were promoted, and vegetable production was encouraged. This entailed considerable interaction with the food industry. To support the program, much effort went into the training of health personnel, teachers, and community leaders. Table 17–4 shows the results of these efforts over 5 and 10 years. Small but meaningful gains were made in hypertension control, serum cholesterol levels (in men), and cigarette smoking (in men). Thus, this study also demonstrates the feasibility of changing the theoretical IHD risk of a whole population.

Salonen and colleagues compared IHD mortality trends in North Karelia to the rest of Finland over 10 years of follow-up (Salonen et al, 1983), using death certificate information. For the whole of Finland, there were 12 and 26 percent reductions in mortality for men and women, respectively. However, for North Karelia, corresponding figures were 24 and 51 percent. This rate of decline was significantly greater than the rest of Finland for both men and women. As compared to the immediately adjacent reference county of Kuopio, the rates of decline were higher in North Karelia, but significantly so only for women.

This does not prove that the intervention accounted for this more rapid change in North Karelia, as the counties were inevitably not comparable at baseline with respect to many characteristics, including IHD mortality. Consequently this quasi-experimental design is not optimal to answer the question of mortality trends, but the results are compatible with the hypothesized effect.

An Industrially Based Study

The World Health Organization enrolled 49,781 men in a randomized trial of multifactorial intervention for IHD (WHO European Collaborative Group, 1980, 1982, 1983). Those men worked at 66 factories in the United Kingdom, Belgium, Italy, and Poland. Rather than individuals, factories were randomized, as it was impossible to intervene on only some individuals at a particular location. Interventions involved posters, brochures, personal letters, progress charts, and group discussions directed toward changes in diet, smoking, weight reduction, exercise, and drug control of "hypertension."

The success of risk factor change seemed to correlate with the ratio of professional staff to patients. Risk factor changes were modest and of the same order as those observed in northern California and North Karelia. Although the overall intervention and control groups were well balanced at baseline, there was considerable variation in both baseline values and risk factor changes for different countries. Changes were most successful in Italy and Belgium and least successful in the United Kingdom and Poland. Over 6 years, differences in IHD events between intervention and control also varied widely between countries but correlated broadly with the degree of risk factor change achieved for that country (the Polish results have not yet been reported). For instance, there was a non-significant 5 percent increase in events with the minimal intervention achieved in the United Kingdom, but a significant ($P < 0.03$) 24 percent decrease in events within the more successful intervention in Belgium (Kornitzer et al, 1983). Results appeared equally encouraging in Italy, but small numbers made significance difficult to achieve.

All these studies leave some important questions unanswered; however, health professionals should be reassured that these interventions appear safe for all. An exception may be thiazides for some (Whelton, 1985). We still do not have final proof that the health of whole communities can be improved by community-wide multifactorial interventions, although risk factors clearly can be changed for the better across major segments of communities. This may surprise some clinicians. There are four studies under way in the United States now that aim to provide further answers: the Minnesota Community Prevention Program (three pairs of intervention and control communities), the Pawtucket Heart Health Program, the Stanford Five-Community Program, and the Pennsylvania County Health Improvement Program. Together, they should furnish valuable information.

Summary

1. It is possible to bring about important changes in dietary habits of high-risk men by appropriate advice, education, and encouragement. The Oslo Study suggests that in hypercholesterolemic, normotensive men with normal resting electrocardiograms, this is effective prevention of IHD. There may also have been some effect of a limited smoking intervention, but the results did not clearly support this in this study.

2. The Multiple Risk Factor Intervention Trial demonstrated the feasibility of substantially altering smoking behavior and of improving the effectiveness of hypertension control measures in high-risk men. This was largely within the context of the usual medical model. Changes in diet and serum cholesterol were more modest but were somewhat in line with the relatively modest dietary goals during much of the study period.

3. The overall MRFIT result could not prove benefit of these interventions in relation to mortality. The result suggests the need for further study of certain subgroups of high-risk men. For most subgroups, reduced mortality of the predicted magnitude was observed (although statistical significance was not achieved). A notable exception was the group of hypertensives with abnormal electrocardiograms at baseline who seemed to react adversely to the intervention. Subgroups appearing to respond particularly well were those with an ischemic treadmill stress test at baseline, and the subgroup of hypercholesterolemic normotensive men with normal resting electrocardiograms at baseline (similar to the subjects of the Oslo study).

4. The Stanford and North Karelia studies have demonstrated the feasibility of changing the risk in whole communities. Other similar studies that will try to decide whether the theoretical health gains are realized have not yet been concluded, but are under way.

5. An industrially based study conducted in four countries found substantial reduction in IHD mortality in the two countries where risk factors were most effectively changed.

18

The Natural History of Ischemic Heart Disease and Surgical Attempts to Change It

It is well established from many follow-up studies that persons who survive a myocardial infarction until hospital discharge have a first-year mortality of 8 to 15 percent (Kuller, 1979; "Prognosis After Myocardial Infarction," 1979). In subsequent years mortality is 3–5 percent, and most deaths (50–60 percent) are sudden. Men who have uncomplicated angina pectoris as the only manifestation of IHD also have a 3–5 percent mortality per year (Weinblatt et al, 1973). By contrast, the Framingham Study has shown that the mortality for women under 60 years of age with only uncomplicated angina pectoris is very low (Kannel and Feinleib, 1972). Most prognostic information after a myocardial infarction relates to those infarctions recognized clinically during the acute phase, yet 11–25 percent of myocardial infarctions are clinically unrecognized (Margolis et al, 1973; Medalie and Goldbourt, 1976a; Rosenman et al, 1967). The Framingham data indicate that these clinically unrecognized infarctions may have a worse outlook as compared to those recognized (Kannel et al, 1979).

Once disease is established, other risk factors are more important than those traditionally considered for primary prevention, and most of these relate to the clinical status of the patient, particularly the impairment of cardiac function caused by the disease. Thus, myocardial pathophysiology becomes the most powerful determinant of subsequent events, although there is evidence that the traditional risk factors remain significant.

Traditional Risk Factors

Several problems emerge when investigating traditional risk factors in post-infarction patients. Two of the classical risk factors can be changed by the infarction. Blood lipids fall for a period of 1 to 2 months before normalizing, and blood pressure may fall permanently, particularly after a severe infarction. So it would not be surprising to find that the association between high blood pressure and subsequent mortality is weakened (see below). People often change their life-style after the onset of symptomatic IHD, yet it may be their previous habits that still determine risk for some time, and they are no longer observable.

The evidence that the level of serum cholesterol is a risk factor after infarction is not entirely consistent, but the larger studies with long-term follow-up usually find that it retains predictive value. The Coronary Drug Project (Schlant et al, 1982) followed 2789 men who had had at least one myocardial infarction 3 months or more before entry to the study. They were aged 30–64 years at intake and were of New York Heart Association functional class I or II (i.e., exercise tolerance normal or symptomatic only on moderate exertion). The follow-up period was for 5 years. A list of 40 variables, the majority noninvasive clinical variables, was studied in relation to mortality. Serum cholesterol emerged as a significant predictor (Table 18–1), and even after adjustment for electro-cardiographic, historical, and physiologic variables, it retained independent significance.

Another large prospective study of men, the Western Collaborative Group Study, also demonstrated a significant relationship between serum cholesterol levels (not measured during hospitalization) and risk of recurrent IHD events (CD Jenkins et al, 1976). Persons experiencing no recurrence showed an average serum cholesterol level of 241.64 mg/dl compared to 254.52 ($P = 0.03$) for those experiencing a recurrence. A study of a large population of persons who were members of the Health Insurance Plan of Greater New York also showed a rela-tionship between serum cholesterol and further events in women, but not in men (Weinblatt et al, 1973).

A Finnish rural population of 1711 men was followed for 15 years, being reexamined each 5 years (Heliovaara et al, 1982). It was possible to divide the cohort into those with no IHD, those with IHD but no history of infarction, and those with a history of infarction. These assessments were made at the beginning of each 5 year period. The interesting result was that the estimated relative risks of coronary death associated with hypercholesterolemia were very similar for all three groups of patients, even though the absolute risks were much higher for the two groups with established disease. These results were

Table 18–1 Five-year percentages of deaths by lipid findings at entry

Serum cholesterol (mg/dl)	Age group	Number of men	Deaths (%)
<250	<55	792	16.8
≥250	<55	799	19.5
<250	≥55	663	22.8
≥250	≥55	535	28.2

Source: Adapted from RC Schlant et al: The natural history of coronary heart disease: Prognostic factors after recovery from myocardial infarc-tion in 2789 men. *Circulation* **66**:401, 1982, by permission of the American Heart Association, Inc.

statistically significant for those with no IHD and those with IHD but no infarction.

The effect of diet on established coronary atherosclerotic lesions is of fundamental interest. A group in Leiden, the Netherlands, has shown in a preliminary report that over a 2-year follow-up of 39 angina patients, there was a highly significant association between serum cholesterol levels and changes in coronary artery luminal diameters (Arntzenius et al, 1983). The patients were placed on a vegetarian diet, and those who had values of serum total cholesterol/HDL cholesterol in a lower range had clearly less progression of coronary atheroma. One-third of these patients showed increased coronary artery diameters on follow-up. Great attention was given to the comparability of angiographic technique at baseline and at 2 years. Scoring was performed by two independent cardiologists and also by computer. The correlations using both scoring systems were almost identical. The National Heart, Lung and Blood Institute's type II study investigated the effect of cholestyramine on coronary lesions with quite similar results and is described in more detail in chapter 20.

Recall that diet not only alters serum cholesterol but has other effects on cardiovascular physiology, particularly platelet function. As yet, few investigators have analyzed platelet function for prognostic value, but Heptinstall and co-workers (1980) report that enhanced platelet reactivity in acute infarction patients predicts a worse outcome during the hospital phase and over the next year. Whether previous diet influences platelet function in the peri-infarction period is unknown.

Because dietary change as secondary prevention is controversial, all the relevant experiments using a control group that could be found are compiled in Table 18–2. Others, comparing dietary adherers to nonadherers could be cited, all suggesting substantial benefit to the dieters, but these may well be biased by the good adherers having a lower initial risk status, as has been found in similar trials of physical activity. The six studies included in Table 18–2 do not have this problem. Starting in 1946, Morrison studied 100 consecutive patients with proven myocardial infarction within the previous 6 months and alternatively assigned them to control or experimental diets. The experimental diet was relatively low in fat and cholesterol. The patients were intensively observed for 3 years, but 8- and 12-year follow-up results were also reported. Although formal matching between the two groups was not attempted, the method of assignment and statistical testing should have allowed for any baseline differences between the two groups. Significantly lower mortality was found among dieters (Table 18.2).

Leren and colleagues conducted a trial involving 412 men aged 30–64 years, who entered the study 1–2 years after a first myocardial infarction. They were randomly allocated to a control diet or an experimental diet low in saturated fat and higher in polyunsaturates. Good matching was achieved with respect to clinical and other risk factors. Detailed counseling and follow-up were performed over a period of 5 years, with a less intensive effort for another 6 years. Serum cholesterol dropped substantially in the dieters. Table 18–3 shows the

Table 18–2 Controlled clinical trials assessing diet as a means of secondary prevention of ischemic heart disease

Study	Design	Number of men Diet	Number of men Control	Years following	Diet[a] TF D	TF C	S D	S C	P D	P C	Serum cholesterol difference	Attack rates Diet	Attack rates Control	P	Syndrome
LM Morrison et al, 1960	Randomized controlled trial	50	50	3 / 8 / 12	60 g	?	(1500 calories 25 mg cholesterol)				? / ? / ?	14% / 44% / 62%	30% / 76% / 100%	0.06 / 0.001 / 0.0001	Death
GA Rose et al, 1965	Randomized controlled trial	28	52	2	50%	33% / 46% (Corn oil gave 29% of calories in dieters)	Two control groups				11%	12/28	15/52	n.s.[b]	Sudden death, definite or probable infarction
London Research Group, 1965	Randomized controlled trial	132	132	3.5	40 g	110 g	(No added P)				6%	4 cases / 27 cases	7 cases / 27 cases	n.s. / n.s.	Probable MI / Definite MI
Medical Research Council Research Committee, 1968	Randomized controlled trial	200	200	4	110 g	120 g	P/S 2:1 cf. 1:6 (80 g soybean in diet)				15%	39 cases	40 cases	n.s.	MI
Bierenbaum et al, 1970	"Controlled" trial	100	100	5	61 g	62 g	12 g	21 g	31 g	7 g	6%	18 cases	25 cases	0.02 (<45 age only, else n.s.)	MI
Leren, 1970	Randomized controlled trial	206	206	11	39%	?	8.5%	?	21%	?	14%	32 / 2 / 79 / 52	57 / 7 / 94 / 53	0.004 / n.s. / 0.097 / n.s.	Fatal reinfarction / CHF death / Total CHD mortality / Sudden death

[a] Where possible, reported as percentage of calories; otherwise in grams. Abbreviations: TF, total fat; S, saturated fat; P, polyunsaturated fat; D, diet group; C, control group.

[b] Not significant.

Table 18–3   Five-year results of a randomized trial of
dietary therapy

	Diet	Control
Number of men at risk	206	206
Fatal myocardial reinfarction	10	23
Sudden death	27	27
Nonfatal myocardial reinfarction	24	31
Major CHD relapses[a]	61	81
Total cardiovascular mortality[b]	38	52
Total mortality[c]	41	55

Source: From P Leren: The Oslo Diet–Heart Study. *Circulation* **42**:935,
1970, by permission of the American Heart Association, Inc.

[a] $P=0.05$.

[b] $P=0.09$.

[c] $P=0.13$.

results after 5 years of intensive intervention. There was a significant advantage
for dieters with regard to major IHD relapses, as well as suggestive differences in
the same direction for total cardiovascular mortality and total mortality.
Results at 11 years still favored the dieting group (Table 18–2), although dietary
assessment and risk factor status were not tabulated beyond 5 years.

The three British studies of Table 18–2 do not show significant differences,
but all had some design problems. One used a very high total fat, high polyunsaturated fat experimental diet, which is not the diet that epidemiologic evidence would favor. There is no natural experience with a diet approaching the
quality of that used in this study. The other two British studies accepted patients
to the study immediately after infarction at a time when powerful determinants
of subsequent events are the hemodynamic and arrhythmic consequences of the
recent infarct. All had relatively short follow-up periods.

Several reports, mostly anecdotal or describing uncontrolled experiments,
suggest that drastic dietary changes may improve symptoms such as frequency
of angina and treadmill performance in cardiac patients. Patients with IHD at
Nathan Pritikin's Longevity Center in California, for instance, have experienced symptomatic benefits and also improved exercise tolerance and marked
improvement in traditional risk factors—all apparently because of the stringent
diet, exercise, and weight loss residential program (Diehl and Mannerberg,
1981). Long-term adherence to the program seemed quite good even after 5
years (Barnard et al, 1983). However, clinical inference is difficult in the absence
of a control group.

Two short-term experimental studies with control groups have investigated
the effects of marked dietary intervention in angina patients where symptomatic

and functional end points were used. Hartley et al (1981) followed patients for 12 weeks, using a high complex carbohydrate, low-fat (less than 15 percent of calories) experimental diet. The reference group had the identical program, but diet was not controlled. Ornish and coinvestigators (1983) followed 46 patients for 24 days, half of whom were randomized to a program of stress management and vegan diet. Both studies found statistically significant improvement in anginal symptoms as well as substantially greater improvement in treadmill performance for the dieting groups.

In summary, much more evidence is needed, but the efficacy of diet in retarding symptoms and reducing events is clearly suggested by several data sets. Most of the studies have small numbers, hence low statistical power, so the number of studies with positive results is impressive.

Cigarette smoking seems well established as a continuing risk factor after infarction. Several investigators have compared quitters to continuing smokers after an infarction. Mulcahy et al (1977) followed 213 patients for 5 years after their first attack of acute coronary insufficiency or myocardial infarction. Of the 190 initial smokers, 89 stopped, 42 reduced, and 59 continued to smoke. Those who continued to smoke had IHD rates twice as high as those who quit (Table 18–4). Similar results come from the Framingham Study (Sparrow et al, 1978). Of 202 cigarette smokers who survived a myocardial infarction, 56 quit and 139 continued to smoke (7, missing data). There were no important baseline differences between these two groups with respect to number of cigarettes smoked, relative weight, blood pressure, serum cholesterol, or percentage with a history of diabetes or angina pectoris. The results showed a significant advantage for the ex-smoker in terms of total mortality and a nonsignificant advantage for reinfarction or IHD death. In a Swedish study of 405 smokers who had experienced one myocardial infarction, 174 continued to smoke and 231 quit

Table 18–4   Effect of cigarette smoking status at 5-year follow-up on CHD and overall mortality, 188 initial smokers (and 2 ex-smokers who resumed)

Cigarette smoking status	Number of cases	CHD deaths		Total deaths	
		No.	%	No.	%
Stopped	89	11	12.4	13	14.6
Reduced	42	6	14.3	6	14.3
Continued	59	17	28.8	17	28.8
Total	190	34	17.9	36	18.9

Source: From R Mulcahy et al: Factors affecting the 5-year survival rate of men following acute coronary heart disease. *Am Heart J* **93**:556, 1977, with permission.

(Wilhelmsson et al, 1975). Over 2 years of follow-up 9 percent of the quitters had a reinfarction, compared with 18 percent of the continuing smokers ($P < 0.05$). Five percent of the quitters died from cardiovascular causes, while 10 percent of the continuing smokers died ($P < 0.05$).

Mulcahy (1983) reviews about eight studies of broadly similar design and finds consistent results that continued smokers on average suffer about twice the mortality after infarction than quitters. Somewhat less information is available to assess risk of reinfarction, but trends appear similar.

There is evidence that smoking aggravates the status of angina patients. Aronow (1978) has shown that even passive smoking precipitated exercise-induced angina earlier. Normal volunteers smoked in ventilated or unventilated rooms. Angina patients exercised in the same room either with the smokers or without, but did not themselves smoke during the study. It took 181 and 146 seconds before angina developed when they were exposed to smoking in ventilated or unventilated rooms, which was 51 and 88 seconds less, respectively, than when not exposed to smoking ($P < 0.001$).

Blood pressure continues to have predictive ability postinfarction, but less impressively than for risk of first onset of IHD (chapter 9). The 5-year follow-up findings from the Coronary Drug Project showed a modest but significant all-cause mortality advantage for postinfarction patients with systolic blood pressures less than 130 mm Hg or diastolic pressures less than 85 mm Hg. A trend persisted but was not clearly significant for cardiovascular mortality (Schlant et al, 1982). The Health Insurance Plan Study (Weinblatt et al, 1973) found an impressive and significant univariate and multivariate advantage for normotensive men, but no such difference between normotensive and hypertensive women who had a previous myocardial infarction or a current diagnosis of angina. Other smaller studies have usually confirmed the continuing importance of blood pressure, at least in men (Luria et al, 1979; Pell and D'Alonzo, 1964).

For Framingham men who survived an infarction, there was no overall relationship between blood pressure after infarction and subsequent survival (Kannel et al, 1980a). However, blood pressure before infarction was distinctly related to survival after infarction. The greater the decrease in pressure post-infarction (no doubt related to the severity of the infarction), the greater the mortality. Excluding those who experienced a reduction of greater than 10 mm Hg, men with hypertension after infarction had a fivefold mortality increase as compared to normotensive men after infarction. The two opposing relationships of higher blood pressures being associated with less myocardial damage, so improving prognosis but also the increased risks associated directly with those higher blood pressures, explain the lack of an overall relationship between blood pressure and mortality in this population.

The evidence that the type A behavior pattern remains a risk factor after myocardial infarction is conflicting. The follow-up results of the Western Collaborative Group Study indicated that in this population of mainly white-collar workers, type A behavior was associated with a significantly increased risk of recurrent IHD events (CD Jenkins et al, 1976). The measuring instrument used in this study was the Jenkins Activity Scale. Those with no recurrence had a mean score of 0.55, compared to 4.39 ($P < 0.005$) for those who suffered IHD recurrence. This remained significant after adjusting for smoking and serum cholesterol. By contrast, recently reported findings from the Aspirin Myocardial Infarction Study (AMIS) did not show any relationship between the risk of recurrent event and type A–B score (Shekelle et al, 1983). Similar negative findings are reported by Ruberman et al (1984) from 2320 males involved in a psychosocial substudy of the β Blocker Heart Attack Trial (BHAT).

Marital status is still an important predictor of both early and late survival after an infarction. Chandra and colleagues (1983) followed 1401 patients with an acute myocardial infarction. In-hospital case fatality was 19.7 and 26.7 percent ($P < 0.05$) for married and unmarried males, respectively, and similarly, 23.3 and 37.4 percent for females ($P < 0.05$). The reasons for this and the relationship to the values of traditional risk factors are unknown.

The recent substudy of BHAT males by Ruberman and colleagues (1984), provided important new information about the impact of social support and stress in the postmyocardial infarction period. They found clear evidence that education was inversely associated with both total mortality and sudden IHD death during a follow-up period spanning three years. Moreover, it was clear from further multivariate analyses that social isolation (such factors as lack of memberships in clubs, church groups, hardly ever visiting friends or relatives in their homes, not asking medical personnel about the need for life changes) and high levels of life stress (such factors as retired but preferred to be working, relatively low-status job as last occupation, patient did not enjoy his work, recent violent assault or family disruption causing patient to be upset) powerfully predicted risk of total or sudden death and probably explained the effect of education. Those with more education were much less likely to be either socially isolated or under high stress. These effects were independent of the presence of ventricular ectopy and an index of myocardial function. The estimate was of a relative risk of death from any cause or sudden IHD death of 4.56 and 5.62, respectively ($P < 0.001$), comparing persons who had both social isolation and high stress to those who had neither. It should be pointed out that these male BHAT participants were not entirely typical of all male post-MI patients as they satisfied the entry criteria for the trial and also that this substudy contained only persons who survived at least 2 to 3 months after the heart attack. It also is not clear whether traditional risk factors such as blood pressure and smoking may explain some of the excess risk associated with these psychosocial variables.

The last of the traditional risk factors that needs to be considered is physical inactivity. As this is a prominent component of most cardiac rehabilitation programs, its role in secondary prevention will be discussed in chapter 19.

Measures of Existing Disease as Predictors of Future Events

It is not surprising that measures of current clinical status of IHD patients are the most powerful predictor of future events. Existing physiologic abnormalities often imply severe underlying disease. The literature relating values of bedside clinical, pathologic, and functional variables to prognosis is vast. As many of these variables cannot be changed by behavioral or other forms of therapy, our discussion will only briefly overview the evidence, focusing first on pathologic, then on physiologic variables, and finally, on indices that combine both.

Pathological Variables as Risk Factors in the Ischemic Heart Disease Patient

It has been demonstrated that anterior infarction has a worse prognosis than posterior or inferior infarction (Davis et al, 1979; Luria et al, 1979). Davis showed that there was about an 84 percent as compared to a 90 percent survival between the two locations at 40 months follow-up.

The severity of coronary artery disease is also known to predict subsequent risk in IHD patients. Most of the information comes from coronary angiographic studies (Bruschke et al, 1973; Detre et al, 1977; Humphries et al, 1974). Bruschke and colleagues followed up 590 consecutive nonsurgical cases of ischemic heart disease. These were persons referred for angiography at the Cleveland Clinic, usually suffering from chest pain. Only those persons with at least 50 percent reduction of luminal diameter in one or more of the major coronary arteries were included in the study. Severity was expressed as the number of vessels with significant lesions. On average, the more severe the obstructive disease, the worse the outlook for survival (Fig. 18–1). Similar findings have

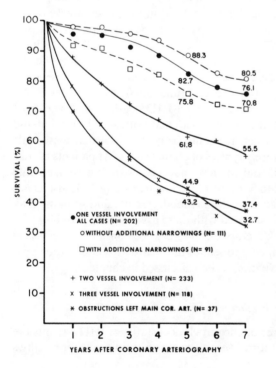

Figure 18–1 Survival curves for individual arteriographic categories. Cases with one-vessel involvement were divided in cases with and without additional moderate (>30 and <50%) narrowings. For cases with one-vessel disease without additional narrowings the survival curve for cardiac death only is also given (interrupted line); in the other cases the influence of noncardiac deaths was practically negligible. Adapted from A Bruschke et al: Progress study of 590 consecutive nonsurgical cases of coronary disease followed 5–9 years. *Circulation* **47**: 1147, 1973, by permission of the American Heart Association, Inc.

been reported from the medically treated groups in large randomized studies comparing medical and surgical treatment of stable angina (European Coronary Surgery Study Group, 1982; Takaro et al, 1976).

The tendency is toward pathologic progression of the disease. Bruschke et al (1981) investigated this over a period ranging up to 6 years using repeated coronary catheterizations. They analyzed an average of about 23 segments of the coronary tree in each of 256 non-surgically treated patients undergoing angiography. The results indicated that the disease progresses in all but a few patients and that the severer the initial disease, the greater the rate of progression (Fig. 18–2). Only 4.7 percent of patients experienced any regression of disease. This, of course, was without any structured intervention on risk factors. The analyses of JR Kramer and colleagues (1983) confirm these findings for both occlusive

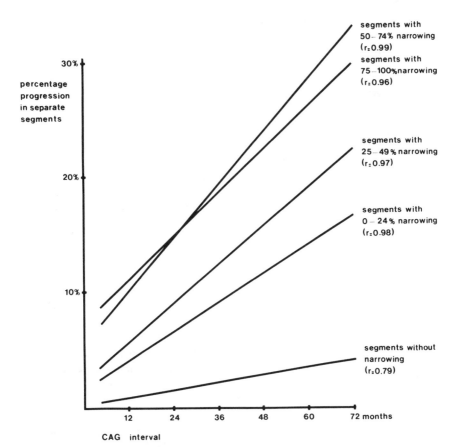

Figure 18–2 Progression in separate segments grouped according to the degree of initial narrowing. CAG, coronary arteriography. From A Bruschke et al: The anatomic evolution of coronary artery disease demonstrated by coronary arteriography in 256 nonoperated patients. *Circulation* **63**:527, 1981, by permission of the American Heart Association, Inc.

and nonocclusive lesions. Interestingly, time was a factor only for degree of nonocclusive progression. The lack of relationship between follow-up time and progression to total occlusion suggests that this often occurs suddenly.

Physiologic Variables as Risk Factors in the Ischemic Heart Disease Patient

Myocardial perfusion as measured by the thallium stress test has excellent ability to predict subsequent events in patients with chronic symptomatic IHD (Silverman et al, 1980; Staniloff et al, 1982). Some find it a better prognostic indicator than coronary angiography (Brown et al, 1983; Gibson et al, 1983).

Another powerful indicator of prognosis is left ventricular function. This can be measured accurately by invasive techniques and can be approximated by many common clinical measurements. Simple clinical observations of cardiac function in the coronary care unit have important predictive value. These include the finding of pulmonary vascular congestion on the chest x-ray film, significant pulmonary rales, pitting edema, a third heart sound, and a history of digitalis or diuretic therapy not given for hypertension (Davis et al, 1979; Helmers and Lundman, 1979). The Coronary Drug Project's 5-year follow-up of 2789 men who had suffered at least one previous myocardial infarction showed that cardiomegaly on the chest roentgenogram, functional status according to the New York Heart Association classification, and diuretic use (usually for heart failure or hypertension) were all among the most powerful predictors of mortality (Schlant et al, 1982). The effects of these variables were independent, each adding a significant amount of new information.

Systolic time intervals correlate significantly with invasively measured ejection fractions. Weissler and colleagues (1981) found that this measure of left ventricular performance in postinfarction patients predicts survival even better than a knowledge of coronary anatomy. An estimate of left ventricular function is also provided by exercise radionuclide ventriculography, which measures the change in left ventricular ejection fraction with submaximal exercise. This differed significantly between groups of post-MI patients defined according to whether or not they experienced major cardiac events on follow-up (Corbett et al, 1981; Multicenter Postinfarction Research Group, 1983). The epidemiologic picture of congestive heart failure from the Framingham Study gave a dismal outlook for these patients with poor left ventricular function (McKee et al, 1971). Sixty-two percent of the men and 42 percent of women were dead within 5 years.

The resting electrocardiograph provides information on myocardial ischemia, electrical instability, and conduction disturbances that has prognostic value. In the medically treated group of the Veterans Administration randomized study of men with stable angina, the variable that predicted 5-year survival best was depression of the ST segment on the resting electrocardiogram probably indicating myocardial ischemia (Detre et al, 1981). Similarly, in the Coronary Drug Project control group of postmyocardial infarction men, ST depression was the most powerful predictor of 5-year survival (Coronary Drug

Project Research Group, 1974). ST changes induced by the stress of exercise on a treadmill or bicycle are also well known predictors of future events. This is so even when testing occurs before discharge after acute infarction (Theroux et al, 1979; Starling et al, 1980; Davidson and DeBusk, 1980). Theroux and colleagues found in 210 consecutive patients that 1-year mortality varied from 2.1 percent to 27 percent according to the presence of ST segment depression ($P < 0.001$). Exercise-induced angina also has prognostic value (Starling et al, 1980). The presence of bundle branch block after infarction, particularly left bundle branch block, is a bad prognostic sign (Woo, 1979).

Electrical instability of the myocardium as indicated by both supraventricular and ventricular arrhythmias is associated with a worse prognosis in the post-myocardial infarction patient. Luria et al (1979) followed 126 such patients for a period of 5 years and found those who had supraventricular ectopic beats, atrial flutter, atrial fibrillation, or other atrial arrhythmias in the coronary care unit suffered higher mortality. They also found that the recording of ventricular ectopic beats (VEB) by 8-hour halter monitor later in the hospital stay had prognostic significance even for rates as low as 0.5 ectopic beats per hour.

Many others have also demonstrated the prognostic importance of such premature ventricular contractions (JW Smith, 1980). The experience of Moss et al (1979), who followed 940 post-MI patients for up to 45 months, is instructive. During the last 3 days of hospitalization, patients had 6 hours of cardiac electrical activity recorded by halter monitor. Ventricular ectopic beats were classified as complex or simple. Complex VEBs included bigeminal and multiform patterns, as well as repetitive ectopics and those showing the R-on-T phenomenon. The results clearly indicated that simple and particularly complex VEBs are associated with a worse prognosis in the presence of established ischemic heart disease (Fig. 18–3). Some have managed to find a relationship between frequency of ventricular ectopic beats and subsequent risk even when the arrhythmias have been those documented only by the brief standard resting ECG (Coronary Drug Project Research Group, 1974).

An interesting subgroup are persons who experience ventricular fibrillation outside the hospital and who are resuscitated. Baum et al (1974) found that those whose ventricular fibrillation was associated with a transmural myocardial infarction had a 2-year mortality of 14 percent. By contrast, the group with no evidence of infarction in association with the cardiac arrest had a 2-year mortality of 47 percent (mostly sudden deaths), presumably because of an electrically unstable myocardium.

There is evidence that left ventricular function, electrical instability, and myocardial ischemia, the major classes of variables discussed above—particularly the first two—tend to be correlated and to some extent measure each other. Despite this, it is clear that all three have some independent effect (Coronary Drug Project Research Group, 1974; Moss et al, 1979).

An interesting analysis of the medically treated stable angina group from the V.A. Cooperative Study of stable angina combined invasive and noninvasive parameters in a risk assessment. It was found that a noninvasive score based on

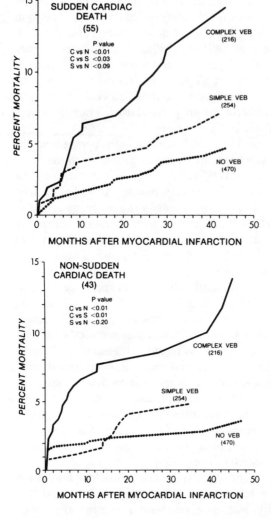

Figure 18–3 Cumulative sudden and nonsudden cardiac mortality for patients with complex (C), simple (S), and no (N) ventricular ectopic beats (VEB). From AJ Moss et al: Ventricular ectopic beats and their relation to sudden and nonsudden death after myocardial infarction. *Circulation* **60**: 998, 1979, by permission of the American Heart Association, Inc.

ST depression in the resting electrocardiogram, history of previous myocardial infarction, history of hypertension, and New York Heart Association functional status predicted outcome independently of (and thus complementary to) an invasive score based on the number of diseased vessels (> 50 percent diameter reduction) and left ventricular dysfunction (Detre et al, 1981). Moreover, the noninvasive score predicted 5-year mortality just as well as the invasive score. Even in patients with significant left main coronary disease, the noninvasive index showed significant ability to discriminate between subgroups with differing prognoses (Takaro et al, 1982). The lack of correlation between visual interpretation of coronary artery stenoses and their physiologic importance is shown by another recent study (White et al, 1984). Two persons with very similar angiographic findings may have different symptomatic, historical, and electrocardiographic characteristics. Functional measures in such patients add significant prognostic information.

Surgical Revascularization as an Attempt to Change the Natural History of Ischemic Heart Disease

Over the last decade, coronary artery bypass grafting has become a common operation. Each year more than 100,000 of these operations are performed in the United States. Many studies have attempted to evaluate the operation as treatment for angina pectoris, as well as its effect on longevity in people with established ischemic heart disease. Most of these studies were not randomized controlled trials, and a comparison of persons placed on medical therapy for clinical reasons may not be fair, as such patients often represent a sicker group not eligible for surgery. Probably the only appropriate investigation is the randomized controlled trial.

There is little doubt that coronary artery bypass grafting is effective symptomatic treatment for stable angina pectoris, and is superior to medical therapy. However, it is expensive and is associated with a small but not negligible morbidity and mortality ("Brain Damage After Open-Heart Surgery," 1982; "Some Consensus on Coronary Bypass Surgery," 1981). The European Coronary Surgery Study Group (1980) investigated 768 patients with stable angina, significant disease in at least two vessels, and good left ventricular function. Half were randomly allocated to surgical therapy and half to medical therapy. The symptomatic results clearly favored surgical therapy (Fig. 18–4).

The recently reported Coronary Artery Surgery Study (CASS) identified 780

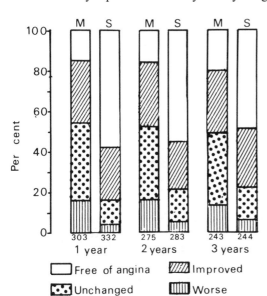

Figure 18–4 Changes in angina pectoris at 1, 2, and 3 years of follow-up in relation to the time of randomization. M, Medical group; S, Surgical group. Number of patients given at bottom of each bar. From European Coronary Surgery Study Group, 1980, with permission.

compliant and eligible patients from 24,959 who underwent coronary angiography at 11 clinical centers in the United States (Fig. 18–5). These were patients with mild angina (not provoked by climbing one flight of stairs or walking two blocks) or well-documented previous myocardial infarction, at least one operable artery with 70 percent reduction of diameter, and ejection fraction of

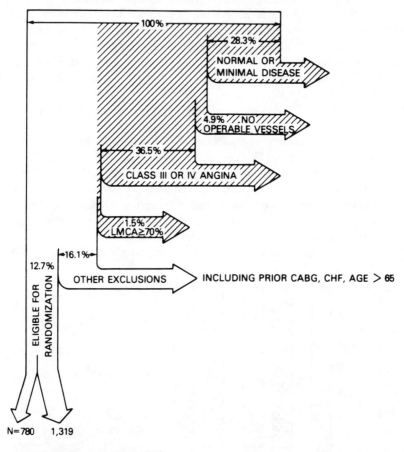

Figure 18–5 Allocation of patients in CASS registry at randomizing sites (*n* = 16,626). Reasons for exclusion of patients from study. LMCA, Left main coronary artery; CABG, coronary artery bypass graft; CHF, congestive heart failure. From CASS principal investigators and associates: Coronary Artery Surgery Study (CASS): A randomized trial of coronary artery bypass surgery. *Circulation* **68**:939, 1983b, by permission of the American Heart Association, Inc.

at least 0.35 (CASS principal investigators and associates, 1983a). Patients with a left main coronary artery stenosis of 50 to 69 percent were also eligible.

Of the 2099 patients eligible for randomization, only the 780 agreed to be randomized. Fortunately, the baseline characteristics and follow-up experience of the randomized and randomizable have been virtually identical, making it unlikely that there were any biases introduced (CASS principal investigators and associates, 1984a). The symptomatic findings, like those of the European Coronary Surgery Study, clearly favored surgery. In addition, the surgical group showed longer duration on follow-up treadmill testing and less ST depression. The use of β-blocking drugs and nitrates was also less in the surgically treated group, although all of these parameters had been comparable between the two groups at baseline.

The CASS also compared the frequency of new Q-wave infarctions among the survivors of the two groups at each time point (CASS principal investigators and associates, 1984b). There was no difference, as shown in Fig. 18–6. This result was unchanged by analyses within subgroups of one, two, or three diseased arteries or with high or low ejection fractions. Other studies have confirmed this result (Rahimtoola, 1982).

The effect of bypass grafting on subsequent mortality in angina patients has received considerable attention, but mostly in nonrandomized studies. The exceptions are the Coronary Artery Surgery Study, the European Coronary Surgery Study, and the Veterans Administration Cooperative Study. The CASS found no definite survival advantage for either the surgically or medically treated groups. Even on extensive subgroup analysis, the two survival curves generally lay very close together. This was true for single-, double-, and triple-

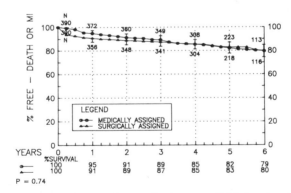

Figure 18–6 Survival and absence of recognized myocardial infarction (MI) in patients with coronary artery disease who were randomly assigned to medical or surgical therapy (life-table method). Probability of remaining alive and free of MI was similar for the two groups. From CASS principal investigators and associates: myocardial infarction and mortality in the Coronary Artery Surgery Study (CASS) randomized trial. Reprinted by permission, *N Engl J Med* **310**:750, 1984b.

vessel disease (Fig. 18–7). The only subgroup that gave some hint of advantage to surgery was where the ejection fraction was less than 0.50. However, this did not quite reach traditional levels of statistical significance and would fall further short of significance if the multiple statistical testing inherent in subgroup analyses is considered. In the European Coronary Surgery Study, stable angina patients who were followed for 5 years had a better survival record after surgery than medical care (Fig. 18–8). Further analyses indicated that much of this advantage accrued to two subsets of patients: those with severe triple vessel disease and possibly those with significant obstruction of the left main coronary artery. Patients with two-vessel disease gained no advantage from surgery, and this study did not include patients with single-vessel disease or severe left ventricular dysfunction.

The Veterans Administration Cooperative Study assigned roughly 680 men to either medical or surgical treatment. These patients had stable angina of at least 6 months' standing, an abnormal resting or exercise electrocardiogram, and at least a 50 percent reduction of luminal diameter of one major coronary artery, with the distal segment suitable for grafting. Patients with recent myocardial infarction, uncontrolled hypertension, or very poor myocardial contractility were excluded. The mortality comparison confirmed the advantage of surgical treatment in patients with significant left main stenosis (Murphy et al, 1977) but like the CASS could not demonstrate a significant advantage of surgery for patients with one-, two-, or three-vessel disease.

The different results for patients with three-vessel disease in the different studies are superficially explained by better survival of the medical group in the CASS and worse survival of the surgical group in the V.A. study, as compared to the European study. It is not clear whether these differences reflect advances in medical therapy in the CASS, poorer surgical techniques during the early years of bypass surgery in the V.A. study, or differences in the characteristics of the patients.

The V.A. Cooperative Study has been criticized for rather high surgical mortality and graft occlusion rates, particularly in the first 2 years (1970–1972). Results during the last 2 years of the study were more acceptable by today's standards. Further analysis of the 91 veterans with significant left main artery disease, who were entered and randomized during these last 2 years of intake, revealed much heterogeneity (Takaro et al, 1982). It was possible to divide them into three risk groups based on noninvasive criteria (New York Heart Association Functional Group, ST depression on the resting electrocardiogram, history of myocardial infarction, history of hypertension). In contrast to coronary angiography, this score will tend to reflect function rather than anatomy. A high noninvasive score includes the combination of all four variables, all combinations of three of these four variables, and also three of the six possible combinations of two of the four variables. A low noninvasive score includes none or one of the four variables but does not include ST depression only.

Surgery markedly improved the prognosis of left main artery disease patients in the high or mid noninvasive risk terciles, but if anything, patients in the low-

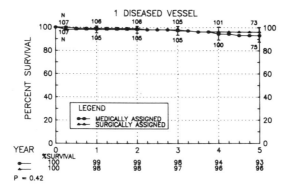

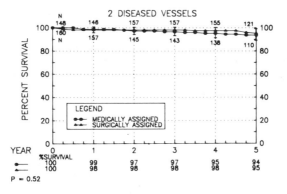

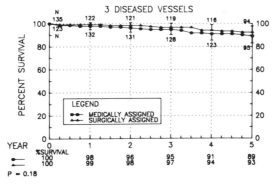

Figure 18–7 Five-year cumulative survival in groups with single-, double-, and triple-vessel disease, with disease being defined as at least 70 percent luminal diameter reduction. From CASS principal investigators and associates: Coronary Artery Surgery Study (CASS): A randomized trial of coronary artery bypass surgery. *Circulation* **68**:939, 1983b, by permission of the American Heart Association, Inc.

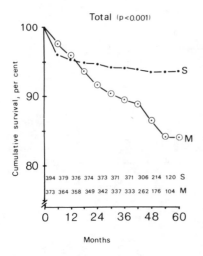

Figure 18–8 Cumulative survival curves for total patient population. M, Medical group; S, Surgical group. Numbers along bottom represent patients at risk at beginning of each 6-month period. Number in parentheses indicates there were six preoperative deaths in the surgical group. From European Coronary Surgery Study Group, 1980, with permission.

risk tercile were slightly worse off (Fig. 18–9). In patients without left main artery disease entered to the study during the latter 2 years of the study, the findings were somewhat similar (Detre et al, 1981). Those in the mid-risk non-invasive tercile did not benefit from surgery, and the low tercile did significantly better with medical therapy. A clear benefit of surgery was seen only in the high tercile of noninvasive risk (Fig. 18–10). The data represented in Fig. 18–10 come from the 10 hospitals with the lowest operative mortality rates (3.3 percent), which should make it more representative of current experience. The apparent advantage of surgery for those with a high noninvasive risk profile may have its counterpart in the CASS, where those with moderate left ventricular dysfunction had a borderline significant advantage with surgery.

Several randomized studies have investigated the effect of coronary artery bypass grafting in unstable angina patients. If the operation takes place when the angina is still unstable, there is no consistent evidence that it improves subsequent rates of mortality or infarction (Bertolasi et al, 1976; National Cooperative Study Group, 1978; Pugh et al, 1978; Selden et al, 1975). However, the numbers of events were small in these studies, and these results cannot answer the question with certainty. Again, most studies have shown a *symptomatic* advantage for the surgical group. One randomized trial investigated the effect of bypass grafting on subsequent mortality in asymptomatic patients who had previously suffered two or more myocardial infarctions (Norris et al, 1981). No difference could be found between the surgically and medically treated groups over 6 years.

Clotting or atheromatous obstruction of bypass grafts or progression of disease in the native vasculature leads to recurrence of anginal symptoms at a rate of 3 to 10 percent per year after bypass grafting. Graft patency is also clearly related to dyspnea and impaired sexual activity (Table 18–5). Fifteen to twenty-five percent of grafts occlude during the first year (those with a low flow

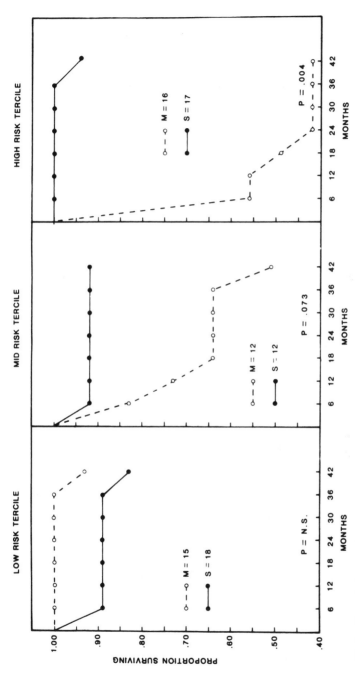

Figure 18–9 Cumulative survival rates in patients with significant left main coronary artery obstruction, by tercile of noninvasive risk: the V.A. Cooperative Study. M, Medical treatment; S, Surgical treatment. From T Takaro et al: Survival in subgroups of patients with left main coronary artery disease. *Circulation* **66**:14, 1982, by permission of the American Heart Association, Inc.

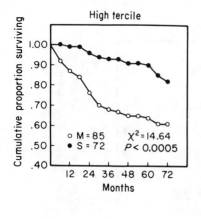

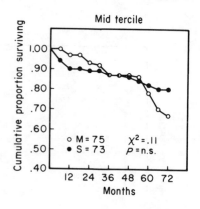

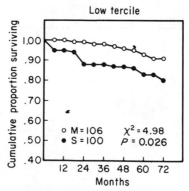

M = medical; S = surgical.

Figure 18–10 Cumulative survival rates in each risk tercile for all 1972–1974 patients without left main disease. Patients with missing data were included in the high-risk tercile, and survival rates were determined by the crossover method. The Mantel–Haenzel chi-square statistic was used to compare survival rates in the two treatment groups at 5 years. Results are shown for the 10 hospitals with low operative mortality rates. M, Medical; S, Surgical. From K Detre et al: Effects of bypass surgery on survival in patients in low- and high-risk subgroups delineated by the use of simple clinical variables. *Circulation* **63**:1329, 1981, by permission of the American Heart Association, Inc.

rate are most vulnerable). Thereafter the occlusion rate is about 2 percent per year (Rahimtoola, 1982).

Consequently, the issue of surgical or medical therapy for symptomatic IHD has become more complicated. Clearly there are many different subgroups, only some of which derive mortality benefit from surgery. They are those with severe left main coronary artery obstruction and possibly persons with moderate left ventricular dysfunction. Whether asymptomatic persons with IHD are helped cannot be answered at present. Surgery has no proven benefit in preventing re-

Table 18–5 Variables showing a significant linear trend across patency categories: Veterans Administration Cooperative Study

	Patency of vein grafts (%)		
	None	Partial	All
Limitation of normal activity			
Angina	72	46	29
Dyspnea	48	47	27
Nocturnal dyspnea	22	15	8
Sexual activity			
Impaired	52	32	29
Associated with angina	36	11	8
Nitroglycerin four times per day	14	5	2
Employment			
None	90	80	65
Full-time	7	17	26

Source: From SH Rahimtoola: Coronary bypass surgery for chronic angina—1981. A perspective. *Circulation* **65**:225, 1982, by permission of the American Heart Association, Inc.

infarction, although future subgroup analyses will be of interest. Finally, there is no doubt that surgery improves anginal symptoms and hence quality of life. The physician must weigh the severity of the symptoms against the cost, discomfort, and small morbidity of the surgery to reach the best conclusion.

Summary

1. After myocardial infarction, first-year mortality is 8–15 percent and thereafter about 3–5 percent per year, similar to patients with chronic ischemic heart disease.

2. The traditional risk factors for primary prevention generally remain as significant predictors of subsequent events. However, their importance is relatively less.

3. Smoking cessation postinfarction is effective in reducing risk of both reinfarction and mortality.

4. Serum cholesterol retains some predictive power postinfarction.

5. Dietary changes may improve outlook and also function in IHD patients. More evidence is needed, but several short- and longer-term studies suggest this possibility.

6. The most important predictors postinfarction are those measuring the cur-

rent cardiac status of the patient—both pathologic and physiologic. The physiologic predictors can be grouped to those measuring left ventricular function, myocardial electrical instability, myocardial perfusion, and cellular ischemia (ST depression on electrocardiogram). All are important.

7. As expected, the severity of obstructive coronary lesions predicts prognosis, although a noninvasive index (perhaps measuring the functional significance of the obstructions) importantly refines this prediction.

8. Coronary artery bypass surgery is excellent symptomatic treatment for stable angina pectoris uncontrolled by medical therapy.

9. Coronary artery bypass grafting has preventive value. Subgroups of patients with stable angina benefit by increased longevity after bypass grafting. These include (a) patients with left main coronary artery disease and a poor or midrange-valued noninvasive risk profile, and (b) possibly patients with at least one significant lesion and a poor noninvasive risk profile. However, there is no evidence that risk of future myocardial infarction is diminished by surgery.

10. Bypass surgery can be viewed as providing some patients extra asymptomatic time in which to employ more easily the usual preventive changes in lifestyle.

19

Cardiac Rehabilitation—A Broad Perspective

The objectives of cardiac rehabilitation are to restore the patient to a maximally productive, active, and satisfying life as soon as possible after the recognition of cardiac disease. This usually involves consideration of not only physical status but also mental status and social circumstances (National Heart and Lung Institute Task Force on Cardiovascular Rehabilitation, 1974). In addition to this process of social and physical integration, most would also include secondary prevention—that is, retarded disease progression, greater longevity, and less morbidity—as an objective. Much of the emphasis in cardiac rehabilitation is on appropriate changes in living habits, as well as the optimization of drug therapy and the teaching of coping skills. Patient compliance with a medical regimen can often be maximized around the time of an acutely threatening event, such as myocardial infarction or coronary artery bypass surgery. Thus, there is an opportunity for secondary prevention that should not be missed. This chapter will not attempt a comprehensive description of program organization, but instead will provide a conceptual overview and a discussion of the efficacy of such programs. Excellent reviews of program organization are available elsewhere (National Heart and Lung Institution Task Force on Cardiovascular Rehabilitation, 1974; Pollock and Schmidt, 1979a; Wenger, 1973).

The population standing to benefit from cardiac rehabilitation is large. About 4 million persons in the United States have symptomatic IHD, and about half of them are under the age of 65 years. Each year well over 1 million heart attacks occur, and more than 670,000 people survive the acute phase. Each year, more than 100,000 persons will undergo coronary artery bypass surgery and so are particularly favorable candidates for a rehabilitation effort. A by-product of the pain relief afforded by this surgery is the greater freedom to effect meaningful changes in exercise habits and so weight control.

Although figures are hard to come by, it is probable that few acute myocardial infarction patients are exposed to more than a 1- or 2-week inpatient experience of education and rehabilitation. Proportionately fewer still of *chronic* IHD patients will be involved in a continuing formal program. There are several reasons for this. Programs with outpatient and maintenance-phase components are available to a minority of patients, often because they are far from a patient's residence after hospital discharge. Many physicians are unfamiliar with exercise prescriptions and still more so with dietary prescriptions. This means that maintenance phase at present must usually be handled by specialists.

A problem endemic to preventive medicine in the United States is inadequate third-party insurance coverage to allow appropriate compensation for the health professional engaged in such programs. Finally, there is the problem of patient disinterest and/or noncompliance over the long run.

Approaches to Cardiac Rehabilitation

Cardiac rehabilitation is often divided into three phases. The first phase spans the period in the coronary care unit and the rest of the hospital stay. The emphasis is on carefully graduated exercise as well as health education. The exercise progresses from passive to active to resistive movement. There has been a tendency toward progressively earlier mobilization for uncomplicated infarction, patients now being encouraged to ambulate within the first 3–4 days. More extended bed rest is known to decrease peripheral muscular efficiency and maximal oxygen uptake (Saltin et al, 1968), and to decrease plasma volume, thus increasing blood viscosity and predisposing patients to thromboembolism (Hyatt et al, 1969; PB Miller et al, 1965). Early mobilization is also associated with less anxiety and depression (McPherson et al, 1967). Health education covers topics such as the physiology and pathology of ischemic heart disease, the rationale and content of a rehabilitation program, dietary instruction, sex and the heart patient, cigarette smoking, and medications for heart disease. Where possible, other family members are involved.

Before discharge, a careful assessment of the patient's exercise capability is made, so as to facilitate progression to the next phase. This usually includes a limited exercise test, which also provides valuable prognostic information. Such variables as the time the patient was able to remain exercising, ST depression on the electrocardiogram, the occurrence of angina, inadequate blood pressure response to exercise, and ventricular ectopy on a halter monitor have prognostic value even this early in the postinfarction period (Corbett et al, 1981; Davidson and DeBusk, 1980; Luria et al, 1979; Starling et al, 1980; Theroux et al, 1979).

Phase II is a period of usually about 8 weeks, during which the exercise prescription is gradually increased. Exercise may be walking, exercycling, cycling, or swimming. By 10 weeks postinfarction, the patient without complications may be walking 3 miles in 72 minutes. Some high-risk patients (e.g., with heart failure or arrhythmias) may make slower progress and need to continue exercising under direct supervision or by telemetry. For this subgroup, phase II exercise may still be entirely supervised. For all others, the program can be home-based with regular clinic visits. In addition to exercise, attention should be given to stopping cigarette smoking and making dietary changes if necessary. However, the emphasis is still on improving physical capabilities.

Phase III rehabilitation involves maintenance of exercise and intensification of the focus on other aspects of life-style change such as weight loss, smoking cessation, and dietary change. The techniques of self-directed behavioral change (chapter 21) are the best available to influence behavior in such patients and should be applied to all components of the program, including exercise, in an effort to ensure long-term compliance. Sometimes this phase is offered through community service organizations, but more often it is unavailable. This is unfortunate, because recidivism is a major problem. Patients spend by far the longest time in phase III, so that it is probably the most important though least adequately handled phase.

A special type of program attempts to deal effectively with phase II and decisively lead into phase III. Particularly in Europe the concept of residential centers for rehabilitation has become popular (Angster et al, 1982; Halhuber, 1977). During their stay, patients are involved in group and individualized therapy for anxiety and depression, training in cooking and menu selection, and help with quitting smoking. In addition, organized exercise, often in outdoor rural settings, is a regular component. There are several similar, often controversial programs in the United States (Diehl and Mannerberg, 1981).

This innovative idea has clear advantages but also some disadvantages. The advantages include the ability to monitor and perform tests at all times during therapy, and to deal with psychosocial problems following heart attacks such as anxiety, depression, denial, and overmotivation. In particular there are advantages with regard to education, motivation to assume a new life-style, teaching new skills, and utilizing group dynamics (Konig, 1978). The "live-in" experience is seen as an intensive start to the outpatient maintenance phase, which then has a more leisurely pace. The effectiveness of such programs in modifying risk factors for the short term has been demonstrated with substantial reductions in body weight, serum cholesterol, and blood pressure (Angster et al, 1982; Diehl and Mannerberg, 1981). Programs range from 3 to 6 weeks in duration (Barnard et al, 1981; Halhuber, 1977).

Problems of the "live-in" approach include high cost and their very artificial environment, which raises the question to what extent behavioral change learned under such circumstances will be carried over to the home situation. Undoubtedly for a sizable subgroup it can be quite effective, and this has been demonstrated (Angster et al, 1982; Barnard et al, 1983). Barnard and colleagues found in 64 IHD patients who had been recommended for bypass surgey before entering a 3-week program, that at 5 years follow-up about half of the gains in serum cholesterol made during the intensive phase were retained. However, there was no control group by which to compare the natural history of cholesterol trends in such patients. Only 12 patients subsequently underwent coronary artery bypass surgery.

As in traditional programs, however, maintenance is often neglected. Patients may live far from the health center, so maintenance depends on the often-nonexistent professional and social support mechanisms in the local community. Hence the potential for recidivism is considerable, even following such a residential program, unless a clear maintenance support mechanism is identified.

Another approach to phase II and III rehabilitation involves regular office visits with a physician and also the dietitian, exercise physiologist, or behavioral psychologist, as necessary, with lengthening intervals between visits for the fore-seeable future. The philosophy behind these visits is to provide regular clinical care (interim medical history, physical examination, review of drug therapy) but with greater emphasis on continuing behavioral change (or maintenance of such change) in order to modify risk factors (Angster et al, 1982; Fraser et al, 1984; Kallio, 1982; Salonen and Puska, 1980). The physician has a critical role to play in the behavioral change process (Stone, 1979). Providing support during re-habilitation will give credibility to the efforts of the other clinic staff and will enable the physician to judge clinical progress effectively and report this back to the patient—an important stimulus to continued behavioral change (chapter 21). An additional advantage is that insurance coverage is available for physi-cian visits and often also for dietary counseling occurring under the supervision of and at the request of the physician.

The Efficacy of Exercise Alone as Cardiac Rehabilitation and Secondary Prevention

Exercise receives the greatest emphasis in most rehabilitation programs and in much rehabilitation research. Many investigators have demonstrated that ap-propriate physical activity by IHD patients without congestive heart failure can indeed improve work capacity. Table 19–1 reports the results of several studies that used the product of heart rate and systolic arterial pressure, or heart rate, systolic pressure, and ejection time as indirect indices of cardiac work. The car-diac work needed to support the same external workload is consistently reduced after the training programs, implying an adaptation of peripheral musculature to require less oxygen. Supporting this conclusion are studies like that of Doba and colleagues (1983), who exercised 60 patients (48 with previous myocardial infarction and 12 with angina pectoris) for 12 weeks. The average interval since infarction was 5 months. One result (Fig. 19–1) was a 32.7 percent increase in the time that patients could walk on a treadmill before symptoms or other reasons necessitating a halt ($P < 0.001$). This is demonstrated in the figure, as the regression line lies well above the diagonal that would represent no change. Thus, the likelihood of developing angina pectoris is decreased until higher external workloads are imposed. The evidence that exercise therapy actually im-proves myocardial perfusion is controversial (Ferguson et al, 1978; Froelicher et al, 1980; Sim and Neil, 1974; Verani et al, 1981).

Regular physical activity in cardiac patients probably has psychologic bene-fits (Gentry, 1979). This may extend to an improved self-image, greater self-confidence, and less anxiety or depression. There is no consistent evidence that the improved physical capacity of patients undergoing rehabilitation results in improved rate of return to work (Krasemann and Jungmann, 1979; Mayou, 1983).

Regular physical activity has the potential to change risk factors in cardiac patients as it does in others (chapter 12). It is well known that regular exercise is

Table 19–1 Indirect indexes of myocardial oxygen demand before and after exercise training in cardiac patients

Study	n	Age (years)	Index	Same workload Before	After	Δ%
Redwood et al, 1972	7	48	TP^a	4300	3521	−18
Frick and Katila, 1968	7	47	DP^b	262	242	−8
Clausen et al, 1969	9	52	DP	204	166	−19
Hellerstein, 1968	100	49	DP	248	193	−22
Detry et al, 1971	12	49	DP	166	137	−17
Kasch and Boyer, 1969	11	50	DP	—	—	—
Clausen and Trap-Jensen, 1976	29	55	DP	222	202	−9
Sim and Neill, 1974	8	50	DP	175	206	+18
Detry and Bruce, 1971	14	50	DP	179	155	−13
Bjernulf, 1973	21	53	DP	196	172	−12
Ferguson et al, 1978	10	46	DP	152	124	−18
Letac et al, 1977	15	50	DP	312	261	−16
Kentala, 1972	61	53	DP	189	174	−8

Source: Adapted from WL Haskell, in *Heart Disease and Rehabilitation*, ML Pollack and DH Schmidt (ed). Houghton-Mifflin, 1979, with permission.

[a] TP = heart rate (beats/min) × systolic arterial pressure (mm Hg) × ejection time (seconds).

[b] DP = heart rate (beats/min) × systolic arterial pressure (mm Hg)/100.

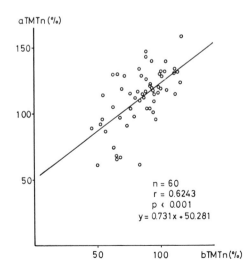

Figure 19–1 Correlation between normalized treadmill times before (bTMTn) and after (aTMTn) training. From N Doba et al, 1983, with permission.

an effective aid to obesity control and prevention (Brownell, 1982a). Systolic blood pressure may drop slightly in exercising cardiac patients, although the evidence is not entirely consistent (Pollock and Schmidt, 1979b, p. 286). Some believe that persons who exercise regularly are more likely to quit smoking, but the evidence is anecdotal and conflicting (Shephard, 1979). Of course, many patients quit smoking after a myocardial infarction in the earliest phase of rehabilitation, and so this cannot be clearly related to exercise. The effect of exercise to elevate HDL cholesterol applies also to IHD patients, and may also extend to lower LDL cholesterol levels (Hartung et al, 1981; Heath et al, 1983).

Exercise as rehabilitation can relieve symptoms, but does it reduce morbidity and mortality? Many studies have addressed this question, but to date there is no clear answer. Although many older studies produced positive results (Leon and Blackburn, 1977), they should be viewed with suspicion as most did not involve random assignment to "exercise" and "no-exercise" categories. *Voluntary* exercisers probably differ in several ways from those preferring not to exercise, for example in clinical status, health consciousness, obesity, and cigarette smoking.

Three studies involving random assignment have been completed (Rechnitzer, 1979; Rechnitzer et al, 1983; Shaw, 1981; Wilhelmsen et al, 1975). None showed clear evidence of reduction in either mortality or morbidity. One serious problem plagued all three: noncompliance with the exercise assignment over the several years of follow-up. This is particularly well documented by the Swedish trial (Wilhelmsen et al, 1975).

The National Exercise and Heart Disease Program, a multicenter study in the United States (Shaw, 1981), randomly allocated about 650 men with myocardial infarction within 3 years, to either an exercise or a no-exercise program. Before randomization, those men had demonstrated likelihood of good adherence by complying well with a 6-week low-intensity exercise program. Compliance was nevertheless a problem over the 3-year follow-up, but for purposes of analysis the subjects were left in their original groups, regardless of adherence. This retained the random allocation, thus balancing potential confounding factors. However, it did tend to bring the two groups closer with respect to average exercise status, thus biasing toward the null hypothesis of no difference. Mortality data seemed to favor the exercise group (Table 19–2), although no hint of benefit was seen for nonfatal events (Table 19–3). None of the mortality or morbidity results were statistically significant, given the multiple testing employed. This study lacked statistical power, and the possibility that the nonsignificant results reflect this should be considered.

A similar program in the Canadian province of Ontario studied 678 male postinfarction patients for at least 3 years. These men were randomly allocated to low- and high-intensity exercise. There was a slight mortality and reinfarction advantage for the group allocated to the low-intensity exercise control group (Rechnitzer, 1979). The Swedish study by Wilhelmsen and colleagues (1975) randomly assigned 315 postinfarction patients to exercise or control groups. Adherence was a problem over the 4-year follow-up, but a difference in exercise

Table 19-2 Mortality in post-myocardial infarction patients randomly allocated to exercise or control status over a 3-year follow-up

Events counted	Control group (n = 328)		Exercise group (n = 323)		Statistical significance (P value)
	n	%	n	%	
All deaths	24	7.3	15	4.6	0.22
Cardiovascular deaths					
Acute myocardial infarction	8	2.4	1	0.3	0.047
Other definite[a]	6		5		
Subtotal	14	4.3	6	1.9	0.13
Sudden deaths[b]	6		8		
Total	20	6.1	14	4.3	0.40
Indeterminate cause	4		1		

Source: From LW Shaw: *Am J Cardiol* **48**:39, 1981, with permission.

[a] Includes six deaths from arrhythmias, two from congestive cardiac failures, one from cardiogenic shock, and two from cerebrovascular accidents.

[b] Within 1 hour.

Table 19-3 Morbidity experience of post-myocardial infarction patients randomly allocated to exercise or control status, over 3 years of follow-up

Events counted	Control group (n = 328)		Exercise group (n = 323)		Statistical significance (P value)
	n	%	n	%	
Cardiovascular deaths	20	6.1	14	4.3	0.40
Nonfatal infarctions	11		15		
Subtotal	31	9.5	29	9.0	0.95
Suspected infarctions	2		3		
Other events	25		25		
Total	58	17.7	57	17.6	1.0
All recurrent myocardial infarctions	23	7.0	17	5.3	0.46
Total hospitalizations for reasons other than myocardial infarction	90	27.4	92	28.5	0.86

Source: From LW Shaw: *Am J Cardiol* **48**:39, 1981, with permission.

did persist between the two groups. Although analysis slightly favored the exercisers in general, no comparisons achieved statistical significance.

Thus, the overall results are not very promising, although the ideal study with good statistical power has not yet been conducted.

Problems Encountered in Cardiac Rehabilitation

Compliance is a major problem in a long-term exercise program, particularly when organized exercise sessions are at some distance from the participant's home. In the Ontario Multicentric study, Oldridge and colleagues (1978, 1983) analyzed characteristics of compliers and noncompliers with fascinating results. The subjects in this study were randomly allocated to either "high-intensity" or "low-intensity" exercise. The high-intensity exercisers met twice weekly for a 25- to 35-minute session of walking or jogging, 5–10 minutes of cycle ergometry, and 10–20 minutes of volleyball or badminton. They were also expected to exercise on their own at least twice weekly at a slightly lower intensity. The low-intensity exercisers engaged in such activities as relaxation, bowling, and yoga, which were designed to minimize training effects. Of the 678 subjects who could have participated for at least 3 years, 46.5 percent dropped out. Noncompliance was defined as missing eight consecutive supervised activity sessions. There was no difference in dropout rates between high- or low-intensity exercisers. In fact, the curves of cumulative dropout rate with time were almost identical.

There was a significant difference in compliance between smokers and nonsmokers: smokers were 2.46 times more likely to drop out than nonsmokers. In addition, blue-collar workers were 1.66 times more likely to drop out as compared to white-collar workers, and subjects with cough or phlegm were 1.6 times more likely to drop out than others (Fig. 19–2). Subjects with angina but no reinfarction were also more likely to drop out. All these results were statistically significant.

A separate analysis of the 163 men who were in the program at MacMaster University divided noncompliance within the first 1 year into early and late, defining early noncompliance as starting before the end of the first month and late noncompliance as occurring between 1 month and 12 months (Oldridge et al, 1978). About 46 percent of the noncompliance was early, and the reasons given were classified as psychosocial, "unavoidable," and medical (Fig. 19–3). The analysis of results from the MacMaster subjects further indicated that *early* noncompliers were more likely to display the type A behavior pattern, to be inactive during their leisure time, to be smokers, and to have had more previous myocardial infarctions. Consequently, men leaving an exercise program early may be a particularly high-risk subgroup for further events—a group that rehabilitation efforts certainly should strive to include.

It has been stated that program factors associated with noncompliance include (1) the duration of the program, (2) the degree of behavioral change required, and (3) the complexity of the regimen (Haynes, 1976a). In cardiac

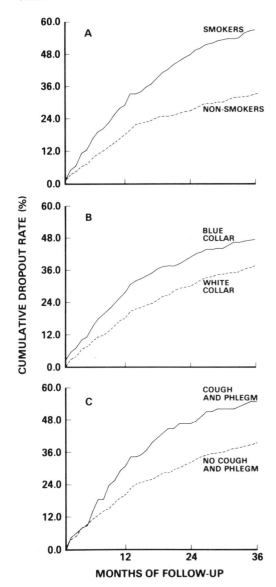

Figure 19–2 An analysis of compliance with an exercise program according to smoking habits, occupation, cough, and phlegm. From NB Oldridge et al: *Am J Cardiol* **51**:70, 1983, with permission.

rehabilitation, the duration of the program needs to be lifelong; however, the other two factors allow some flexibility. The degree of behavioral change can be suggested, but should not be required for continuing participation. Often the apparent degree of behavioral change can be minimized by making it progressive over many months. To decrease the complexity of the program, it can be made home-based and less structured as soon as this is safe.

The safety question revolves in particular around the possibility of serious arrhythmias occurring away from medical supervision. Given the available re-

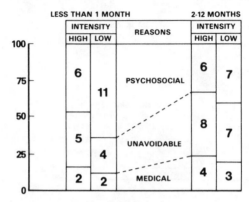

Figure 19–3   Reasons given for leaving physical conditioning program before 1 month or between 2 and 12 months by men exercising at high or low intensity after suffering a myocardial infarction. *Unavoidable*: conflicts with subject's working schedule, financial inability to pay costs, moving away; *psychosocial*: lack of interest, motivation, as well as personal problems involving family. From NB Oldridge et al: *Canad Med Assoc J* **118**: 361, 1978, original publisher.

sources, it seems inevitable that most phase III rehabilitation will take place away from medical supervision. Clearly certain precautions are appropriate for nonsupervised activity by cardiac patients. Probably the intensity of the exercise should be less than that prescribed while under supervision. If premature ventricular contractions (PVCs) occur frequently on halter monitor or a submaximal stress test, these should be controlled by drugs where possible. Most PVCs in cardiac patients undergoing rehabilitation appear to occur during *normal* activities rather than during the rehabilitation exercise. It does not seem possible to predict the occurrence of serious arrhythmias by exercise testing, whereas the 24-hour halter monitor is apparently quite sensitive but nonspecific (Simoons et al, 1980). The most practical course is to exclude from exercise programs patients with severe left ventricular dysfunction, particularly those with an inadequate heart rate or blood pressure response to exercise, very low physical capacity (Simoons et al, 1980), or uncontrollable arrhythmias. All patients should be taught to recognize warning signs and to measure their own pulse rates periodically during exercise.

This issue of unsupervised exercise as cardiac rehabilitation has recently been reviewed by RS Williams et al (1981), who arrived at essentially these conclusions. The rationale of unsupervised exercise is that with appropriately selected patients and lesser exercise intensities, rates of cardiac arrest (most of whom will not be resuscitated) will be lower and so such programs can be acceptably safe.

Table 19–4 Average number of hours to find one event during exercise training of cardiac patients[a]

	Nonfatal	Fatal	Total
Cardiac arrest	38,801	203,704	32,593
	(42)[b]	(8)	(50)
Myocardial infarction	325,927	814,816	232,805
	(5)	(2)	(7)
Other		497,408	407,408
		(4)	(4)
Total	34,673	116,402	26,715
	(47)	(14)	(61)

Source: From WL Haskell: Cardiovascular complications during exercise training of cardiac patients. *Circulation* **57**:920, 1978, by permission of the American Heart Association, Inc.

[a] Number of patient-hours of participation per event—average for all 30 programs surveyed with total of 1,629,634 patient-hours of participation.

[b] Number of events for each classification.

Sooner or later almost all patients will need to graduate to programs largely unsupervised and home-based.

Haskell (1978) has examined the occurrence of complications during *medically supervised* rehabilitation exercise, in which rapid cardiopulmonary resuscitation is possible. He reviewed 30 programs involving 13,570 patients and 1,629,634 patient hours of exercise. The minimum time following myocardial infarction or cardiac surgery before a patient was allowed into these exercise programs ranged from 2 to 12 weeks. Sixty-one major cardiovascular complications occurred (Table 19–4), and of these, 44 occurred during the warm-up or cool-down phases of the exercise sessions. Notice that 84 percent of cardiac arrests were successfully resuscitated. Haskell calculated that in these programs the risk of dying actually while exercising was no higher than the overall mortality for post-myocardial infarction patients during the first several years following hospitalization. Thus, supervised exercise in cardiac patients seems relatively safe.

Simultaneous Multifactor Intervention as Cardiac Rehabilitation and Secondary Prevention

Very few papers have been published on the effectiveness of multiple interventions in postinfarction patients. A multivariate program has the disadvantage of making it difficult to dissect the relative contributions of the components in producing any observed change, but it has the advantage of potentially increasing the magnitude of the effect. Such interventions may address smoking, diet,

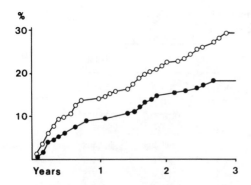

Figure 19–4 Cumulative percentage of deaths from coronary heart disease in the multiple factor rehabilitation (●) and control (○) groups of post-myocardial infarction patients (*P* = 0.02). Circles denote monthly cumulative mortality, not number of individual cases. From V Kallio et al, 1979, with permission.

blood pressure control, and exercise. The reader will recall that there is observational evidence that cigarette smoking and hypertension continue as risk factors in the postinfarction patient. The same is true of serum cholesterol, and there are also several dietary intervention studies, some showing a significant reduction in subsequent IHD events, and others reduction of angina and improved exercise tolerance in the short term. Serum cholesterol levels have also been associated with the rate of progression of coronary atherosclerotic lesions in IHD patients (chapter 18).

In Finland, Kallio and colleagues (1979) combined diet, smoking, and exercise interventions. A total of 375 consecutive patients below 65 years of age who had had an acute myocardial infarction were randomly assigned to a rehabilitation or control group. The two groups were well matched according to several clinical and risk factor variables. The intervention group's program started 2 weeks after the hospital discharge and consisted of a medical examination by an internist at least monthly for 6 months, and thereafter at least every 3 months. Other staff included a social worker, psychologist, dietitian, and physical therapist. Advice was given on diet and smoking cessation, and an individualized exercise program was prescribed. Most exercise was done under supervision. The follow-up period was 3 years. Subjects in the control group were followed by their own doctors and were seen by study personnel annually. At 1, 2, and 3 years there were significant differences in body weight, serum cholesterol, triglycerides, and systolic and diastolic blood pressures favoring the rehabilitation group, although physical working capacities were similar. Deaths from IHD were significantly reduced in the rehabilitation group, and this was largely due to a decrease in sudden death (Figs. 19–4 and 19–5). Total mortality was 21·8 percent in the intervention and 29.6 percent in the control group (*P* <0.10). This result contrasts with the studies of exercise alone.

Further evidence comes from a controlled trial at the postinfarction clinic in Göteborg, Sweden where post-myocardial infarction patients in the program were compared to the control group of patients who were referred to other physicians for follow-up (Vedin et al, 1976). The program included traditional medical care (which presumably included careful blood pressure control) and also vigorous antismoking measures. Intensive dietary or exercise interventions

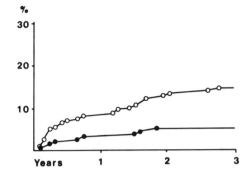

Figure 19–5 Cumulative percentage of sudden deaths in the multiple factor rehabilitation (●) and control (○) groups of post-myocardial infarction patients ($P = 0.01$). Circles denote monthly cumulative mortality, not number of individual cases. From V Kallio et al, 1979, with permission.

were not used. Over a 2-year period, examinations at the postinfarction clinic took place every 6 weeks, many being carried out by a specially trained nurse. No patient in this group was treated with β blockers, nor were antiarrhythmic agents, lipid-lowering drugs, or anticoagulants used. As compared to the control group, there was a significant reduction in nonfatal reinfarction and new coronary events but no difference in mortality. Possible explanations include the optimal traditional medical therapy and that 60 percent of smokers quit. It also seems possible that the frequent visits with professional personnel may have had the effect of repeatedly sensitizing the patients to their condition, provoking some self-motivated educational efforts and increased efforts to improve health habits.

Summary

1. Rehabilitation is usually considered in three phases: (I) the in-hospital phase, (II) a period immediately following discharge of increasing exercise and other behavioral changes, and (III) maintenance of changes in health habits and functional capacity.

2. Traditionally rehabilitation has mostly focused on exercise, although some dietary advice, stress control, and vocational guidance is usually given.

3. Alternative or supplementary approaches are being explored particularly for phases II and III. Phase III is often ineffective or nonexistent in many situations. Part of the problem in instituting phase III rehabilitation is poor patient compliance when programs are highly structured over prolonged periods.

4. Home exercise for selected patients is one reasonable solution. This should be combined with other appropriate behavioral changes, such as smoking cessation and dietary interventions, which can be supervised during outpatient visits.

5. Exercise therapy clearly reduces angina (probably largely through peripheral muscular adaptation) and may improve psychologic well-being. These are the major justifications currently for traditional rehabilitation efforts. There is no convincing evidence that IHD morbidity or mortality is reduced.

6. Long-term rehabilitation programs emphasizing diet, smoking cessation, social support, and exercise are probably most effective in reducing IHD mortality, although more evidence is needed.

20

Drugs as Prevention and Cause of Ischemic Heart Disease

Physicians often find it more convenient to write a prescription than to become involved with the complexities of life-style and the difficulties of changing entrenched habits. Most patients are more willing to accept the notion of drug side effects (which usually happen to someone else) than to expend energy breaking old and establishing new ways of eating, exercising, and perhaps socializing.

Most drugs are designed for the treatment of recognized disease. Although there has often been a hope that they would serve for *secondary* prevention, little effort has been made to demonstrate the validity of such preventive action until recently. In fact, some of the standbys of traditional cardiologic therapy (e.g., digoxin, quinidine) have often been used to improve test values or clinical signs with little evidence that they improve quality of life or longevity. There have been several large clinical trials concerning the role of various drugs in preventing occurrence or recurrence of myocardial infarction or IHD death over the last decade.

In this chapter a common study design is the randomized trial, frequently placebo-controlled and double-blind. While this is a very powerful design, often permitting strong conclusions, some precautions need to be exercised in interpretation. Many of the trials have somewhat restrictive inclusion and exclusion criteria for study participants. This may be because of possible clinical contraindications to drug use, or to maximize the power of the study yet minimize costs by selecting those persons likely to be most responsive. Often there are age–sex limitations, and the white race may be largely represented. Compliance with medications may be a problem, as may crossover from one treatment group to the other for overwhelming clinical reasons. Dropouts partway through the study can lead to inequality between the two comparison groups, as may deaths where the end point is a physiologic or pathologic measure. For these reasons, the clinician will often find the trial does not exactly match the patient across the office desk or the specific question to be answered, so judgment is still necessary. It is important in this chapter to distinguish carefully between investigations of primary and secondary prevention as several of these drugs have been tested for both.

Studies of Lipid-Lowering Agents

Many agents have been used to lower both serum cholesterol and serum triglycerides with the hope of both primary and secondary prevention. These include clofibrate, thyroxine, estrogens, nicotinic acid, neomycin, cholestyramine, colestipol, probucol, and gemfibrozil, acting by a variety of mechanisms such as increasing fecal steroid excretion, decreasing hepatic cholesterol synthesis, or altering peripheral utilization of lipids.

The Coronary Drug Project Research Group (1975) designed its study to test the safety and efficacy of estrogens (two dosages), thyroxine, clofibrate, and niacin as compared to a lactose placebo in ameliorating the natural history of ischemic heart disease. The subjects were men who had had a myocarcial infarction and were not selected according to lipid levels. The study included 53 clinical centers and a total of 8341 patients who were randomly assigned to the six treatments. The patients entered the study between the years 1966 and 1969 at various times postinfarction, and the follow-up for clofibrate, niacin, and placebo averaged 76 months. The groups allocated to estrogens and thyroxine therapy were terminated prematurely because of early indications of adverse effects. The study was double-blind, neither staff nor patients knowing which drug patients were using. Side effects from the medications were monitored and adherence was good—only a 10 percent dropout rate for niacin and 7 percent for clofibrate and placebo. There were clear reductions in both serum cholesterol and triglyceride levels for both the clofibrate and niacin groups (Fig. 20–1) The association between these drugs and a large number of cardiovascular and noncardiovascular outcomes was analyzed (Table 20–1). No evidence of any reduction in all causes, all cardiovascular, or even coronary heart disease mortality was found. Although there was a significant advantage for niacin takers with respect to definite nonfatal myocardial infarction (a 26 percent reduction compared to placebo takers), this was counterbalanced by an *increased* propensity to atrial fibrillation, other arrhythmias, and a variety of skin disorders. Clofibrate use had no advantages and was associated with an *increase* of definite and suspected pulmonary emboli, intermittent claudication, angina pectoris, certain arrhythmias, and gallstones. Side effects as indicated by symptoms, signs, and changes in biochemical values were also analyzed. Both drugs were clearly associated with multiple side effects and biochemical changes. In summary, it seems quite likely that any beneficial effects from the lowered serum cholesterol levels were counterbalanced by side effects of the drugs.

Whereas the Coronary Drug Project dealt with secondary prevention in men unselected by serum cholesterol, the World Health Organization Clofibrate Trial (Committee of Principal Investigators, 1978) evaluated clofibrate as primary prevention in relatively hypercholesterolemic men. Of the 55,519 male volunteers who were screened for admission to this study, 15,745 were admitted and 10,703 completed 5 years in the trial. The men were initially divided into tertiles by serum cholesterol values, and those in the upper tertile were randomly assigned to clofibrate treatment (1.6 gm daily, group I) or to an olive oil placebo

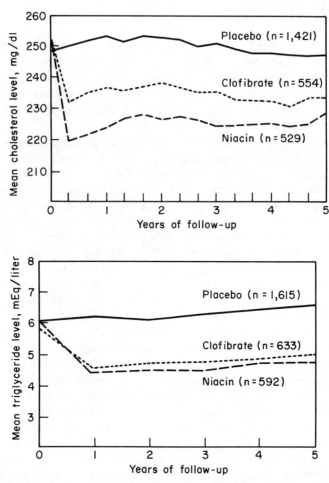

Figure 20–1 Mean levels of serum cholesterol (upper) and serum triglyceride (lower) at baseline and 4-month (for cholesterol) or annual (for triglyceride) intervals, for cohorts of men observed for at least 5 years with no missing determinations. From Coronary Drug Project Research Group: Clofibrate and niacin in coronary heart disease. *JAMA* **231**:360, copyright © 1975, American Medical Association.

(group II). A random half of the men in the lowest cholesterol tertile also received the olive oil placebo and so formed an additional low-cholesterol control group (group III). Groups I and II had virtually identical average ratings for a large set of physiologic and life-style risk factors, but they differed considerably from group III. Group III subjects were a little younger and tended to have a superior risk profile for most variables.

The active phase of the trial was between 1965 and 1976. During this period

Table 20–1 Deaths and nonfatal events by cause occurring since entry, 5-year rates

	Percent with event		
	Clofibrate	Niacin	Placebo
Death			
All causes	20.0	21.2	20.9
All cardiovascular	17.3	18.8	18.9
All noncardiovascular	2.1	2.1	1.5
Coronary heart disease	14.1	15.9	16.2
Sudden cardiovascular	8.4	10.5	9.6
All cancer	0.6	0.6	0.6
Definite, nonfatal myocardial infarction	11.6	8.9[a]	12.0
Definite or suspected fatal or nonfatal pulmonary embolism or thrombophlebitis	5.2[a]	3.9	3.3
New angina pectoris	52.2[a]	38.1	44.7
Congestive heart failure	24.1	22.3	21.2
New hypertension	24.2	21.2	23.3
New intermittent claudication	21.0[a]	16.1	16.9
Stroke	2.3	2.3	2.9
Atrial fibrillation	3.9	4.7[a]	2.9
Other arrhythmias	33.3[a]	32.7[a]	28.2
Any of above	81.3[a]	74.6	75.8

Source: Adapted from Coronary Drug Project Research Group: Clofibrate and niacin in coronary heart disease. *JAMA* **231**:360, copyright © 1975, American Medical Association.

[a] $P < 0.05$ as compared to placebo, using $z = 2.58$ as a critical value because of the multiple statistical testing.

there was a 20 percent reduction in first major coronary events ($P < 0.05$) in the clofibrate group as compared to group II. The incidence of *non-fatal* myocardial infarction was reduced by 25 percent, but there was no reduction in fatal first MI or mortality from IHD. Unfortunately, mortality from all causes was significantly higher in the clofibrate group ($P < 0.05$). This persisted even after the end of the trial in a follow-up through 1978, even though only 2 percent of those in group I continued to take clofibrate after the trial ended (Committee of Principal Investigators, 1980). The excess in mortality from all causes appears very nonspecific, and the pathophysiology is unknown. Specifically, there was no evidence of excess cancer mortality in the clofibrate group; rather, there was a *nonsignificant* excess in the low-cholesterol control group. As in the Coronary Drug Project, an increase in gallstones and cholecystectomies was documented (Committee of Principal Investigators, 1978).

The investigators concluded that despite some evidence of reduction in IHD events, side effects and particularly the increase in mortality from all causes favors the use of dietary intervention, particularly in that this can cause reduc-

tions in serum cholesterol of similar magnitude to those associated with clofibrate use (Committee of Principal Investigators, 1979).

The Coronary Primary Prevention Trial (CPPT) has shown conclusively that
serum cholesterol lowering is effective primary prevention of IHD (Lipid
Research Clinics Program, 1984a,b). This study was a double-blind placebo
trial of the bile acid sequestrant resin, cholestyramine, an effective cholesterol-
lowering agent. Goal dosage was 24 gm (six packets) per day. An advantage of
this drug is that its primary action is confined to the bowel lumen as it is not
absorbed. It has also shown that bile sequestration results in increased activity
of cell receptors that remove LDL. Side effects are minimal, with occasional
constipation and abdominal bloating being the most noteworthy. The study
population were 3806 men aged 35–59 years with a plasma cholesterol of
265 mg/dl or greater. Those with triglycerides greater than 300 mg/dl were
excluded. Thus, this was a study of type II primary hypercholesterolemia. The
men were mainly college or high-school-educated whites with a mean age of
47.8 years. No participant had evidence of IHD at baseline.

The participants were randomly allocated to receive drug or placebo with a
follow-up of 7–10 years. Both drug and placebo groups were prescribed a mild
cholesterol-lowering diet, which in accord with design lowered blood cholesterol by 10–12 mg/dl in both groups. The clinical end point was the combination
of definite IHD death and/or definite non-fatal myocardial infarction. Hence
this was a trial of primary prevention by the use of cholestyramine.

The resin effectively lowered serum total and LDL cholesterols, there being,
respectively, average 8.2 (20.7 mg/dl) and 12 percent (22.3 mg/dl) differences
between drug and placebo groups. Adherence to the medication was acceptable
at about four packets/day on average. Thirty IHD deaths and 130 definite nonfatal infarctions occurred in the cholestyramine group during follow-up.
Corresponding figures for the placebo group were 38 and 158. The analysis estimated that the incidence rate of IHD was 19 percent lower in the cholestyramine group ($P < 0.05$) (Fig. 20–2). The reduction in all-cause mortality was
proportionately lower, as would be expected. There was no increase in cancer
deaths with cholestyramine, the only increase being in violent and accidental
deaths, which was presumably a chance finding. Although not primary end
points, there were 25, 20, and 21 percent lower rates, respectively, of positive
exercise tests, angina, and coronary bypass surgery in the cholestyramine group.

A valid question is whether the effect was due to the cholesterol lowering or
some other effect of the drug. However, clearly the effect was due to the cholesterol lowering. Multivariate analyses within the cholestyramine group found, as
expected, a significant relationship between the number of packets of resin per
day and the incidence of IHD after adjustment for levels of other risk factors at
baseline. Of greater interest is that when the change in serum cholesterol was
added to the model this was a highly significant predictor of IHD incidence, but
the packet count was no longer even close to significance. This indicates that it
was specifically the cholesterol reduction and not some other effect of ingesting
cholestyramine that was effective. Although this study did not directly check the

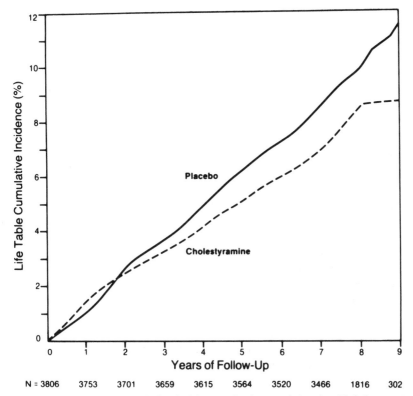

Figure 20–2   Life table cumulative incidence of primary end point (definite coronary heart disease death and/or definite nonfatal myocardial infarction) according to cholestyramine treatment status. From Lipid Research Clinics Program, 1984a, with permission.

effect of diet in reducing IHD, there is an implication here suggesting that diet can probably be effective. If the effect of the cholestyramine is through cholesterol reduction, any other means of cholesterol lowering without side effects, such as the prudent diet, should be equally effective.

These multivariate analyses within the cholestyramine group indicated that for each percentage point of lowering of serum total cholesterol, there is about a 2 percent reduction in IHD incidence (Table 20–2). It should be pointed out that such analyses within one group have lost the advantage of randomization in balancing other risk factors, and it is theoretically possible that those who took more cholestyramine were lower risk due to the unknown and therefore unadjusted factors. However, this is made most unlikely by the observation that those in the placebo group more compliant in taking placebo did not have any significant reduction in IHD incidence.

It is interesting to note that the achieved difference in IHD events between drug and placebo groups is consistent with estimates of effect from multivariate

Table 20–2   Relation of reduction in LDL and total cholesterol to
reduction in ischemic heart disease risk

	Cholesterol reduction (%)		Reduction in IHD risk (%)
	Total	LDL	
Study average	8	11	19
Full cholestyramine dose	25	35	49

Source: From Lipid Research Clinics Program: *JAMA* **251**:365, 1984b, with permission.

analyses relating cholesterol changes to IHD within each group separately.
Also, the predicted effect of the achieved cholesterol lowering, using the major
observational studies such as Framingham, Seven Countries Study, Western
Electric Company Study, is close to that actually observed in CPPT. Thus, there
is both internal and external consistency of the results of this study, which very
effectively provides the last experimental link needed to establish not only the
causality of the cholesterol–heart link, but the preventive potential of cholesterol-lowering intervention.

Although the average reduction in serum cholesterol in the CPPT was modest
and so the overall reduction in IHD incidence modest, those who took the prescribed 24 gm of cholestyramine daily had much greater reductions of serum
cholesterol and an average predicted 49 percent reduction in IHD incidence.
Patients and their physicians, not blinded as in this trial and so knowing post-
treatment values of blood lipids, should frequently be able to maintain substantial lipid lowering by using full-dosage cholestyramine combined with a more
rigorous diet than that used in the CPPT. The CPPT results strictly apply only
to men who have levels of serum cholesterol greater than 265 mg/dl. However, it
is important to notice that this study population gave no hint of being an
unusual response group. The reduction in events was very much in accord with
expectations from statistical models based on the major observational studies of
generally normolipidemic individuals.

Another trial with several similarities to the CPPT is the National Heart,
Lung, and Blood Institute (NHLBI) Type II Coronary Intervention Study
(Brensike et al, 1984; Levy et al, 1984). This again was a randomized double-
blind trial of the effect of cholestyramine. The differences were that the patient
population consisted of hypercholesterolemic men and women with presump-
tive evidence of coronary artery disease (previous myocardial infarction,
angina, positive exercise stress test, or coronary calcification on fluoroscopy).
Also, the end point was angiographic progression of atheromatous coronary
obstruction rather than disease events. There was considerable attention given
to the validity of the angiographic measurements. Unfortunately, the investigators were able to recruit only 143 patients, whereas 250 were required to give
adequate statistical power according to design. Despite this, there was more

progression of disease in the placebo group than the cholestyramine group over 5 years, although this was statistically significant only when definite and probable progression were included together.

The investigators were able to show a significant dependence of pathologic progression on changes in serum lipid values, adjusting for baseline values of several risk factors. Although disease progression was significantly related to dosage and compliance with cholestyramine therapy, it was related only to the lipid changes and not cholestyramine dosage when both were included in the same statistical analysis. Hence the effect was due to lipid reduction and not some other effect of the medication. Those who had progression tended to have less increase or a decrease in the HDL/total cholesterol ratio compared to those with no progression.

Platelet-Active Drugs

Given the recent interest in platelet activity and IHD, it is natural to investigate the effects of drugs altering platelet function to reduce IHD. Some years ago it was noted that patients taking large doses of aspirin for rheumatic complaints seemed to suffer very little IHD. It is now known that aspirin deactivates prostaglandin synthetase, but the relative effects of this on levels of thromboxane A_2 and prostacyclin I_2 are controversial (JB Smith et al, 1980). Several randomized controlled trials have addressed the potential of aspirin ingestion as a secondary preventive measure (Braunwald et al, 1980). Genton (1980) reviewed the results of these studies and, as Table 20–3 shows, they are generally consistent and in some cases statistically significant in suggesting a reduction in nonfatal MI. No significant effect on mortality, or sudden death in particular, was seen. It seems reasonable to conclude that there is about a 20 percent reduction in the chances of *reinfarction* among aspirin users ("Aspirin After Myocardial Infarction," 1980b). The conflicting evidence regarding sudden deaths and total mortality is all the more perturbing in that the studies showing no hint of reduction of fatal events for the aspirin users (AMIS and PARIS) were the largest of those reviewed. Among other unanswered questions is that of the most appropriate dosage, which has varied substantially in the clinical trials. There is evidence that aspirin should be administered in low doses (40–80 mg), as it may then inhibit platelet prostaglandin synthetase and so thromboxane formation, but not the production of prostaglandin I_2 by the arterial wall (Hanley et al, 1981; Packham and Mustard, 1980). Another question is whether female users of aspirin postinfarction have an increased mortality (Table 20–4).

Aspirin (324 mg/day) also protects against death or acute myocardial infarction in patients with unstable angina as documented by a Veterans Administration Cooperative study involving 1266 men at 12 centers, over a 12-week follow-up period (Lewis et al, 1983). This was a double-blind placebo-controlled trial. The criteria for unstable angina were new onset or sudden worsening of angina without increased physical activity, manifested by a frequency of one or more episodes per day, duration of longer than 15 minutes, or

Table 20–3 Summary of results of aspirin therapy in post-myocardial infarction randomized trials

| | | | | Percent reduction (treated vs. control) | | |
Trial[a]	Drug	Dose (mg)	Number of patients	Mortality	Sudden death	Myocardial infarction (nonfatal)
Elwood I	Aspirin	300	1239	24	—	—
CDPA	Aspirin	972	1529	30	19	5
German–Austrian	Aspirin	1500	1060	18	36	27
AMIS	Aspirin	1000	4524	11[b]	35[b]	22[c]
Elwood II	Aspirin	900	1725	17	—	35[c]
PARIS	Aspirin	972	2026	18	27[b]	29
	Aspirin + dipyridamole	972/ 225		16	16	19

Source: From E Genton: A perspective on platelet-suppressant drug treatment in coronary artery and cerebrovascular disease. *Circulation* **62**(suppl 5):111, 1980, by permission of the American Heart Association, Inc.

[a] Abbreviations: CDPA, Coronary Drug Project Aspirin; AMIS, Aspirin Myocardial Infarction Trial; PARIS, Persantine–Aspirin Reinfarction Study; Elwood I, see Elwood et al, 1974; Elwood II, see Elwood and Sweetnam, 1980; German–Austrian, see Breddin et al, 1979.

[b] Mortality higher in treated group.

[c] $P > 2$ standard errors of the difference.

Table 20–4 Aspirin in post-myocardial infarction trials—mortality outcome by sex

| | % reduction (treated vs. control) | |
Study[a]	Male	Female
German–Austrian	30[b]	30[c]
AMIS	8[c]	60[c]
Elwood II	21	5[c]

Source: From E Genton: A perspective on platelet-suppressant drug treatment in coronary artery and cerebrovascular disease. *Circulation* **62** (suppl 5):111, 1980, by permission of the American Heart Association, Inc.

[a] Abbreviations: See Table 20–3, note a.

[b] Statistically significant.

[c] Mortality higher in treated group.

occurrence at rest or with minimal activity. In addition, evidence of coronary artery disease historically, by ECG or angiogram, with no evidence of acute myocardial infarction, was required. Notice that these criteria included relatively mild cases of unstable angina.

Of 7312 patients meeting these criteria only 18 percent were admitted to the study, because such factors as recent ingestion of aspirin or other platelet-active drugs (19.2 percent), recent infarction or bypass surgery, contraindications to aspirin therapy, other severe illness, or patient refusal resulted in the exclusion of others. The results were impressive, indicating that death or acute myocardial infarction was 51 percent lower in the aspirin group ($P < 0.0005$). Nonfatal acute infarction was also 51 percent lower ($P < 0.005$). There was no difference in gastrointestinal blood loss or other side effects between the two groups.

Sulfinpyrazone, a uricosuric agent, is known to lengthen platelet survival in a reversible fashion (Packham and Mustard, 1980). An American randomized, double-blind, multicenter trial compared the effect of sulfinpyrazone (200 mg qid) to placebo in reducing IHD mortality postinfarction (Anturane Reinfarction Trial Research Group, 1980). Of the 1629 eligible patients enrolled, about 70 percent completed the protocal as planned. Randomization yielded two equivalent groups at baseline. The initial follow-up lasted only 8.4 months, when the study was prematurely stopped because of "clear evidence of benefit." The question then arose whether the benefit persisted longer than this, and the study was restarted with follow-up for another year. The reported reduction in cardiac mortality was 32 percent and in sudden death 43 percent. Most of the reduction occurred between the second and seventh months postinfarction, and there was no further benefit beyond this point. The study has been criticized for its diagnostic criteria, exclusions from the study after randomization, and the unusual result that all except one of the 106 deaths were of a cardiac cause. The question whether this study is believable or not is unresolved (Anturane Reinfarction Trial Research Group, 1978, Mitchell, 1980; Relman, 1980).

A study of quite similar design is reported from Italy (Anturane Reinfarction Italian Study, 1982) but with apparently more attention to some of the details for which the American trial was criticized. A group of 727 post-infarction patients were recruited and randomized to receive either placebo or sulfinpyrazone (400 mg bid) within 5 to 25 days of infarction. Follow-up over 2 years found a highly significant 56 percent reduction in reinfarction (Fig. 20–3). There was no suggestion of difference in either sudden death or all cardiac deaths—an interesting contrast with the American study—although numbers of such cases in Italy were small. It is unclear whether the effect is due to the action of sulfinpyrazone on platelet function or to some other mechanism.

The Effect of Drug Control of Hypertension on Subsequent Mortality and Morbidity

Several randomized, controlled trials have used drugs to treat hypertension and have then followed the intervention and control groups to observe disease mor-

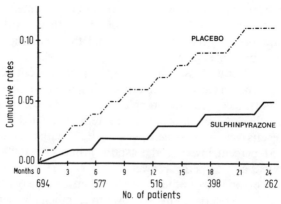

Figure 20–3 Cumulative rates of total reinfarction with either sulfinpyrazone or placebo therapy. From Anturane Reinfarction Italian Study, 1982, with permission.

bidity and mortality. Three of the largest such trials were community-based, and the other described here involved a population of hypertensive U.S. war veterans. Although all give somewhat consistent results, it is possible that different drugs may have different effects on IHD end points.

One of the earliest trials was that of the U.S. war veterans. Patients were admitted to the study according to criteria involving diastolic blood pressure levels and end-organ damage. If averaged diastolic blood pressure levels were less than 90 or greater than 129 mm Hg, these individuals were excluded as being either not clearly hypertensive or too severely hypertensive to be ethically in an untreated control group. A prerandomization phase excluded persons who were potentially poor adherers to the medication regime. This was accomplished by prescribing two placebo tablets, one containing 5 mg of riboflavin, which fluoresces under ultraviolet light. Patients were excluded if on either of two visits the urine did not fluoresce under ultraviolet light, if they did not attend either clinic appointment, or if pill counts in returned bottles showed 10 percent or more in excess remaining than should have been.

The 523 remaining male subjects were randomized to drug therapy (hydrochlorothiazide, reserpine, hydralazine) or placebo. Comparison of the two groups shows a good match on most risk factors, including duration of known hypertension, but cigarette smoking was not documented. There were two separate reports, one for patients whose diastolic blood pressures before randomization averaged between 115 and 129 mm Hg (V.A. Cooperative Study Group, 1967), the other for milder cases between 90 and 114 mm Hg (V.A. Cooperative Study Group, 1970).

The drug-treated group of the more severe hypertensives had a sharp drop in

Table 20–5 Trends of diastolic blood pressure during the V.A. cooperative randomized trial

	Placebo		Active	
Time of observation	Number of patients observed[a]	Average diastolic (mm Hg)	Number of patients observed	Average diastolic (mm Hg)
Prerandomization	70	121	73	121.2
At 4 months	57	118.5	68	93.1
8	50	120.3	64	92.2
12	44	118.8	58	91.6
16	33	118.5	47	92.1
20	27	115.2	40	89.4
24	23	119.7	32	91.5

Source: V.A. Cooperative Study Group on Antihypertensive Agents: Effects of treatment on morbidity in hypertension. I. *JAMA* **202**:1028, copyright © 1967, American Medical Association.

[a] The decline in the number of patients observed is due primarily to the fact that patients were admitted over a 2½-year period. Hence, many were not in the study long enough to be observed at the longer time periods.

blood pressure, while the placebo group had a very small one (Table 20–5). The end points documented were (1) death, (2) severe complications requiring removal from protocol drugs or placebo and substitution of more intensive antihypertensive therapy (class A events), (3) events similar to class A, except that such diagnoses had not been written into the protocol (other treatment failures), and (4) morbid events not judged to warrant discontinuation of protocol (class B events). Typical class A events included dissecting aneurysm, malignant hypertension, and resistant congestive heart failure. Typical class B events included cerebral thrombosis and myocardial infarction. The study of severe hypertensives was terminated after an average of about 18 months follow-up, because results at that time clearly favored the treatment group (Table 20–6). The 21 terminating events that occurred in the placebo group were aortic aneurysm dissection or rupture (three cases), fundal hemorrhages or exudates (nine cases), sudden death (one case), deterioration in renal function (three cases), cerebrovascular accident (two cases), and markedly elevated basal diastolic pressure (three cases). The one terminating case while under treatment had hyperglycemia and depression. The nonterminating events in the placebo group were myocardial infarction (two cases), congestive heart failure (two cases), and cerebrovascular thrombosis or transient ischemic attacks (three cases). The one event on active therapy was a cerebrovascular thrombosis. It is clear that treatment resulted in great savings of morbidity and mortality in these severe hypertensives.

Table 20–6 Incidence of mortality and morbidity in the placebo and active group of the more severely hypertensive participants of the V.A. Cooperative Study

	Placebo-treated patients	Actively-treated patients
Deaths	4	0
Class A events	10	0
Subtotal	14	0
Other treatment failures	7	1
Total terminating events	21	1
Class B events (nonterminating)	6	1
Total	27	2

Source: V.A. Cooperative Study Group on Antihypertensive Agents: Effects of treatment on morbidity in hypertension. I. *JAMA* **202**:1028, copyright © 1967, American Medical Association.

For the milder hypertensives a similar protocol was used with follow-up over 5 years. Again, the treatment lowered blood pressure in the intervention group very effectively. The causes of death and the terminating and nonterminating events can be seen to involve the same organs as before (Table 20–7). The effect

Table 20–7 Summary of assessable events for the control and treated milder hypertensives of the V.A. Cooperative Study

	Control group		Treated group		Percent effective-ness[b]
	No.	%	No.	%	
Terminating morbid events[a]	35	18.0	9	4.8	73
Nonterminating B events	21		13		
Total morbid events	56	28.9	22	11.8	59
Terminated on account of elevated blood pressure	20		0		
Total assessable events	76	39.2	22	11.8	70
Number of patients randomized	194	100.0	186	100.0	

Source: V.A. Cooperative Study Group on Antihypertensive Agents: Effects of treatment on morbidity in hypertension. II. *JAMA* **213**:1143, copyright © 1970, American Medical Association.

[a] Includes cardiovascular deaths, class A events, and treatment failures except those due to diastolic levels > 124 mm Hg.

of the treatment is again dramatic. However, numbers are too small to decide any benefit for specific diagnostic end points. In particular, it is not possible to make any statement from these data regarding ischemic heart disease events. Recall also that the participants were not representative of the whole community but were veterans selected for good compliance.

The largest trial of drug therapy in hypertension reported to date is the Hypertension Detection and Follow-up Program (HDFP) (HDFP Cooperative Group, 1979a,b, 1980). The study was started in 1972 to answer the following specific questions:

- Is a systematic, aggressive approach to hypertension effective in reducing mortality for hypertensive adults in the community setting?
- Can a substantial proportion of all hypertensives detected in the general population be brought under medical management aimed at reducing blood pressure to normal levels, and can they be kept under management?
- Do the benefits of hypertension treatment exceed possible toxicity, especially in the case of patients with so-called mild hypertension?
- Is antihypertensive therapy effective in young adults and women, and equally effective in blacks and whites?
- Can mortality from coronary heart disease be reduced by antihypertensive therapy?

The study design was a randomized controlled trial, and the participants were hypertensives detected through community screening. Fourteen U.S. communities were involved in the study; 178,009 persons aged 30–69 were identified, and 89 percent completed the first screening (three readings using a standard mercury sphygmomanometer). One spin-off of this study was the large amount of descriptive data on blood pressure generated by this screening process (Hypertension Detection and Follow-up Program Cooperative Group, 1977a,b, 1978). If the mean diastolic pressure of the second and third readings was greater than 95 mm Hg, they were invited to attend an HDFP center for a second screening. This applied to 22,978 or 14.5 percent of those first screened. Seventy-six percent of these persons (17,476) attended the second screening. At this time, if an average of two random zero sphygmomanometer readings was greater than 90 mm Hg, they were enrolled into the study (10,940). As can be seen, the determination of hypertension was far from that based on a casual blood pressure reading, and clinicians should bear this in mind in interpreting the results. These enrollees were then randomized to treatment or referred-care status. The latter was not a true control group, as these patients were referred to their own doctors for whatever treatment they might receive. The follow-up period was 5 years, and the two groups were shown to be comparable with respect to other risk factors at study baseline.

Each patient received a diastolic blood pressure goal of less than 90 mm Hg if they entered with a diastolic blood pressure greater than 100 mm Hg, or else a fall of greater than 10 mm Hg if the entry diastolic pressure was between 90 and

100 mm Hg. A stepped-care regime of drugs was used as follows, progressing from weaker to stronger drugs:

Step 1: Thiazides (or less commonly triamterene or spironolactone)
Step 2: Reserpine or methyldopa
Step 3: Hydralazine
Step 4: Guanethidine

These steps were progressively traversed until goal blood pressure was obtained. Thus, the most commonly used drugs were the thiazides, as most people were mild hypertensives.

The major end point was overall mortality. It is difficult to assess more specific nonfatal end points because of different frequencies and intensities of observation between the two study groups. Data relating to nonfatal ischemic heart disease events has not yet been reported. Another potential problem was the narrowing of the magnitude of the treatment difference between the two groups due to nonadherence by some stepped-care individuals and increasingly effective care of hypertension by the community doctors who cared for the comparison group. Despite this, there was a consistent difference between groups in the percentage of cases being treated and the percentage below the HDFP study goal throughout the follow-up (Table 20–8). Notice the increasing proportion of stepped-care patients achieving goal status as time progressed, but notice that

Table 20–8 Percentage of stepped-care and referred-care participants at or below HDFP goal DBP by year of follow-up[a]

Year	HDFP goal status	Stepped-care total	Referred-care total
1	At or below goal	51.8	29.4
	Not at goal	42.2	62.6
	Unknown	6.0	8.0
2	At or below goal	56.7	33.7
	Not at goal	38.6	59.4
	Unknown	4.7	6.9
4	At or below goal	61.7	40.7
	Not at goal	31.3	47.2
	Unknown	7.0	12.1
5	At or below goal	64.9	43.6
	Not at goal	29.9	47.5
	Unknown	5.2	8.9

Source: Adapted from HDFP Cooperative Group: *JAMA* **242**:2562, 1979a, with permission.

[a] HDFP, Hypertension Detection and Follow-up Program; DBP, diastolic blood pressure.

some less pronounced changes are also seen in the referred-care group. The effectiveness of the stepped-care approach in lowering blood pressure was documented for males and females, for blacks and whites.

Mortality from all causes dropped by 16.9 percent in the stepped-care group ($P < 0.01$) as compared to the referred-care group. This mortality reduction was fairly consistent across different age, sex, and racial groups, although the study was not designed to look at subgroups effectively. The mortality reduction was seen to be greatest in those who had baseline pressures between 90 and 104 mm Hg (20.3 percent reduction) and least in those who had baseline pressures > 115 mm Hg (7.2 percent reduction). This unexpected result of maximum benefit for the mildest hypertensives may be explained as a consequence of using a "referred-care" rather than a placebo control group. The effectiveness of treatment of the severely hypertensive in the referred group came rather close proportionately to the effectiveness of treatment in the stepped-care group. However, substantial proportionate treatment differences persisted for the milder hypertensives. The result does not indicate that the mortality benefits of treating hypertensives diminish in severe hypertensives. The Veterans Administration Study suggests that the reverse is likely. A death-by-cause classification (Table 20–9) for both the total group and also the milder hypertensives (stratum 1) showed that in many cases the number of events was relatively small. Nevertheless, it is impressive to find a 45 percent reduction in cerebrovascular disease mortality and a 46 percent reduction in mortality ascribed to acute myocardial infarction in the stepped-care group.

The study results promise a significant mortality reduction with appropriate therapy in a very common disease. The HDFP "required the efforts of hundreds of workers and has so far cost over $60 million, but if its promise can be realized, it will represent one of the great health bargains of our time" ("Mild Hypertension: No More Benign Neglect," 1980).

The Australian Mild Hypertension Trial (Australian National Blood Pressure Study, 1980) is another randomized controlled trial that was conducted in Melbourne, Perth, and Sydney. Mild hypertension was defined as a mean of four diastolic pressures between 95 and 110 mm Hg with systolic pressures averaging less than 200 mm Hg. The stepped-care regime was similar to the HDFP study, but an important difference was the use of a true control group of mild hypertensives who were given placebo tablets. Of the 104,171 subjects who were screened, 3427 were finally selected for the study. Follow-up averaged 4 years, and at the close of the study about two-thirds of each group were adhering to the study protocol. The final report showed a significant reduction in both fatal and nonfatal end points that included cardiac and cerebrovascular events, as well as retinal hemorrhages, hypertensive encephalopathy, and renal failure (Fig. 20–4). However, it was not possible to be confident of a reduction in IHD end points, perhaps because of the small numbers. The number of cases, respectively, in the active and placebo groups for fatal ischemic heart disease were 5 versus 11, for nonfatal myocardial infarction 28 versus 22, and for total IHD events 98 versus 109.

Table 20-9 Number of deaths by cause, stepped care, and referred care participants, total and stratum 1: HDFP[a]

Cause of death (ICDA codes)[b]	Total		Stratum 1 (DBP, 90–104 mm Hg)	
	SC	RC	SC	RC
Total	349	419	231	291
All cardiovascular diseases	195	240	122	165
Cerebrovascular diseases (430–438)	29	52	17	31
Myocardial infarction (410)	51	69	30	56
Other ischemic heart disease (411–413)	80	79	56	51
Hypertensive heart disease (402)	5	7	5	5
Other hypertensive diseases (400–401, 403–404)	4	7	2	3
Other cardiovascular diseases (390–458 exclusive of above)	26	26	12	19
All noncardiovascular diseases	154	179	109	126
Renal diseases (580–599)	15	10	7	5
Diabetes mellitus (250)	5	10	4	8
Neoplastic diseases (140–239)	61	74	45	57
Breast cancer (174)	(2)	(5)	(2)	(4)
Gastrointestinal diseases (530–537)	11	20	9	15
Respiratory diseases (460–519)	13	17	9	10
Infectious diseases (000–136)	6	3	4	2
Accidents, suicides, and homicides (800–999)	26	25	20	17
Other diseases	17	20	11	12

Source: From HDFP Cooperative Group: *JAMA* **242**:2562, 1979a, with permission.

[a] DBP, diastolic blood pressure; SC, Stepped care; RC, referred care.

[b] From death certificates. ICDA Codes indicates International Classification of Diseases Adapted Codes.

A Scandinavian study (Berglund et al, 1978) began by screening nearly 10,000 men. This represented a random third of all men born during the period 1915–1922 and 1924–1925 living in Göteborg, Sweden. Of these men, 1229 were hypertensive at first screening, defined as systolic blood pressure greater than 175 mm Hg, or diastolic blood pressure greater than 115 mm Hg, or currently on antihypertensive treatment. Those not receiving treatment had their blood pressure checked again in 2 weeks. Men whose results were positive for *both* screens and those taking antihypertensive medications and who had elevated pressures at the single screen formed the treatment group (635 men), and they were admitted to the hypertension clinic. The untreated control group consisted

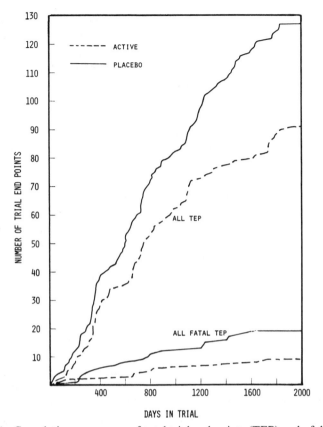

Figure 20–4 Cumulative occurrence of total trial end points (TEP) and of deaths from all causes in 1721 subjects of the active antihypertensive and 1706 of the placebo group while adhering to trial regimen. Difference between active and placebo group was significant for all trial end points ($P < 0.01$) and all deaths ($P < 0.05$). From Australian National Blood Pressure Study, 1980, with permission.

of 391 persons who were not on medication and who were hypertensive at the first screen but not at the second check. This rather unusual design then biases *against* a favorable result for treatment, as the severer cases were in the treatment group. Although this study was not a randomized trial, other risk factors appeared similar between the two groups. β-blockers were the primary treatment, and thiazides or hydralazine were added if necessary. The few noncompliers were retained within the groups to which they were originally assigned for purposes of analysis; the follow-up period averaged 4.3 years. The treatment group had a significantly lower total mortality (3.3 vs. 6.1 percent, $P < 0.05$). Ischemic heart disease events were also significantly lower ($P < 0.03$) when fatal and nonfatal events were combined. Stroke incidence was lower but not significantly so (numbers were small).

Thus, there is clear evidence that drug therapy decreases total mortality, but some consider the evidence inconclusive for IHD end points. Results from the HDFP and the Berglund trials give impressive evidence of IHD mortality reduction, but these were the non-placebo-controlled studies so doubts remain. It has been suggested that the lack of unequivocal evidence is due to the unfortunate metabolic effects of thiazides on lipid and glucose metabolism (Ames, 1983).

Left ventricular hypertrophy (LVH) is a serious risk factor for all manifestations of IHD, including death (chapter 9). It has been demonstrated that hypertension is the most common cause of LVH. Consequently, there is interest in the possibility of preventing and reversing LVH by the use of antihypertensive drugs.

About 70 percent of the men with initial diastolic blood pressures between 90 and 114 in the Veterans Administration Cooperative Trial had 12-lead electrocardiograms before treatment and again 1 year after randomization (Freis, 1983). All follow-up conditions were similar for the two treatment groups of this placebo-controlled trial, and differences in the frequency of development of ECG changes consistent with LVH in men with normal baseline electrocardiograms are impressive. Increased voltages and ST-segment depression in 25 and 19.3 percent, respectively, of the control group, but only 6.6 and 3.8 percent of the treated group (both $P < 0.005$). For those patients with voltage criteria for LVH at baseline, this reverted to normal in 74.4 percent of the treated patients as compared to 24 percent of the control group ($P < 0.005$).

The HDFP has reported qualitatively similar findings, although the differences were of less magnitude, perhaps due to the partially treated state of the "usual-care" control group (Hypertension Detection and Follow-up Program Cooperative Group, 1982). The ECG is a relatively insensitive detector of LVH, but echocardiography is more accurate. Several studies have also confirmed the regression of LVH in drug-treated hypertensives using echocardiography to measure changes (Rowlands et al, 1982; Wollam et al, 1983). Some believe that the development of LVH is more likely in association with increased catecholamine activity (Tarazi, 1983), and it is of interest that Wollam and colleagues found regression of LVH when treatment was with β-blockers or methyldopa but could not demonstrate such with thiazide therapy. However, numbers of patients were small.

Recommendations for the evaluation of raised blood pressure levels have been made by the Joint National Committee on Detection, Evaluation, and Treatment of High Blood Pressure (1984). Two or more measurements should be taken at each visit and averaged. Treatment should not be started based on a single reading. As shown in Table 20–10, except for the severest cases, a confirmation visit is generally required.

There has been controversy over the practical application of the results of these trials, particularly in reference to the range of mildest hypertension with diastolic pressures between 90 and 100 mm Hg. The Australian Mild Hypertension Trial could not demonstrate significant benefit of drug therapy for those with diastolic pressures less than 100 mm Hg. In contrast, a substantial benefit

Table 20–10 Suggested follow-up criteria for first-occasion blood pressure measurement and at confirmation visits

Range (mm Hg)	Recommended follow up[a]
First occasion	
Diastolic	
<85	Recheck within 2 years.
85–89	Recheck within 1 year.
90–104	Confirm promptly (not to exceed 2 months).
105–114	Evaluate or refer promptly to source of care (not to exceed 2 weeks).
>115	Evaluate or refer immediately to a source of care.
Systolic, when diastolic BP is >90	
<140	Recheck within 2 years.
140–199	Confirm promptly (not to exceed 2 months).
>200	Evaluate or refer promptly to source of care (not to exceed 2 weeks).
Confirmation visits	
Diastolic	
<85	Recheck within 2 years.[b]
85–89	Recheck within 1 year.
>90	Evaluate or refer promptly to a source of care.
Systolic, when diastolic BP is <90	
<140	Recheck within 1 year.
>140	Evaluate or refer promptly to a source of care.

Source: Adapted from Joint National Committee on Detection, Evaluation, and Treatment of High Blood Pressure: *Arch Intern Med* **144**:1045, 1984, with permission.

[a] If recommendations for follow-up of diastolic and systolic BPs are different, the shorter recommended time period supersedes and a referral supersedes a recheck recommendation.

[b] Rechecking within 1 year is recommended for persons at increased risk of progressing to higher BPs, including family history of hypertension or cardiovascular event, weight gain or obesity, black race, use of an oral contraceptive, and excessive ethanol consumption.

(34 percent mortality reduction) was seen for those with diastolic pressures of 90–94 mm Hg in the HDFP trial (Gifford et al, 1983). Neither of these studies was designed to be able to draw conclusions within subgroups such as 90–100 or 90–94 mm Hg for diastolic pressure. Different patterns are likely to be only chance fluctuations. However, it is theoretically true that those with milder abnormalities probably stand to benefit less, and we need to be concerned that the benefits outweigh the risks of therapy in a relatively low-risk population (chapter 15).

The HDFP study had been criticized because the nonplacebo control group had less intense and different clinical contacts, which in theory could affect outcomes. Extensive analyses of the data have shown that well over half of the excess risk in the control group could be attributed to factors directly related to hypertension treatment such as blood pressure levels, goal blood pressure, and medication status (Hardy and Hawkins, 1983).

Based on these observations, and also results of the Multiple Risk Factor Intervention Trial (MRFIT, chapter 17), recent recommendations of the National Heart, Lung, and Blood Institute (1983) for treatment of mild hypertension are as follows:

- Initiate treatment of mild high blood pressure, particularly in the range of 90 to 94 mm Hg diastolic, with nonpharmacologic measures as long as this treatment is effective in maintaining normal blood pressure. (It should be noted that the efficacy of nonpharmacologic treatment *on a large-scale basis* has not yet been demonstrated.)
- Pharmacologic treatment, as used in the HDFP, should be considered when other treatments are not effective in maintaining blood pressure control, even in those subgroups with abnormal resting ECGs.
- In general, it is prudent medical therapy to use the lowest dosage of any drug effective in maintaining control. Regarding diuretics, a dosage of 50 mg daily of hydrochlorothiazide (or its equivalent) should probably not be exceeded.
- In the subgroups of patients with resting ECG abnormalities, addition or substitutions of other approved antihypertensive agents may be warranted if diuretics in low dosage (e.g., hydrochlorothiazide 25–50 mg daily) are not adequate to control the blood pressure.
- Appropriate monitoring of serum potassium levels is warranted, as always.

There are some clear indications that detection and control of hypertension in our communities have greatly improved even over the past decade. As an example, in Minneapolis–St. Paul the results of a 1980–1981 survey of risk factors was compared to a 1973–1974 survey conducted in one suburb within the same area of the later study (Folsom et al, 1983). The suburb studied in the earlier survey closely resembled the metropolitan area of the later study in age, race, employment, education, and income. Comparison of the two studies showed significant drops in mean blood pressure by 1980–1981. The prevalence of hypertension and/or need for anti-hypertensive medications was unchanged; however, whereas in 1973–1974 only 40 percent of hypertensives were adequately controlled, in 1980–1981 the figure was 76 percent. In 1973–1974 25.5 percent had previously undetected hypertension, but by 1980–1981 this was true of only 6.6 percent.

β-Blockers, Calcium Channel Blockers, and Secondary Prevention of Ischemic Heart Disease Events

Over the decade since 1974, several randomized studies have compared the effectiveness of various β-blocking drugs to placebo in preventing either death or reinfarction in coronary patients. Some of these studies encompassed small numbers of events, so that they had low statistical power and variable results from one to another (JT Anderson et al, 1979; Barber et al, 1975; Wilhelmsson et al, 1974). However, five large randomized, double-blind, placebo-controlled clinical trials have been reported. These provide conclusive evidence that β-blockers reduce subsequent mortality and possibly morbidity in postinfarction patients. The drugs involved were practolol, propranolol, timolol, sotalol, and metoprolol. The randomization process produced reasonably comparable groups, but as usual those finally enrolled often represented only a fraction of all myocardial infarctions, due to various clinical and administrative exclusion criteria. Usually there was no reason to suspect that the final study groups would be unusual with regard to response to the β-blockade.

The practolol study (KG Green et al, 1977) showed a significant reduction in mortality and a suggestive reduction in nonfatal reinfarction in the treated group, but practolol has subsequently been withdrawn from the market because of ocular and dermatologic side effects. The timolol study (Norwegian Multicenter Study Group, 1981) randomized 1884 patients to treatment of 10 mg twice daily or placebo, starting 7–28 days after infarction. Through a follow-up period of up to 33 months, there was a 39 percent reduction in overall mortality, and the reductions in sudden deaths and reinfarction were both statistically significant. The metoprolol study (Hjalmarsen et al, 1981) involved nearly 700 patients and a relatively short follow-up period of about 3 months. Treatment began on admission to hospital with intravenous metoprolol followed by 100 mg twice daily. The result was a 36 percent reduction in overall mortality for the treated versus control group during this 3-month period. A placebo-controlled trial in Britain randomized 1456 patients (5–14 days after infarction) to either placebo or 320 mg/day of sotalol (Julian et al, 1982). At 1 year there was a nonsignificant 18 percent reduction in mortality and a significant 41 percent reduction in definite myocardial reinfarction. The Beta Blocker Heart Attack Trial (BHAT) randomized 3837 patients to either propranolol 40 mg three times daily or placebo for periods of up to 30 months. The average time between infarction and start of treatment was nearly 14 days. Reduction in overall mortality and nonfatal reinfarction for the treatment group was 26 and 15.6 percent, respectively (Beta Blocker Heart Attack Research Group, 1981, 1982, 1983). [A smaller trial of propranolol in Norway also showed good effect (Hansteen et al, 1982).] The survival curves from the BHAT study, which are similar in form to those of other studies, are shown in Fig. 20–5.

Although the reduction in mortality seems to lie between about 25 and 40 percent when expressed as a percentage of the rate in the placebo group, this figure becomes somewhat less impressive when applied to the total population; the reduction in absolute mortality is then closer to 1 fewer death per 100 persons at risk per year. (Of course, equivalent observations could be made for the results of the cholestyramine, aspirin, and sulfinpyrazone trials.) The optimal time for starting the β blockade after infarction is not clearly established. In the metoprolol study and a smaller alprenolol study (MP Andersen et al, 1979), therapy began on hospital admission; in the rest of the studies it started several days

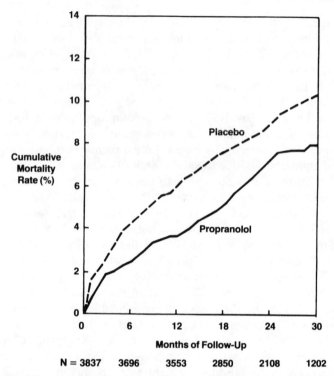

Figure 20–5 Life table cumulative mortality curves for propranolol hydrochloride and placebo groups. From Beta Blocker Heart Attack Study Group: The Beta Blocker Heart Attack Trial. *JAMA* **246**:2073, copyright © 1981, American Medical Association.

later. In view of the possibility of complications in the first few days, some suggest caution until the safety and efficacy of using these medications immediately after admission is proven. The duration of effectiveness is also open to question. From most of the survival curves it appears that maximal benefit was gained within the first year after infarction, but it is unclear whether there is a subgroup that continues to benefit beyond this period or whether side effects may develop in the longer term. In any event, the advantage is still clear up to about 3 years, and the medications can be safely continued for this period. The syndrome particularly affected by these medications appears to be cardiac death (particularly sudden death), although some studies give some hint of reduction in reinfarction also. There is some disagreement as to the consistency of effect for the two sexes, for different ages, according to presence of cardiac failure, and for different sites of infarction. Several studies suggest that the beneficial effect extends to all of these subgroups. The mode of action is also uncertain. Possible mechanisms include reduction of arrhythmias as suggested by the BHAT, metoprolol, and sotalol studies (Lichstein et al, 1983), limitation of infarct size (Hjalmarson and Herlitz, 1983), and possibly limitation of the ability of platelets to generate thromboxane (J Mehta and P Mehta, 1982).

Little information is available yet from large trials as to the effects of calcium channel blockers on subsequent morbidity and mortality of IHD patients. However, one double-blind placebo-controlled trial of 138 patients tested the effect of nifedipine added to conventional β-blocker and nitrate treatment of unstable angina patients, as prevention of persistent angina, sudden cardiac death, myocardial infarction, or the need for coronary bypass surgery (Gerstenblith et al, 1982). Participants initially had chest pain at rest and transient ST elevation, depression, T-wave changes, or arrhythmias on the ECG. The results showed marked and statistically significant ($P < 0.03$) benefit to the nifedipine group, this being especially apparent in the subgroup with ST elevation during baseline unstable angina. The greatest portion of the overall benefit was in reduction of need for coronary bypass surgery.

Possible mechanisms of good effect include reduction in myocardial oxygen demand, reduction in coronary vascular tone and so a potential increase in perfusion, and also reduction of platelet aggregation, as calcium ions are involved in platelet activation (Ikeda et al, 1981; Johnsson, 1981).

Antiarrhythmic Drugs as Prevention

Ectopic ventricular beats in otherwise fit young people are very common. There is a little evidence that such people have a slightly increased risk of developing ischemic heart disease, in particular sudden death (Rabkin et al, 1981). In a 7-year follow-up of 72 such individuals, Horan and Kennedy (1981) found that this was a relatively benign syndrome. When IHD is present, however, frequent premature beats have prognostic significance (chapter 18), and it is common practice to administer antiarrhythmic drugs. The discussion below will be restricted to the efficacy of these drugs in reducing mortality when used in the nonacute situation.

In the few randomized studies of antiarrhythmics that have been conducted, patient numbers have been small. This requires that the drugs be very effective if statistical significance is to be achieved. In a study by Kosowsky et al (1973), long-term oral procainamide did not show a statistically significant mortality advantage, and indeed only 8 of 39 patients remained on the drug at 18 months, as a result of side effects. Long-term phenytoin administration also showed no mortality advantage (Lovell, 1978; Peter et al, 1978). Mexiletine was used in a randomized study of high-risk postinfarction patients (Chamberlain et al, 1980), and again no advantage was demonstrated. A randomized study of aprinidine in the Netherlands found a nonsignificant difference between the two groups after 1 year (Van Durme and Bogaerts, 1980).

Several of these studies were able to demonstrate improved arrhythmia control. While more information is needed, the findings so far give little encouragement regarding any effect on mortality. It is possible that ventricular premature beats reflect underlying cardiac damage and dysfunction (associated with sudden death) rather than having a direct causal link with sudden death. Maybe we are treating the electrocardiogram rather than the patient in some instances. However, there may be subgroups who benefit from the suppression of such arrhythmias, and few would argue with the prudence of treating *complex* ventricular premature beats (couplets, ventricular tachycardia, multiform, R on T). Exercise-induced ventricular ectopy may also be in a separate category (Goldschlager et al, 1979), although Simoons et al (1980) found that ectopy during normal activities was more predictive of cardiac arrest in patients with IHD.

Antihypertensive Agents and Serum Lipids

Both total cholesterol and triglyceride levels are raised by the use of thiazide diuretics or the related diuretic chlorthalidone. Goldman et al (1980) found that hypertensives being treated with chlorthalidone showed an overall 10-mg/dl increase in total cholesterol as compared to the placebo group (Table 20–11), the increase being particularly evident in younger individuals. This was entirely explained by the change in LDL cholesterol. Results from the MRFIT study (Kuller et al, 1980; Lasser et al, 1984) are roughly similar, except in indicating that VLDL cholesterol was the major cause of the cholesterol rise. Perhaps the fact that MRFIT involved both hydrochlorothiazide and chlorthalidone may account for the difference in the lipid fraction. Grimm and colleagues (1981) performed a randomized study to investigate the effect of both hydrochlorothiazide and chlorthalidone on blood lipids. They found that both VLDL and LDL cholesterols appeared to be raised by both drugs as compared to placebo. There was no evidence of change in HDL cholesterol. Furosemide may also elevate LDL cholesterol (Gluck et al, 1978).

β-blockers have come into question on related grounds. In a small crossover study, Leren et al (1980) used 23 hypertensives as their own controls, placing them on an increasing dose of propranolol (up to 80 mg bid) over 3 weeks. The drug therapy was associated with a 13 percent reduction in HDL cholesterol and a 16 percent increase in triglyceride levels, and had no effect on LDL cholesterol. A report from the Beta Blocker Heart Attack Trial stated that of 2874 survivors of recent myocardial infarction, those randomized to propranolol therapy had HDL cholesterol levels 4 and 3 mg/dl lower in men and women, respectively, than the control group ($P < 0.01$). At baseline there had been no significant differences (Shulman et al, 1983). This effect of propranolol on HDL was also found for females in the Lipid Research Clinic Study (Wallace et al, 1980). Other small studies have shown a similar effect (Day et al, 1979; Helgeland et al, 1978). By contrast, there is some evidence from several studies that prazocin therapy raises HDL cholesterol, and so improves the LDL/HDL ratio (Kokubu et al, 1982; Leren et al, 1980; Velasco et al, 1982; Zanchetti, 1984).

One possible conclusion is that we may be "robbing Peter to pay Paul" when we treat hypertensives with thiazides. Using estimates of effect from the

Table 20–11 Changes in lipid concentrations after 1 year of treatment with chlorthalidone

Lipid	n	lipid (mg/dl), mean ± SE	
		Baseline	Change
Total cholesterol			
Active group	302	203.1 ± 2.0	9.9 ± 1.5[c]
Placebo group	308	196.5 ± 2.0	−0.1 ± 1.1
Difference	—	6.6 ± 2.9[a]	10.0 ± 1.8[c]
Triglycerides			
Active group	297	152.2 ± 5.8	14.5 ± 3.8[c]
Placebo group	308	128.8 ± 5.0	4.7 ± 3.6
Difference	—	23.4 ± 7.6[b]	9.8 ± 5.2[d]
HDL cholesterol			
Active group	89	43.7 ± 1.1	1.1 ± 0.6
Placebo group	100	44.3 ± 0.9	1.0 ± 0.6
Difference	—	−0.6 ± 1.4	0.1 ± 0.8
LDL cholesterol			
Active group	89	125.8 ± 3.2	12.6 ± 2.7[c]
Placebo group	99	123.7 ± 3.1	0.0 ± 2.0
Difference	—	2.1 ± 4.5	12.6 ± 3.4[c]

Source: From V.A. Cooperative Study Group on Antihypertensive Agents: Serum lipoprotein level during chlorthalidone therapy. *JAMA* **244**:1691, copyright © 1980, American Medical Association.

[a] $t > 1.96$; $P < 0.05$.   [c] $t > 3.29$; $P < 0.001$.

[b] $t > 2.58$; $P < 0.01$.   [d] $t = 1.89$; $P = 0.06$.

Framingham Study, Grimm et al (1981) found that the lipid-raising effect counterbalances the risk reduction producted by the hypotensive action. This is clearly not true for *all-cause* mortality over a 5-year period, but it may be one reason why the V.A. Study and the Australian Mild Hypertensive Trial do not show statistically significant reductions for IHD events. These lipoprotein changes should not prevent us from treating hypertension by drugs, as the balance of risk and benefit still favors treatment. Hypertension, of course, is treated to prevent morbidity and mortality from other causes than IHD. However, it is probably prudent to emphasize the control of hypertension by lifestyle changes more forcefully, especially in persons with a poor lipid profile ("Antihypertensive Drugs, Plasmo Lipids, and Coronary Disease," 1980).

Oral Contraceptives, Postmenopausal Estrogens, and Cardiovascular Disease

Oral contraceptives have been suspected of producing myocardial infarction, among other side effects. Not all studies have shown such a relationship, but the

Table 20–12 Mortality rate per 100,000 woman-years from cardiovascular causes by oral contraceptive use[a,b]

| | Mortality (number of deaths) | | Ratio of rate in ever-users to controls |
Cause	Ever-users	Controls	
All diseases of the circulatory system	25.8 (24)	5.5 (5)	4.7[c]
Nonrheumatic heart disease and hypertension	10.4 (11)	2.5 (2)	4.0[d]
Cerebrovascular disease	13.2 (10)	2.8 (3)	4.7[d]
Woman-years of observation	91,880	91,521	

Source: Adapted from Royal College of General Practitioners Oral Contraceptive Study Group, 1977, with permission.

[a] Because the rates for each cause are standardized separately, there are small discrepancies between the sum of the individual rates and the "total" rates.

[b] Pregnancy excluded and standardized for age at entry, parity, social class, and smoking.

[c] $P < 0.01$.

[d] $P < 0.05$.

largest and best designed have found a significant increase in these events. As myocardial infarction in young women is rare, numbers of cases have usually been quite small, affecting the statistical power to find a significant result.

A large prospective study in the United Kingdom followed 46,000 women of childbearing age and compared the health experience of those who were taking oral contraceptives with those who were not. Called the Royal College of General Practitioners Oral Contraceptive Study (1977), its report covered about 200,000 woman-years of experience. Contraceptive users were at a clear disadvantage with respect to mortality from "non-rheumatic heart disease and hypertension" as well as cerebrovascular disease (Table 20–12). This was adjusted for any concurrent effect of cigarette smoking. The relative risk represented a fourfold difference. There appeared to be a relationship between duration of therapy and risk of mortality from diseases of the circulatory system (Table 20–13). As this was not an experiment but an observational study, it is possible that oral contraceptive users differed from nonusers in variables apart from those adjusted for, but there is no evidence for this. Most studies have shown that risk increases with age (Krueger et al, 1980; Mann et al, 1976), but the *relative* risk is high also for young women. The possible mechanisms include alterations in blood lipids, in blood pressure, and also in the viscosity and coagulability of blood. In addition, there is evidence that oral contraceptive users have higher levels of blood glucose and insulin (Ostrander et al, 1980).

That oral contraceptive use elevates blood pressure is clear. This increase averages 6–8 mm Hg systolic and 1–2 mm Hg diastolic (Fisch and Franks, 1977;

Table 20–13 Mortality per 100,000 woman-years from diseases of circulatory system by duration of continuous oral contraceptive use

| Duration of oral contraceptive use (months) | Mortality (number of deaths) | | | Ratio of age-standardized rates to that of controls |
| | Age (at time of death) | | Age standardized[a] | |
	15–34	35–49[a]		
0	3.7 (2)	7.9 (3)	5.2 (5)	1.0
1–59	8.5 (3)	33.0 (4)	17.5 (7)	3.4
60+	0.0	113.8 (9)	50.5 (9)	9.7

Source: From Royal College of General Practitioners Oral Contraceptive Study Group, 1977, with permission.

[a] Tests for linear trends, $P < 0.01$.

Weir et al, 1971, 1974). Although in most women the elevation is modest, in a few women it can be very important. Fisch and colleagues analyzed data from over 13,000 women in the Kaiser Permanente Medical Care Program. As can be seen in Fig. 20–6, mean blood pressures were significantly higher for current contraceptive users. Expressed a little differently, 8 percent of users versus 3.2 percent of never-users had systolic hypertension (> 140 mm Hg), and 10 percent of users versus 7.2 percent of never-users had diastolic hypertension (> 90 mm Hg). The elevations prove reversible on stopping these medications (Fig. 20–7). The mechanism is uncertain, and different studies have suggested that both estrogen or progestagen may be responsible (Khaw and Peart, 1982). Blood viscosity, which is increased by oral contraceptive use, is one determinant of blood pressure levels (Letcher et al, 1981).

The reader will also recall the startling estimate of relative risk of myocardial infarction in women who were oral contraceptive users and also heavy smokers (> 25 cigarettes/day). This relative risk was estimated at about 39-fold (95 percent confidence interval 22 to 70), apparently demonstrating an interaction between smoking and oral contraceptive use in producing myocardial infarction (Shapiro et al, 1979).

The issue of oral contraceptive use and blood lipid levels has been quite confused. In particular there is a difference between the effect of post-menopausal estrogens and combination oral contraceptives. Oral contraceptive users in general have higher levels of serum total cholesterol (Lipid Research Clinics Program Epidemiology Committee, 1979; Wynn et al, 1979), but evidence suggest that all oral contraceptives are not alike in this regard. It has been known for many years that estrogens tend to elevate HDL and depress LDL cholesterol (Fig. 20–8), whereas androgens do the opposite (Heiss et al, 1980a). As several of the progestagens in oral contraceptives have anti-estrogenic or androgenic

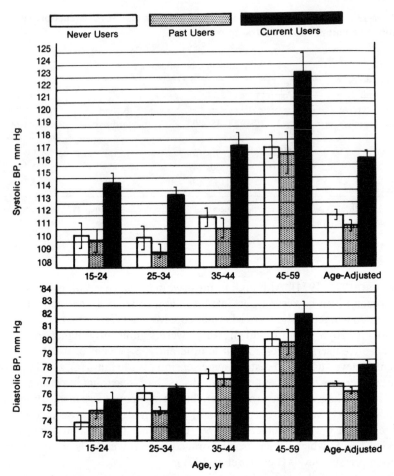

Figure 20–6   Mean blood pressure (BP) by age and oral contraceptive use (95 percent confidence intervals). From IR Fisch and J Frank: Oral contraceptives and blood pressure. *JAMA* **237**:2499, copyright © 1977, American Medical Association.

effects, the effect on blood lipids depends on the type of progestagen and the relative dosages of estrogen and progestagen in the oral contraceptive preparation (Bradley et al, 1978).

Blood viscosity is believed to be one determinant of blood pressure and also the likelihood of thrombosis. It is generally elevated in women taking oral contraceptives—probably largely because hematocrit levels are higher, at about male levels. This may be a result of decreased menstrual blood loss and consequently less iron deficiency (Table 20–14). There may also be small increases in blood fibrinogen levels contributing to the increased blood viscosity. Abnormal types of fibrinogen can be detected in the plasma of 27 percent of oral contraceptive users but only 6 percent of nonusers according to Alkjaersig et al (1975).

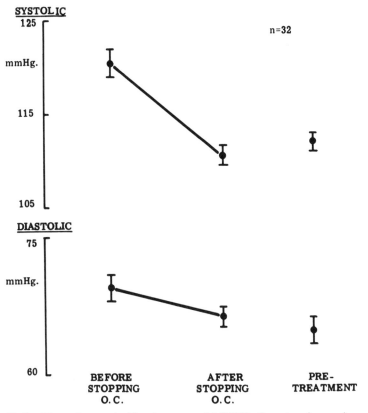

Figure 20–7   Mean changes in blood pressure (± SEM) after stopping oral contraceptives. From RJ Weir et al: *Br Med J* **1**:533, 1974, with permission.

These abnormal fibrinogen constituents indicate enhanced activation of the fibrin-forming system and correlates highly with the presence of clinically silent thrombi. The major plasma inhibitor of thrombin is anti-thrombin III, and the activity of this enzyme is apparently lowered by oral contraceptive use in some women (Stadel, 1981).

The effect of postmenopausal estrogen administration on cardiovascular risk needs further research, but available evidence suggests a contrast with the oral contraceptives. One case–control study was unable to find any hint of increased cardiovascular risk in postmenopausal women taking estrogens after controlling for several other risk factors (Rosenberg et al, 1976). In a younger group of women aged 30–49 taking noncontraceptive estrogens, there was again no evidence of increased risk of myocardial infarction (Rosenberg et al, 1980b). Another case–control study conducted in a Los Angeles retirement community involved 146 females who died of ischemic heart disease over a 5-year period (Ross et al, 1981). Compared with living or deceased matched control groups,

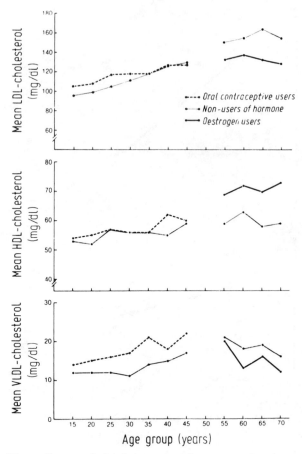

Figure 20–8 Plasma lipoprotein levels in users and nonusers of oral contraceptives and estrogens. From RB Wallace et al, 1979, with permission.

those who had used conjugated estrogens had relative risks of dying from IHD of only 0.43 (*P* <0.01) and 0.57 (*P* <0.05), respectively. Duration of estrogen use or whether menopause was natural or surgical were not analyzed. Women who undergo oophorectomy before menopause may have a higher risk of developing ischemic heart disease (Higano et al, 1963). The beneficial effect of such therapy on the lipoprotein profile has already been noted (Fig. 20–8), but this may be partially offset by effects on blood coagulability or blood pressure. Although the evidence is sparse, it suggests that non-contraceptive estrogens may not place users at higher risk of IHD events.

Table 20–14 Blood viscosity and hematocrit before and during administration of sequential oral contraceptives: Average values for five patients

	Overall average blood viscosity[a]	
	Overall average	Hematocrit (%)
Before	6.01	37.9
After three menstrual cycles	7.76	41.7
After six menstrual cycles	8.93	44.6

Source: Adapted from HB Aronson et al: Effect of oral contraceptives on blood viscosity. *Am J Obstet Gynecol* **110**:997, 1971, with permission.

[a] In centipoises, averaged across five different shear rates (per second).

Summary

1. There are no grounds for the use of clofibrate or niacin unless serum cholesterol is severely elevated. Even here cholestyramine is probably a better first choice. Side effects seem to more than counterbalance any preventive effect from serum cholesterol lowering for postinfarction men, unselected as to serum cholesterol levels, or in relatively hypercholesterolemic men without IHD.

2. The user of cholestyramine in patients with type II hyperlipidemia, and thus moderately or severely elevated levels of serum cholesterol, protects against the development of IHD.

3. Aspirin in low dose is probably modestly beneficial in preventing reinfarction in men with a previous infarction, and very effective in preventing death and infarction in patients with unstable angina.

4. Treatment of severe and also mild hypertension with drugs clearly decreases overall mortality. There is some controversy regarding therapy of the mildest group of hypertensives, and most workers recommend an initial trial of reduction of salt, alcohol, and body weight.

5. Drug therapy of hypertension can prevent the development of left ventricular hypertrophy and also often cause regression of established left ventricular hypertrophy.

6. β blockers are beneficial as secondary prevention—particularly of sudden death. Their relative effectiveness in various demographic and clinical subgroups is controversial, as is the optimal time for commencement of therapy postinfarction. Overall benefit seems to persist for at least 3 years.

7. There is no good evidence that *chronic* antiarrhythmic drug use in IHD patients affects mortality or morbidity. It is probably still prudent to treat complex ventricular ectopy until more evidence is available.

8. Thiazide diuretics and chlorthalidone raise serum cholesterol values, whereas β-blocking agents lower HDL cholesterol and raise serum triglycerides. Prazocin probably raises HDL cholesterol.

9. Estrogens raise HDL cholesterol and lower LDL cholesterol. Androgens and certain progestagens do the reverse. Oral contraceptives are associated with a reversible rise in blood pressure and an increase in blood viscosity. Oral contraceptive users have higher mortality from cardiovascular events, but there is no evidence of increased IHD risk with noncontraceptive estrogen use.

21

Behavioral Change in the Office Setting*

Since behavior and life-style are strongly associated with the development of IHD (Breslow, 1978), the emphasis in this chapter is on *personal* hygiene. As opposed to some models in which physicians prescribe and patients are passively compliant, in this approach individuals take greater responsibility for making desired behavior changes. They are taught effective methods of making healthful alterations in habits, with the behavioral change process being *self-directed* (Karoly and Kanfer, 1982). The techniques we will discuss give *patients* the decision-making role and assist them to reach their own objectives. An important preliminary issue involves the right of health professionals to try to change other people's ways of living. If people *want* to change but are having difficulty, this is no problem. Even for others, the physician can be involved in teaching the health benefits of life-style changes, thus increasing motivation to change.

Adherence to Regimens Advocating Behavioral Change

There is no completely validated model of determinants of health-related behavior, but the Health Belief Model as originally proposed by Rosenstock and modified by Becker and Maiman (1975) is a useful framework. The full model is rather complex and is shown in simplified form in Fig. 21–1.

Patients and Their Environment

While it is not yet possible for a clinician to predict reliably who will or will not adopt healthy behaviors or carry out therapeutic instructions, some information is available. Pirie et al (1982) have recently reported findings suggesting that there are persons who for unknown reasons are more prevention-oriented and are more likely to participate actively in a variety of such activities such as moderate diet, exercise, regular examinations, and seat belt use. Thus, the therapist may find an assessment of other preventive habits informative.

Social support for change can be a vital factor influencing adherence. A per-

* I would like to thank Dr. James Sallis, Ph.D. (University of California, San Diego) for supplying most of the material for this chapter and for offering constructive criticism on its organization.

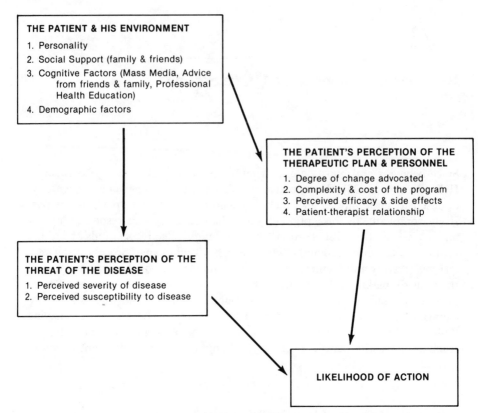

Figure 21–1 Selected portions of the health belief model predicting likelihood of action.

son who has a supportive family is more likely to be successful in many areas of health behavior change (Dunbar and Agras, 1980; Haynes, 1976a), and conversely, single persons are disadvantaged in their ability to comply (Archer et al, 1967).

In the past it was felt that knowledge of risk factors and the benefits of change would constitute sufficient stimulus for action. However, any therapist knows that individuals indulge knowingly in imprudent behaviors, especially when social support for such behaviors is strong. Initiation of teenage smoking is a case in point. Most teenagers who start smoking have a good appreciation of the risks. There is much evidence that health education alone will not result in substantial reduction of risky behaviors in most individuals (Croog and Richards, 1977; RB Haynes, 1976b; Sackett et al, 1975). However, there are some for whom the educational approach is very motivating (perhaps those with the so-called "internal locus of control"), and few would deny that this is one important variable in the interplay of many, resulting in health behavior change.

The limitations of traditional health education alone was highlighted in a study of men at high risk for heart disease (Meyer and Henderson, 1974). All received a 20-minute physician consultation during which behavior changes were prescribed. One group received no other intervention, while a second group received 9 individual sessions with a health educator. A third group participated in 12 group sessions with their wives, in which behavior change was practiced and reinforced. Only the latter group showed improvements in weight control, physical activity, plasma cholesterol, and plasma triglyceride, compared to the control group, at the 3-month follow-up.

The source of health information is important in determining a person's response to the information. Figure 21-2 points out that although mass media are effective in promoting awareness, it is friends, family, and neighbors who have the greatest influence on adoption of the behavior (Yarbrough and Klonglan, 1974). Nevertheless, the Stanford Three-Community Study (chapter 17) has shown that mass media can effect some change—possibly by creating positive social forces as well as educating. Where a *whole community* is being exposed effectively to persuasive information, beginning to adopt some changes no longer appears socially eccentric. The presence of numerous models of healthy behavior in the person's environment has an effect on knowledge, attitudes, and motivation.

Demographic factors such as age, sex, social class, and race are in general poor predictors of compliance with a therapeutic regimen for *established disease*. RB Haynes (1976a) found that of 32 studies of compliance, only 5 found any association with age; of 26 studies only 6 found any association with

Awareness	Interest	Evaluation	Trial	Adoption
Learns about a new idea or practice	Gets more information about it	Tries it out mentally	Uses or tries a little	Accepts it for full-scale and continued use
1. Mass Media—Radio, T.V., Newspapers, Magazines	1. Mass Media	1. Friends and Neighbors	1. Friends and Neighbors	1. Friends and Neighbors
2. Agricultural Agencies, Extension Vo-Ag, etc.	2. Dealers and Salesmen	2. Dealers and Salesmen	2. Dealers and Salesmen	2. Dealers and Salesmen
3. Friends and Neighbors—Mostly Other Farmers	3. Agricultural Agencies	3. Agricultural Agencies	3. Agricultural Agencies	3. Agricultural Agencies
4. Dealers and Salesmen	4. Friends and Neighbors	4. Mass Media	4. Mass Media	4. Mass Media

Personal experience is the most important fact in continued use of an idea.

Figure 21-2 Rank of importance of information source in promoting that stage of the behavioral change process. From P Yarbrough and GE Klonglan, 1974, with permission.

sex; of 24 studies only 3 found an association with education; and of 10 studies only 2 found an association with socioeconomic class. However, as shown in Table 21–1, there *are* demographic factors involved in the likelihood of adoption of *preventive* health measures. Better educated and higher socioeconomic status persons are more likely to quit smoking, to exercise, and to eat a prudent diet. But the physician is encouraged to assume that changing risk factors is a challenge for all patients, and that behavioral counseling is needed in all life-style change efforts.

The Patient's Perception of the Threat of the Disease

People are most likely to be motivated to change health behaviors if the probable consequences of not doing so are perceived as serious, that is, the perceived threat is high (Becker, 1976). Notice it is the *patient's* perception of the disease severity, not the physician's, that is important. The correlation between the physician's and the patient's perception may be rather low, unless the physician is prepared to spend time communicating with the patient.

It has been found by several investigators that excessive degrees of perceived threat and anxiety may be immobilizing and counterproductive (Blackwell, 1973; Joyce et al, 1969; Leventhal et al, 1965). Moderate levels of perceived threat tend to motivate a person to perform self-protective actions, without producing severe arousal, which hinders rational functioning. The importance of this perceived threat is illustrated by the enhanced probability of behavioral change in persons who have already experienced a heart attack. The likelihood of dietary change, smoking cessation, and regular exercise is then markedly increased (Croog and Richards, 1977). Nevertheless, acquainting the patient with the threat is not useful unless there is at the same time a clear and credible plan of action presented to the patient.

The Patient's Perception of the Physician and the Therapeutic Plan

As may have been expected, the more complex the therapeutic plan, the smaller the likelihood of adherence (RB Haynes, 1976b). A program that consists of one main therapeutic modality, or one that at least attempts intervention with only one variable at a time, is more likely to be successful. Unfortunately, in preventive cardiology our recommendations are often quite complex, such as changing dietary, exercise, and smoking patterns.

A procedure that can simplify the sometimes overwhelming nature of complex recommendations is goal setting (Mahoney, 1974; Martin and Dubbert, 1982). A few (or perhaps one) clear goals should be specified in writing. Goals must be realistic and capable of being achieved within a few weeks. This will often necessitate the setting of *interim* goals, giving a progressive nature to the program. A combination of verbal and written instructions is more effective than verbal alone to improve compliance with a drug regime (Dickey et al, 1975). It is also important to teach skills, thus minimizing the hardship in learn-

Table 21–1 Determinants of adherence to recommendations of health experts: A summary of literature

Variable	Following prescribed medical regimen	Staying in treatment	Taking recommended preventive measures
1. Social characteristics			
(a) Age	0	+	−
(b) Sex	0	0	+(fem.)
(c) Education	0	0	+
(d) Income	0	0	+
2. Personality dispositions			
(a) Intelligence	0	0	0
(b) Anxiety	−?	−	?
(c) Internal control	0?	0	+
(d) Psychic disturbance	−	−	?
3. Other psychological dispositions			
(a) Beliefs about threat to health	+	+	+
(b) Beliefs about efficacy of action	+	+	+
(c) Knowledge of recommendation and purpose	+	+	+
(d) General attitudes toward medical care	0	0	0
(e) General knowledge about health and illness	0	0	+?
4. Situational demands			
(a) Symptoms	+	+	NA
(b) Complexity of action	−	−	−
(c) Duration of action	−	−	−
(d) Interference with other actions	−	−	−
5. Social context			
(a) Social support	+	+	+
(b) Social isolation	−	−	−
(c) Primary group stability	+	+	+
6. Interactions with health care systems			
(a) Inconvenience	−	−	−
(b) Continuity of care	+	+	+
(c) Personal source of care	+	+	+?
(d) General satisfaction	0	0	0
(e) Supportive interaction	+	+	?

Source: Adapted by IL Janis, 1983, from JP Kirscht and IM Rosenstock, 1979.

Note: Adapted from Kirscht and Rosenstock, 1979, p. 215. The entries show whether the evidence from all pertinent studies generally supports a positive association (+), a negative association (−), no definite association (0), uncertainty (?), or is not applicable (NA). Kirscht and Rosenstock point out that "the entries are judgmental and oversimplified but are intended to convey a view of the current status of knowledge concerning adherence." Many of the 0 entries represent inconsistent findings; in the case of education, for example, there are positive relationships to medication compliance in several studies but not relationships in many others.

ing the new life-style. Obviously the patient's perception of the efficacy of the therapy will influence the likelihood of compliance (Ley, 1977). Perceived efficacy can be enhanced by both goal setting and teaching of skills, as the patient then has achievable and measurable outcomes and also the reward of goal attainment.

Perhaps the most important factor of all in determining compliance is the quality and quantity of the relationship between the patient and the therapist. Adherence is more likely if the patient sees the same therapist on each occasion (JJ Alpert, 1964; Becker, 1976), particularly if the therapist is warm, empathetic, and noncontrolling (Francis et al, 1969; Gordis et al, 1969). A therapist who takes time to express genuine concern, and to understand the patient's life circumstances and how the behavioral recommendations impinge on these, is more likely to be successful (Shmarak, 1971). Korsch and Negrete (1972) found better adherence also when patients participated in the design of their regimens. It is important that the therapeutic instructions are transmitted in an understandable manner and that any misconceptions about the disease and the treatment are identified and addressed. To accomplish this, it is advisable to use the following techniques:

1. Stress the importance of instructions.
2. Use short words and short sentences.
3. Give specific concrete advice, rather than general principles.
4. Repeat instructions whenever possible.
5. Document them in writing.
6. Ask the patient to restate the instructions.
7. Ask for negative feedback so that anticipated obstacles to implementation can be discussed.

The Ideal Intervention Situation according to the above Model and Evidence

A summary of the evidence from many studies of adherence to recommendations of health care providers is presented in Table 21–1. Thus, the ideal patient is mentally well balanced, is favorably inclined to other preventive activities, and has a good family relationship, in particular a supportive spouse. The family should be willing to be involved in the intervention process. The patient should be acquainted with the basic anatomy, physiology, and nature of the disorders, and should be taught the seriousness of the condition or risk, but should not be inordinately fearful.

The ideal therapeutic program should clearly specify the recommended changes verbally and in writing. If the total intervention is complex, it should be taken in simple stages and considerable attention given to teaching the necessary skills, including actual demonstrations. The physician should try to recommend simple behavior changes that will produce noticeable improvements in symptoms. Whenever reasonable, optimism as to the efficacy of the program should be displayed. Any likely side effects should be discussed and explained ahead of time. The therapist should take time to get to know the patient and family, and to express understanding and support rather than disappointment or condemnation regardless of the rate or amount of progress.

Unfortunately this ideal situation cannot always be attained, but considerable elements of the above are under the control of the therapist and/or patient. The techniques of self-directed behavioral change address many of the concerns and needs of the therapeutic program suggested by the above model.

Self-Directed Behavioral Change

Achieving Initial Changes

In contrast to traditional behavioral therapy of psychiatric patients or retardates, the patient here must be motivated to change; otherwise there will be no self-direction. Health education and other persuasive influences provided by the physician or the mass media clearly have a role in this initial motivating process.

Self-management techniques are of three main types:

1. Observation and *recording* of one's own behavior, and the circumstances or stimuli that prompt it
2. Making changes in the environment to change those cues or stimuli producing inappropriate behaviors; often referred to as *stimulus control*
3. Altering the consequences of behavior to try to make undesirable behaviors have "immediate" undesirable consequences and to make the desirable behaviors more enjoyable and rewarding; called *contingency management*

RECORDING   Patient self-observation of personal behavior is an important preliminary step, but it also needs to be continued intermittently *throughout* the program so that goal achievement and successes in avoiding or dealing with problem environmental stimuli can be appreciated. Usually this is accomplished by having the participant record, every time he or she avoids or succumbs to the relevant behavior (e.g., smoking a cigarette, eating a beef steak pie, taking a walk). Both the physical and social circumstances should be recorded. It is important for the patient to monitor the target behavior for about a week before any change effort so as to identify patterns. Recording the behavior during the program will highlight progress or the need for altering the therapy. Often a prepared diary or notebook can make this task easier. While self-monitoring is not sufficient treatment in itself, it is a necessary component. For example, smokers who were instructed either to self-monitor their smoking or to follow a nicotine-fading procedure (changing to lower nicotine brands) were generally unsuccessful in quitting (Foxx and Brown, 1979). However, those who practiced both together had high abstinence rates even at the 18-month follow-up (Fig. 21-3). Others have also found that the simple act of recording habits daily is important

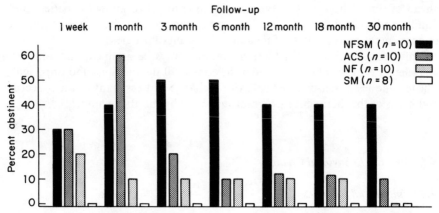

Figure 21–3 An investigation of nicotine fading and self-monitoring in reported rates of abstinence during a smoking cessation program. Groups NFSM, nicotine fading and self-monitoring; NF, nicotine fading; SM, self-monitoring; ACS, American Cancer Society. During the 12-month follow-up, three ACS subjects could not be located. At the 18-month follow-up, two ACS subjects and three SM subjects could not be located. From RM Foxx, and RA Brown: *J Appl Behav Anal* **12**:111, 1979, with permission.

in smoking cessation (Rozensky, 1974) and also for weight reduction (Romanzcyk, 1974).

STIMULUS CONTROL   Stimulus control seeks to *change the environment* to minimize the risk of encountering a stimulus that may cue unhealthy actions. If cigarette smoking is associated with sitting in a favorite chair or watching TV after supper, then after-supper habits should be changed. If cigarette smoking usually occurs around other smokers, do not sit next to a smoker and do choose nonsmoking locations when there is a choice. If obesity is the problem, then do not buy high-calorie foods. A refrigerator full of favorite but unhealthy foods is difficult to resist in moments of weakness. Initially, stimulus control may have to involve some changes in social patterns, but when new habits become entrenched, previous cues for unhealthy behavior can be overcome. The patient should anticipate awkward social situations and rehearse a coping plan with the therapist.

CONTINGENCY MANAGEMENT   Altering the consequences of health-related behaviors is known as contingency management. There are many ways of accomplishing this, depending on the particular intervention and the patient's particular circumstances. However, some general categories of techniques are mentioned. Goal setting not only simplifies and clarifies objectives but also allows the reward of goal achievement. Goals should be written so as to specify new behaviors rather than changes in physiologic variables such as weight loss or serum cholesterol. The use of interim goals, rather than only final long-term goals is essential. An interesting study by Bandura and Simon (1977) taught overweight persons the skill of bite-counting and then requested that they set goals to reduce the number of bites they took. Those who used short-term (daily) goals rather than long-term (weekly) goals were dramatically more successful in achieving weight loss (Fig. 21–4). It did not seem important whether or not the daily goal occurred with a coexistent long-term (distal) goal. Martin and Dubbert (1982) reported a series of studies on goal-setting for exercise. They found that adherence to exercise was improved if the subjects set the goals rather than the instructor, and that weekly goals were more effective than 6-week goals.

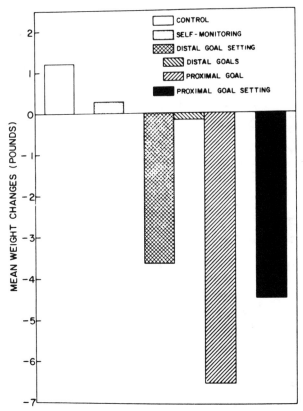

Figure 21–4 Reductions in eating behavior achieved by subjects in self-monitoring and goal-setting conditions. Adherence to distal goals and to improvised proximal subgoals within the distal goal conditions. Adapted from A Bandura and KM Simon: *Cognitive Ther Res* **3**:177, 1977, with permission.

Research has indicated that contracting with important other persons can be important in contingency management (Harris and Hallbauer, 1973). Failure to keep a contract with a spouse, physician, or friend is certainly a negative consequence of the inappropriate behavior. The effect of contracting to increase aerobic exercise has been explored (Wysocki et al, 1979). Subjects put personal items on deposit with the investigators and earned them back if they met their goal of weekly aerobic points. A baseline period preceded the making of the contract, and during this period the participants were actively invited to explore various types of aerobic activity. They were not told ahead of time when contracts would be made but were randomly allocated to two groups with baseline periods of either 1 week (group I) or 3 weeks (group II). The effects over the weeks before and after goal setting can be seen in Fig. 21–5. At 1 year, seven of eight participants were exercising more than at baseline.

Along similar lines, patients should be encouraged to voice their goals and

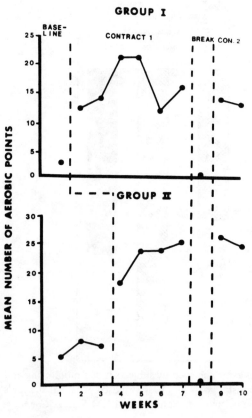

Figure 21–5 The effect of contracting after different baseline periods on exercise habits. Adapted from T Wysocki et al: J Appl Behav Anal 12:60, Fig. 1, 1979, with permission.

plans to friends and family as a means of contingency management. Again this increases the negative consequences of failure and the positive consequences of achievement. The potential influence of friends and family is great, and reinforcement here can mean the difference between success and failure (Mahoney and Mahoney, 1976; Stuart and Davis, 1972). A most striking example of the facilitating role of family support is displayed in Fig. 21–6 (Brownell et al, 1978). If spouses attended weight loss groups with subjects, weight loss was significantly greater than if the spouse did not attend. As another example, Janis and Hoffman (1982) report that subjects in a smoking cessation clinic with high-contact partners had a better immediate reduction–cessation rate than those without such available supports (Fig. 21–7). Further, those with effective support smoked less 10 years later.

Material and financial rewards are of course effective, and several have reported on their use in different circumstances (Harris and Bruner, 1971; Winett, 1973). Commonly, money may be put down at the beginning of a course, to be refunded upon goal achievement, otherwise forfeited (Wysocki et al, 1979). Even symbolic rewards seem to be quite effective (Bellack, 1976). Obese subjects who kept a daily food diary and graded (A, B, C, D, E, or F) the "success" of each meal in writing as self-reinforcement, lost more weight than those who only self-monitored (Table 21–2).

The physician has an important role to play as a reinforcer of appropriate behavioral changes. We are referring here simply to the therapist being quick to praise the patient for any significant achievements. Such positive reinforcement

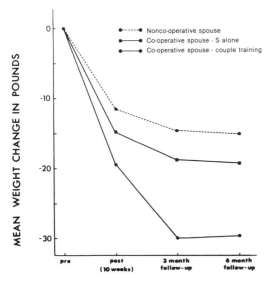

Figure 21–6 Mean changes in percentage overweight according to degree of support from spouse at post-treatment and the 3-month follow-ups. From KD Brownell et al: The effect of couples training and partner cooperativeness in the behavioral treatment of obesity, reprinted with permission, *Behav Res Ther* **16**:323, copyright © 1978, Pergamon Press, Inc.

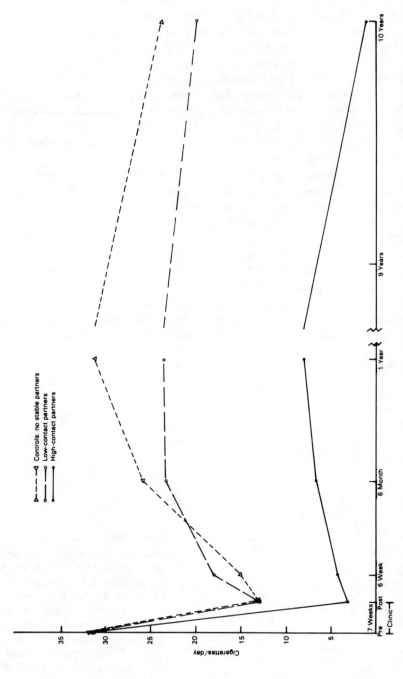

Figure 21–7 Reported number of cigarettes smoked by category of partner support. From IL Janis and E Hoffman, 1982, with permission.

Table 21-2 Changes in weight by treatments including different combinations of self-monitoring and self-reinforcement[a]

Group	Change in pounds		Percentage change in body weight	
	Pre- to post-treatment (7 weeks)	Pretreatment to follow-up (14 weeks)	Pre- to post-treatment	Pretreatment to follow-up
SM, SR—Mail	7.25	7.55	4.92	5.03
SM—Mail	4.69	3.72	2.87	2.26
SM, SR—No contact	7.03	7.67	4.64	5.13
SM—No contact	0.39	3.60	0.04	2.63

Source: Adapted from Bellack, 1976.

[a] SR = self-reinforce; SM = self-monitor only; Mail = participants mailed monitoring record to the investigators.

should be for the *behavior* (e.g., certain social or dietary changes) rather than the physiologic outcome (e.g., weight loss) (Mahoney, 1974). Informing patients at the same time of improvements in serum cholesterol or blood pressure is also rewarding. Aversive reinforcement for inappropriate behaviors has been investigated and generally found to be less effective than positive reinforcement (Mahoney et al, 1973).

Another important aspect of behavioral change and contingency management is the teaching of skills. These are needed so that the patient can change behavior with greater ease, and avoid ridicule and perceived failure. Physicians should be careful to notice such common problems as (a) not knowing how to ask for assistance in quitting smoking, (b) not knowing how to shop for low-fat and low-calorie foods, (c) not knowing how to refuse a cigarette if offered, (d) not knowing how to warm up before exercise, or (e) not knowing how to ask a spouse to serve red meat less often. While lack of needed skills can sometimes be remedied by recommending an appropriate book or referring the patient to a local class or group, physicians can often provide brief and effective training by demonstration. They can role-play asking someone to cook differently or to become an exercise partner, or demonstrate how to refuse a cigarette. Patients can then rehearse these skills with physicians, for instance, telling how they will inspect food labels for low-fat ingredients, or how they plan to refrain from smoking after meals or suggesting a schedule for daily exercise.

A final aspect of contingency management is the use of group sessions. The object of these is not only to provide an efficient means of health education but also to establish a new peer group with similar ideals and objectives (SP Rose, 1977). This, then, to some extent relieves the negative outcome of apparent social eccentricity that may accompany compliance. Group sessions also provide an ideal forum for teaching and discussing skills. In the Meyer and Henderson study (1974), the group sessions were used to teach wives to be supportive, to encourage practice in cooking and shopping, and to teach patients specific exercise skills.

Maintenance of Behavioral Change

Long-term maintenance is perhaps the most difficult and most neglected aspect of behavioral change. Many studies show short-term changes, but recidivism is frequently a major problem. A case in point relates to many of the popular group programs for smoking cessation (see Fig. 21–8). Nevertheless, such programs are successful for a minority and have probably played an important role in community education.

Intensive long-term follow-up is expensive, and few data are available for most interventions. Farquhar's suggestion (1978) is simply a reapplication of the principles described above. This involves periodic reevaluation, that is, self-observation of habits. If the original goals are no longer being achieved, then the patient (with some support from the therapist) should add the stimulus control and contingency management techniques that were originally found beneficial. The familiarity with these techniques and the probable need for a smaller degree of change than originally required should make goal achievement easier. Clearly there also needs be formal periodic reevaluation, so that any tendency to recidivism does not get out of hand. The physician's office is an ideal place for such reevaluation.

One other method of promoting maintenance should be mentioned: relapse prevention training (Marlatt and Gordon, 1980). One relapse episode frequently prompts ex-smokers to return to their habit permanently or dieters to resume uninhibited eating. To help avoid this, relapse prevention training can be carried out by planning how to handle a slip beforehand and then under-

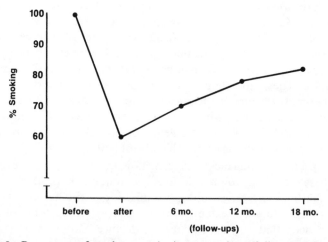

Figure 21–8   Percentage of smokers continuing to smoke at follow-up after a smoking cessation clinic. From RH Pyszka et al, 1973, with permission.

taking a planned relapse. Thus, a patient is told to smoke a cigarette, go off a weight loss program, or miss a scheduled session of exercise. The patient prepares for this test cognitively by learning to distinguish between a "slip" and a "relapse." If the patient genuinely slips at some future date, he or she will not feel so guilty or obsessed with this seeming failure. Learning to talk oneself out of guilt and to try again the next day is effective in preventing a full relapse. Abrams and Follick (1983) found that a group of obese subjects who practiced having a relapse and who were taught to reinstitute behavioral principles maintained their weight loss better than a group that received no such training. King and Frederiksen (1984) found that relapse prevention training significantly improved maintenance of regular physical activity.

The Effectiveness of Behavioral Techniques

Self-directed modification of health behaviors is a relatively young science, and many questions remain to be answered. However, it is clear that this is the best approach available. The intervention model is very broad, and it can and should contain elements of many other models such as values clarification, health education, social learning theory, attitudinal change. The focus is primarily on the behavior, although cognitive elements must not be ignored. There is evidence that behavioral change *produces* attitudinal change (Bandura et al, 1969). Also, behavior is a tangible and manageable focus for the interventionist.

Mazzuca (1982) summarized his review of 320 studies of education and behavioral therapy of chronic diseases by calculating indices of the magnitude of the program effect for "didactic" and "behavioral" programs. Outcome variables were "regimen compliance," "physiologic indicators of therapeutic progress," and "health outcomes." The results (Table 21–3) clearly favor programs with a behavioral emphasis.

The best results at present for smoking cessation, weight control, promotion of physical activity, and improved dietary habits all involve self-directed behavioral techniques. Lando (1977) demonstrated 76 percent abstinence from smoking at 6 months in a group of smokers who attended five sessions and seven maintenance sessions over 2 months. These sessions emphasized aversive smoking (the satiation techniques), behavioral contracts with rewards, suggestions for stimulus control and contingency management, and group discussions. Those who relapsed agreed to undergo booster aversive treatments. By contrast, a group of quitters in the same program who had no maintenance support showed only 35 percent abstinence at 6 months. In a similar program, also with maintenance support, 46 percent reported abstinence at 3 years (Lando and McGovern, 1982). Aversive conditioning (such as rapid smoking or satiation) is an effective adjunct to behavioral smoking cessation programs (Lichtenstein and Rodriques, 1977). However, there is the possible danger in IHD patients of tobacco smoke toxicity if rapid smoking is used (Danaher, 1977). In combination with other portions of a multifaceted program, aversive conditioning is a useful technique—however, hardly suited to office practice. The most successful

Table 21-3 Median improvements in compliance, therapeutic progress, and outcome as a function of patient education, with didactic and behavioral emphasis

	Instructional emphasis		
Dependent variable	Didactic	Behavioral	Total
Regimen compliance	0.26	0.64[b]	0.50[b]
	($n=9$)	($n=21$)	($n=30$)
Therapeutic progress	0.18	0.74[a]	0.30
	($n=13$)	($n=14$)	($n=27$)
Health outcome	0.19	0.31[b]	0.25[a]
	($n=6$)	($n=5$)	($n=11$)
Total	0.23[a]	0.63[a]	0.36[a]
	($n=28$)	($n=40$)	($n=68$)

Source: From Mazzuca, 1982.

[a] Median >0; $P\,0.01$;

[b] Median >0; $P<0.005$.

programs often seem to involve multiple approaches to the problem, also an effective maintenance procedure (Powell and McCann, 1981).

A large number of studies have demonstrated the relative effectiveness of behavioral techniques in weight reduction (Wing and Jeffrey, 1979). Stuart and colleagues (1981) have summarized components that appear to have most value. Typical results are of modest losses such as 9 lb during a 13-week program. Longer-term results show maintenance of the loss but without further weight reduction.

There has been relatively little research conducted on improving adherence to exercise regimens. Information suggests that adherence at 1 year is less than 50 percent for both cardiac patients and nonpatients (Dishman, 1982; Oldridge, 1982). In one study, relapse prevention training resulted in 83 percent adherence to jogging, while in the control group only 36 percent reported regular exercise at follow-up (King and Fredericksen, 1984). Wysocki and colleagues (1979), in a small study, also found contracting effective.

Adherence to fat-modified diets has been shown to produce long-lasting changes in serum lipids (Crouch et al, 1984; Fraser et al, 1984; Meyer and Henderson, 1974). These programs have involved individual and/or group education and behavior modification techniques.

The Role of the Physician as a Behavioral Therapist

While the constraints of their training and lack of time may sometimes place limitations on physicians' effectiveness as behavioral therapists, much of value can be achieved. Physicians are the ideal health educators and motivators as figures of some status in the community. They have the attention of patients when talking about patients' health and can realistically discuss the threat of the disease. Physicians may most often have the opportunity to become involved in secondary prevention as, traditionally, well persons do not go to see the physician. However, this is slowly changing as the concepts of primary prevention gain momentum in the community and in industry. The patient who is already ill, perhaps having suffered the first myocardial infarction, will be greatly impressed by the threat of the disease, so that unhelpful social forces may be somewhat less influential. Where asymptomatic high-risk patients are seen—perhaps incidentally for some other minor malady—the situation is probably a little different. The threat of a disease—often seen by these patients as unlikely for decades—may be unimpressive. Social influences (friends and family) will often be paramount, and the probability of positive social influences should be maximized by involving the spouse or other family members in therapy wherever possible.

The physician's initial role when a patient is found to be at high risk is to inform the patient of his or her risk status. This should be done supportively, but clearly, so that it is understood why recommendations are considered important. Such a message from the physician, coupled with specific behavioral guidelines, provide both the motivation and direction for therapeutic or preventive action.

The physician can easily initiate the self-observation process, particularly if he or she has suitable record-keeping forms and diaries readily available. Self observation is the first step in self-management, but it is a very important step. Set goals in writing, and, if appropriate, make this as a contract where the patient may sign the goal sheet. Table 21–4 shows the information often included in a written goal sheet.

The motivated physician may be able to help the patient with suggestions about how to best modify his or her activities and environment, and so control stimuli promoting inappropriate behaviors. Similarly, the physician may be able to suggest means of effectively rewarding the appropriate behavior. A list of questions helpful to the patient in finding appropriate rewards is shown in Table 21–5. The teaching of skills may often be outside the range of usual physician activities. The help of a dietitian, health educator, consulting psychologist, or exercise physiologist as appropriate is usually invaluable for this purpose. Involvement in group sessions can be fun and rewarding, and can also enhance the physician's reputation in the community. The medical professional's role in positive reinforcement by praise and enthusiasm is natural, easy, and very valuable. By taking a key role in periodic reassessment, counseling, and referral, the physician forms an essential part of the maintenance phase.

The physician should resist the temptation to "excommunicate" problem patients who do not do all that is recommended. Change may be slow and may occur in a different sequence from that which was envisaged and recommended. Many "recalcitrants," with persistence and a caring attitude, can become com-

Table 21–4 A sample contract sheet

What is my long-range goal? _____

_____

When do I want to achieve this goal? Date: _____

List subgoals and time limits   Specify action plans

			Goal
Subgoals	*Date*	*(What, when, where, how, with whom)*	met?
1.	_____	_____	Y N
2.	_____	_____	Y N
3.	_____	_____	Y N
4.	_____	_____	Y N

What my helper will do: _____

Rewards for meeting subgoals: _____

Date: _____ Signed: _____

                       Helper: _____

---

pliers. Finally, physicians should be sure that their own personal life is seen to exemplify the health principles that are being recommended. The reasons are obvious, but it is surprising how often this is neglected.

The Role of the Physician in Smoking Cessation

The first and most essential function of the physician to promote smoking cessation is to communicate clearly to the patient that ceasing smoking will improve his or her health and reduce the risk of future illness. At present, this simple step happens much less frequently than would be desirable. The initial therapeutic session must be spent explaining the strength of the evidence as it relates to that patient's circumstances. Mention of the proven effect of smoking in increasing respiratory infections in children of smokers (Dodge, 1982; Liard et al, 1982) can be an additional motivation for some individuals. Engendering a *modest* perception of threat is probably appropriate. The physical examination can be a learning experience for the patient. Any physical findings such as overexpansion

Table 21–5   How to find suitable rewards for patients

Answering the following questions may help you decide which are the potentially effective rewards that you may use in your problem-solving plans.

1. What kinds of things do you like to have?
2. What are your major interests?
3. What are your hobbies?
4. What people do you like to be with?
5. What do you like to do with those people?
6. What do you do for fun?
7. What do you do to relax?
8. What do you do to get away from it all?
9. What makes you feel good?
10. What would be a nice present to receive?
11. What kinds of things are important to you?
12. What would you buy if you had an extra $10? $50? $100?
13. On what do you spend your money each week?
14. What behaviors do you perform every day? (Don't overlook the obvious.)
15. Are there any behaviors that you usually perform instead of the target behavior?
16. What would you hate to lose?
17. Of the things you do every day, which would you hate to give up?

of the chest, hyperresonance, rales or wheezes, cough, redness of mouth, and postnasal drip, can reasonably be explained to the patient as probable consequences of cigarette smoking. This tool will aid motivation and contingency management by allowing some consequences of reduction or quitting to be shown on follow-up. Preferably the patient's spouse or important other should be present and involved. It is important that the physician should understand the patient's work and home environments, the attitudes of spouse, family, and workmates to the smoking habit, and the patient's need to quit. Will the attempt to quit meet with ridicule or support?

The next step is for the patient to record smoking behavior for 1 week; a sample format for such a diary is shown in Table 21–6 The therapist should review this diary to gain a clearer understanding of the behavioral problem and to help design stimulus control and contingency management strategies. The record will provide clues as to which times and situations "trigger" smoking. The two or three highest-risk situations should be identified. Written confirmation of these high-risk situations and specific suggestions for avoiding smoking at these times should be negotiated with the patient. A list of possible strategies is provided in Table 21–7. The patient should be directed to practice these suggestions in daily life or in imagery, in order to prepare for strong urges.

The physician can assist the patient in preparing to quit by advising a gradual reduction in smoking and the setting of a "quit day." The reduction can be accomplished by stopping smoking in selected situations (e.g., after dinner, while driving, on the phone) or by smoking fewer cigarettes throughout the day.

Table 21–6   Sample diaries documenting smoking, eating, and exercise habits

Name:_____   Date:_____

1. *Smoking*

Number of cigarettes	Time	Situation	Feelings	Urge (on a scale from 1–5)
- -				
- -				
- -				

2. *Eating*

Time	Minutes eating	Food eaten	Amount of food	Location	Other people present	Activity while eating	Thoughts, feelings
- -							
- -							
- -							

3. *Exercise*

Time	Type	Other people present?	Distance or duration	Target heart rate	Heart rate achieved during exercise
- -					
- -					
- -					

After a week or two of gradual reduction, the patient is encouraged to quit "cold turkey" on the specified date. This seems to be the most effective initial strategy (Flaxman, 1978). During the preliminary discussions, it may be helpful to inform the patient that a 4- or 5-day period of mild withdrawal is expected after cessation.

Assuming smoking cessation is successful, the physician should continue to probe regarding the patient's attitude toward smoking and whether he or she still encounters situations where there is the temptation to smoke. An occasional diary to assess this is useful perhaps as far as 1 year into the nonsmoking phase. Recidivism within 3 to 6 months of apparent success is quite common. This frequently occurs at times of emotional stress and/or the use of alcohol.

Table 21–7 Strategies for smoking cessation

Suggestions for the physician

1. Determine smoking status of every patient.
2. Give firm, clear advice to quit smoking.
3. Tag the charts of smoking patients to facilitate follow-up.
4. Follow-up on all anti-smoking advice.
5. Teach patient to use self-monitoring record to help you assess habits, and then direct changes in his or her routine to avoid situations normally associated with smoking.
6. If the spouse smokes, both should quit together, if possible.
7. Model strategies to help the patient to handle high-risk situations.
8. Many patients find it useful to try "nicotine fading"—switching brands to consistently lower nicotine cigarettes, finally smoking a cigarette not enjoyable, before quitting.
9. Train the nurse in smoking cessation counseling methods.
10. Point out any signs or symptoms that may be related to smoking.

Suggestions for the patient

A. *Stimulus control for smoking cessation*

1. Have no cigarettes in the house.
2. Avoid alcohol and be aware of its dangers for loss of control of nonsmoking status.
3. As far as possible, plan to quit during times when stressful circumstances are *not* anticipated.
4. Use nonsmoking areas in public transportation.
5. Breathe deeply and slowly or learn other relaxation techniques.
6. Take a walk when you feel an urge.
7. Prepare for times of tension. Say to yourself, "Even if I feel tense, I'm not going to smoke."
8. Decide not to smoke in certain places, such as in the car or at your desk.
9. Postpone some of your cigarettes for 15 minutes.
10. Buy cigarettes one pack at a time.
11. Change brands every time you smoke.
12. Smoke with the opposite hand.
13. Carry the cigarettes in a different place.
14. Remove all the ashtrays from the house, except one.
15. Avoid acquaintances who smoke, for a few days.
16. Give up coffee while you are trying to quit.
17. Brush your teeth first thing in the morning instead of smoking.

B. *Contingency management for smoking cessation*

1. Ensure that the patient has adequate cognitive understanding of the health problem. This will allow appropriate satisfaction as a reward for goal achievement.
2. Write down reasons for quitting (health, family, social, financial).
3. Patient should proclaim his or her intention to quit to family and friends.
4. Use a written contract with spouse and physician or therapist.
5. A quitting date should be set.
6. The physician should inquire as to the patient's chronic cough, sinusitis, taste, etc., and bring any positive change to the patient's attention.
7. The therapist should compliment the patient on achievement of reduction or cessation of smoking.
8. Suggest that the patient investigate cheaper car insurance available to nonsmokers.
9. The patient may give himself a reward after one week, one month, three months, and six months of quitting (or have someone else give him the reward).
10. Have the patient leave a $50 check with you, made out to a least favorite cause. If patient quits smoking for two months, the check is returned.
11. Use risk slide rule, if appropriate, to visually show the patient the possible gains of quitting for IHD risk.

Where stress can be anticipated, plans for handling it without the use of cigarettes should be developed and written. There is evidence that the likelihood of refraining from smoking for at least 6 months is doubled by supportive follow-up in a physician's office (Wilson et al, 1982).

The smoking intervention program of the Multiple Risk Factor Intervention Trial (chapter 17) achieved an impressive 46 percent quit rate (confirmed by biochemical measures) after 4 years, in a group of 4103 high-risk individuals. Initially there was education, followed by regular office visits with a physician and sometimes a behavioral psychologist, for the duration of the study. There were also intermittent group sessions for continuing smokers. Aversive techniques were generally not used, but monitoring by thiocyanate and exhaled carbon monoxide levels was used for both research and therapy. Monitoring of carbon monoxide levels is particularly recommended, because it provides immediate feedback. The results of this study are important, because these techniques could nearly all be emulated in private practice.

Office-based smoking cessation therapy will be successful in many cases. However, smoking is a very difficult habit to break, and some patients will relapse. If a patient is unable to quit, stress that there is success in "failure." Most people try to quit several times before they become permanent non-smokers. Each quit attempt should teach the patient something that will be helpful on the next attempt. If someone quits for 2 days, 1 week, or 6 months, they have exhibited self-control and reduced their risk. However, additional help may be necessary at times. Thus, the physician should have a list of community resources for smoking cessation, including self-help groups, voluntary agencies, public programs, university programs, private clinics, and reputable practitioners. Useful publications are available for patients (American Heart Association, 1982: *How to Stop Smoking*; Farquhar, 1978; National Cancer Institute, 1983: *For Good*; Office of Cancer Communications, 1982: *Clearing the Air*).

The Role of the Physician in Dietary Management of Obesity and Hypercholesterolemia and Hypertension

These dietary goals are not necessarily independent of each other, as the reduction of serum cholesterol and blood pressure can be markedly aided by concurrent reduction in obesity. Detailed reviews are available on the physiology and treatment of obesity (Brownell, 1982b; Katch and McArdle, 1977), which of course involves regular exercise as well as dietary changes. As with smoking cessation, it is most important to communicate the problem and the potential benefits of dietary change to the patient. If the patient does not cook, it is a great advantage for the spouse or cook to be involved. A dietitian should evaluate the diet, using a food diary or food frequency record. A sample diet diary is shown in Table 21–6. Of particular interest is the analysis of total calories, percentage of calories as fat, saturated and polyunsaturated fat, simple and complex carbohydrates, and also dietary cholesterol. Unfortunately, formal assessment of salt consumption by dietary diary is usually quite inaccurate, but monitoring of foods high in salt is appropriate. Salt consumption is best measured by salt excretion in a 24-hour urine collection. Where relevant, this should be measured initially on several occasions if possible. Interim goals are then set, in collaboration with the patient, using the above information.

As interim dietary goals are set, special attention should be given to monitoring foods involved in these goals. Between occasional full dietary assessments, the patient should record for at least 1 week each month the frequency and portion sizes of certain specific foods that can be related directly to the behavioral goals. These may include red meats, poultry, fish, pastries and pies, eggs, candies, sweet desserts, vegetables, ice cream, fried foods, soups, canned food, pickles, soy sauce. Other foods of interest but specific to that patient will be suggested by the periodic full dietary assessment.

If weight loss is a goal, the patient should be given a weight chart on which to plot weight once each week. More frequent weighings reveal many random fluctuations that may be discouraging. It is helpful to provide realistic expectations about behavioral weight loss. Most people are accustomed to crash diets that produce rapid weight loss. However, when eating habits return to "normal," weight is rapidly regained. Patients should be taught to try to attain 0.5–1.0 lb/ week losses by adhering to their dietary and exercise programs. Weight loss by this method takes longer but is accomplished through changes in behavior that are becoming habitual. Thus, the probability of maintenance is enhanced. Again, a resource list for patients that can direct them to specialized weight loss programs, when needed, should be available.

If lowering of serum cholesterol is a goal, this should be regularly monitored and reported to the patient. However, it is a very variable measure, and the patient should understand that trends can only be discussed when two or preferably three readings are averaged. Single high readings can be very discouraging if this is not understood. The physician should recall that the responsiveness of serum cholesterol to diet is also variable. The Keys equation (chapter 5) describes the responsiveness of the average American male, and your patient may do better or worse. The support given by regular group meetings is useful, especially during the initial stages of dietary change.

When reduction of sodium consumption is a goal, similar ideas apply, but goals involve elimination of salty foods and reduction of added salt during cooking or at the table. Periodic assessment by self-monitoring, by formal dietary recall for important salty foods, and by 24-hour urine collection is important. If the patient is hypertensive, blood pressure should be measured regularly and the levels reported to the patient.

When the final goal is achieved, the physician should become involved in the maintenance phase. The results of periodic dietary analyses, serum cholesterol, blood pressure measurements, and urine sodium levels should be discussed with the patient. Where relevant, present body weight should be related to previous weight charts. If recidivism occurs, the physician can then initiate the return to previously successful behavioral interventions. A list of possible stimulus con-

Table 21–8   Strategies for changing eating habits

Suggestions for the physician

1. Teach the patient to use a self-monitoring record and to use this as a guide for temporarily avoiding friends, locations, and social situations that may involve inappropriate eating habits. Instead, those friends and environments most likely to respect and reinforce the program should be chosen.
2. Model strategies to help the patient handle difficult situations.

Suggestions for the patient

A. *Stimulus control for changing eating habits*

1. Do not purchase or have in the refrigerator forbidden or restricted foods.
2. Change your habits to avoid the high-risk situations, both at home and work.
3. Involve family and close friends in the plans, especially the household cook (if he or she is not the patient).
4. Avoid eating out for the present, or eat out in restaurants with many low-fat, low-calorie choices.
5. Practice responses and ways of handling difficult situations. This can be done with the physician or therapist.

B. *Contingency management for changing eating habits*

1. Ensure that the patient has adequate cognitive understanding of the health problem. This will allow appropriate satisfaction as a reward for goal achievement.
2. Fill out a weight chart, kept in the house. The physician should regularly review plots of weight changes with the patient.
3. Suggest that the patient purchase new clothes smaller than current fit but appropriate to projected weight in the near future.
4. Set written goals as a contract witnessed by therapist and spouse.
5. Consider the use of rewards for goal achievement (e.g., book, clothes, concert, vacation—not food!). A monetary deposit at beginning of program to be returned only on goal achievement.
6. Family and therapist should praise the patient for losses and when appropriate for visual improvement in obesity.
7. Use risk slide rule, if appropriate, to show the patient the possible gains in IHD risk.
8. Regularly review serum cholesterol values (if cholesterol reduction is a goal)—preferably expressed as a running mean of the two or three last values in comparison to the mean of two or three baseline values.
9. Encourage patient to proclaim his or her intention of dieting to family and friends.

---

trol and contingency management strategies for dietary intervention is shown in Table 21–8. To help in the setting of goals, the lipid, cholesterol, sodium, and caloric contents of many common foods are shown in Appendix A.

The Role of the Physician in Promoting Exercise

Exercise therapy is a vital part of cardiac rehabilitation, and equally important in the treatment of obesity (Brownell, 1982a,b). It is important to screen persons adequately before prescribing an exercise prescription. One set of screening criteria is summarized as follows:

1. All patients should have a clinical history (including family history of heart disease), a physical examination, resting electrocardiogram, and also an assessment of blood pressure, blood cholesterol, obesity, and cigarette smoking habits.
2. All patients without manifest heart disease but at high risk, all patients over 35 years of age, and all patients with symptoms or signs suggestive of heart disease should undergo monitored stress testing (American Heart Association, 1972).
3. Ideally, patients with IHD should have supervised activity, but with appropriate screening unsupervised activity can be safe (chapter 19). For a middle-aged or older person with no evidence of IHD, the intensity of the exercise need not be rigidly controlled, but very high-intensity forms of exercise are generally unwise without an extended training period and proof of safety by treadmill testing.

As with other intervention modalities, the physician's opinion needs to be clearly expressed and backed up by a simple statement of the evidence. A preliminary step is to take a simple and approximate exercise history. One should inquire about job activity and leisure-time activity. This can be accomplished by asking about the most physically strenuous activities engaged in over the preceding month, the intensity and amount of regular walking, and any regular sporting activities or hobbies involving physical effort. A more rigorous assessment can be obtained by the use of the Minnesota Leisure-Time Physical Activity questionnaire (Taylor et al, 1978). Having patients record their activity over a 1-week period in a diary will often be very helpful both initially and as therapy progresses. A sample diary for self-recording purposes is shown in Table 21–6.

Graduated exercise goals are essential (Cooper, 1972). Suggested final training heart rates by age for persons without known IHD are shown in Table 21–9, along with some additional instructions for an exercise session. Exercising regularly with spouse or friends is an advantage, and it is useful to distinguish between programmed and routine activity (Brownell and Stunkard, 1980). Programmed activity refers to regularly scheduled "exercise" such as jogging, tennis, calisthenics. Routine activities refers to day-to-day activities such as walking and stair-climbing. Some subjects may initially be most willing to increase the frequency and duration of these routine activities (by taking stairs when the elevator is available or parking the car further away from the work site, etc.) rather than become involved in programmed exercise.

Long-term adherence is a well-known problem in exercise programs (chapter 19; Brownell, 1982b), with dropout rates of up to 50 percent. Unfortunately, there is evidence that persons who need exercise most are just those least likely to adhere. Martin and Dubbert (1982) found that low self-motivation, smoking,

Table 21–9   Steps in an exercise session

1. Take your pulse (standing).
2. Stretching exercises for 5 minutes.
3. Warm up for 5 minutes. (Easy walking)
4. Vigorous exercise for at least 20 minutes.
5. Take your pulse (standing) for 10 seconds. Compare it to target heart rate.

Age	Ideal training heart rate/minutes	Ideal training heart rate/10 seconds
20	146–178	24–30
25	142–173	24–29
30	138–168	23–28
35	134–163	23–27
40	130–158	22–26
45	126–153	21–25
50	122–148	20–25
55	117–143	19–24
60	113–138	19–23
65	109–133	18–22
70	105–128	17–21
75	101–123	17–20

Above are the ideal heart rate ranges that one should train or exercise at. Select a point within the range depending on your condition.

6. Cool down for 5 minutes. (Easy walking)
7. Stretch for 5 minutes.
8. Praise yourself!

inactive leisure-time pursuits, type A behavior patterns, and low social support are all predictors of nonadherence. Very similar results were found by Oldridge et al (1978) in cardiac patients. Evaluation of patients from these perspectives may allow the physician to have more realistic expectations and also act as a guide as to the intensity of planned follow-up. Maintenance must include periodic reassessment, self-monitoring and reinstitution of the goal-oriented approach when necessary. Periodic assessment of physical fitness by treadmill each 6–12 months can be objective reinforcement or can point to reduction of fitness, thus stimulating renewed effort.

Some suggestions for stimulus control and contingency management are given in Table 21–10. To help in the setting of exercise goals, the relative energy expenditures of many different forms of physical activity are given in Appendix B.

Table 21–10 Strategies for improving exercise habits

Suggestions for the patient

A. *Stimulus control for improving exercise habits*

1. Control overwork and fatigue.
2. Develop a regular routine of exercise at the same time each day.
3. Find friends who exercise and join them.
4. Write "exercise" in schedule book.
5. Hang shoes or equipment on door knob.

B. *Contingency management for improving exercise habits*

1. Set a written goal (interim goal) specifying type of activity, frequency, and duration.
2. Specify "some" exercise, not necessarily one particular activity. Be flexible.
3. Arrange a reward for goal achievement with spouse or meaningful other.
4. Self-monitor exercise habits so improvement can be appreciated.
5. Get involved in leisure-time activities with physical content such as hiking or badminton.
6. Expect and note any improved sense of well-being and probably less tendency to depression.
7. Utilize periodic treadmill testing for fitness assessment.
8. Proclaim intention to exercise to family and friends.

These methods for helping patients change their habits are effective and can be very rewarding to use. With a little effort the physician can incorporate them naturally into a traditional medical practice. In many situations, use of other health professionals in supporting roles can greatly enhance the effectiveness of such therapy.

Appendix A
Selected Foods and Nutrients Analysis[a]

		CAL	TFT (gm)	SAT (gm)	LINO (gm)	CHOL (mg)	Na (mg)
1 c	Milk, whole	159	9.4	4.7	0.2	34	122
1 c	Milk, low-fat	145	4.9	2.7	0.1	22	150
1 c	Milk, nonfat	88	0.2	—	—	5	127
1 Tbs	Cream	32	3.1	1.7	0.1	16	6
1 Tbs	Mocha mix	19	1.6	0.3	0.2	—	7
1 c	Yogurt, low-fat, flavored	231	2.5	1.4	0.1	10	133
1 c	Soup, cream	179	10.3	3.5	2.7	27	1054
1 Tbs	Butter	102	11.5	6.3	0.3	32	140
1 Tbs	Margarine, hard	102	11.5	2.1	3.1	—	140
1 Tbs	Margarine, soft	100	11.4	1.0	3.7	—	140
1 Tbs	Margarine, reduced calorie	51	5.7	1.0	1.5	—	140
1 Tbs	Mayonnaise	101	11.2	2.0	5.6	10	84
1 Tbs	Mayonnaise, reduced calorie	65	6.3	1.1	3.2	5	88
1 Tbs	Salad dressing oil-based	88	9.8	1.0	5.2	5	92
1 Tbs	Salad dressing, reduced calorie	22	2.0	0.4	1.0	—	19
1 Tbs	Sour cream	32	3.1	1.7	0.1	15	6
1 Tbs	Oil	120	13.6	1.4	7.2	—	—
1 Tbs	Lard	117	13.0	4.9	1.3	10	—
3 oz	Beef	320	25.8	12.4	0.5	80	36
3 oz	Poultry	154	4.25	1.4	0.9	74	56
3 oz	Pork	308	24.2	8.7	2.2	76	51
1 oz	Hot dog, small	79	6.5	2.2	0.6	23	209
3 oz	Liver	135	3.8	2.0	0.6	300	73
3 oz	Fish	145	4.4	1.1	1.1	42	174
1 c	Beans	218	0.9	—	0.4	—	6
1 oz	Cheese, regular	112	9.0	5.0	0.2	30	196
1 oz	Cheese, imitation	100	8.1	4.5	0.2	—	307
1 oz	Cheese, reduced calorie	56	4.5	2.5	0.1	15	196
½ c	Cottage cheese, regular	130	5.2	2.9	0.2	34	281
½ c	Cottage cheese, low-fat	103	3.6	2.2	0.1	18	348
1	Egg, medium	72	5.1	1.6	0.4	264	54
1	Egg, substitute	38	0.1	—	—	—	134
¼ c	Nuts, seeds	210	18.0	3.9	5.2	—	150
1 Tbs	Peanut butter	94	8.0	1.5	2.3	—	97
3½ oz	Vegetarian meat substitute	180	7.0	0.9	4.0	—	450
1 average slice	Cake, frosted	453	17.1	6.2	2.5	41	282
1 average size	Cookie, chocolate chip	148	6.7	1.9	1.4	9	145
½ c	Pudding	161	3.9	2.2	0.1	21	167
½ c	Ice cream or frozen yogurt	167	9.1	5.1	0.3	27	54
½ c	Ice milk	133	4.5	2.5	0.2	13	60
½ c	Sherbet	130	1.2	0.5	—	—	95
12 oz	Shake or malt	488	20.6	10.2	0.6	55	428
1	Doughnut	176	11.3	2.8	2.5	5	99
1	Candy bar	161	12.4	2.1	1.6	5	17
1 slice	Pizza	153	5.4	2.1	0.5	5	456
10	Chips, potato or corn	114	8.0	2.0	0.4	—	311
2 Tbs	Gravy	48	3.2	1.7	0.1	68	211
1 small	Pancake or waffle	61	2.0	0.7	0.3	5	152

Sources: Adams, 1975; Pennington and Church, 1980.

[a] CAL, Calories; TFT, total fat; SAT, saturated fat; LINO, linoleic acid; CHOL, dietary cholesterol; Na, sodium.

Appendix B
Activities and Intensity Codes[a]

Activity	Intensity code	Activity	Intensity code
Walking for pleasure	3.5	Softball	5.0
Walking to and from work	4.0	Badminton	7.0
Walking during work break	3.5	Paddle ball	6.0
Using stairs when elevator is available	8.0	Racket ball	7.0
Cross-country hiking	6.0	Basketball, nongame	6.0
Backpacking	7.0	Basketball, game play	8.0
Mountain climbing	8.0	Basketball, officiating	7.0
Bicycling to work and/or for pleasure	4.0	Touch football	8.0
Dancing, ballroom and/or square	5.5	Handball	12.0
Home exercise	4.5	Squash	12.0
Health club	6.0	Soccer	7.0
Jogging and walking	6.0	Golf, riding a power cart	3.5
Running	8.0	Golf, walking, pulling clubs on cart	5.0
Weight lifting	3.0	Golf, walking and carrying clubs	5.5
Water skiing	6.0	Mowing lawn with riding mower	2.5
Sailing	3.0	Mowing lawn walking behind power mower	4.5
Canoeing or rowing for pleasure	3.5	Mowing lawn pushing hand mower	6.0
Canoeing or rowing in competition	12.0	Weeding and cultivating garden	4.5
Canoeing on a camping trip	4.0	Spading, digging, filling in garden	5.0
Swimming (at least 50 ft.) at a pool	6.0	Raking lawn	4.0
Swimming at the beach	6.0	Snow shoveling by hand	6.0
Scuba diving	7.0	Carpentry in workshop	3.0
Snorkeling	5.0	Painting inside of house, includes paper	
Snow skiing, downhill	7.0	hanging	4.5
Snow skiing, cross-country	8.0	Carpentry outside	6.0
Ice (or roller) skating	7.0	Painting outside of house	5.0
Sledding or tobogganing	7.0	Fishing from riverbank	3.5
Bowling	3.0	Fishing in stream with wading boots	6.0
Volleyball	4.0	Hunting pheasants or grouse	6.0
Table tennis	4.0	Hunting rabbits, prairie chickens, squirrels,	
Tennis, singles	8.0	raccoon	5.0
Tennis, doubles	6.0	Hunting large game: deer, elk, bear	6.0

Source: Taylor et al, 1978.

[a] Intensity codes are multiples of basal energy expenditure and so are independent of body weight. As basal metabolic rate varies from 50 to 80 cal/hour, these intensity codes often approximate calories per minute of energy expenditure.

References

Abrams DB, Follick MJ: Behavioral weight loss intervention at the work site: Feasibility and maintenance. *J Consult* Clin Psychol **51**:226, 1983.

Acheson RM: The etiology of coronary heart disease. *Yale J Biol Med* **35**:146, 1962.

Adams CF: *Nutritive Value of American Foods in Common Units*, handbook 456. Washington, DC, US Dept of Agriculture, 1975.

Alexander JK, Pettigrove JR: Obesity and congestive heart failure. *Geriatrics* **22**:101, 1967.

Alkjaersig N, Fletcher A, Burstein R: Association between oral contraceptive use and thromboembolism: A new approach to its investigation based on plasma fibrinogen chromatography. *Am J Obstet Gynecol* **122**:199, 1975.

Allison TG, Iammarino RM, Metz KF, et al: Failure of exercise to increase high density lipoprotein cholesterol. *J Cardiac Rehab* **1**:257, 1981.

Alonzo AA, Simon AB, Feinleib M: Prodromata of myocardial infarction and sudden death. *Circulation* **52**:1056, 1975.

Alpert BS, Flood NL, Strong WB, et al: Response to ergometer exercise in a healthy biracial population of children. *J Pediatr* **101**:538, 1982.

Alpert JJ: Broken appointments. *Pediatrics* **34**:127, 1964.

American Heart Association: *Exercise Testing and Training of Apparently Healthy Individuals: A Handbook for Physicians*. Dallas, Texas, AHA Committee on Exercise, 1972.

American Heart Association: *Coronary Risk Handbook*. Dallas, Texas, AHA, 1973.

American Heart Association: Risk factors and coronary disease, committee reports. *Circulation* **62**:449A, 1980.

American Heart Association: *Heart Facts, 1981*. Dallas, Texas, AHA, 1981a.

American Heart Association: *How to Stop Smoking*. Dallas, Texas, AHA, 1981b.

American Heart Association: Rationale of the diet–heart statement of the American Heart Association, committee report. *Circulation* **65**:839A, 1982.

Ames RP: Metabolic disturbances increasing the risk of coronary heart disease during diuretic-based antihypertensive therapy: Lipid alterations and glucose intolerance. *Am Heart J* **106**:1207, 1983.

Anastasiou-Nana M, Nanas S, Stamler J, et al: Changes in rates of sudden CHD death with first vs. recurrent events, Chicago Peoples Gas Co. Study. *Circulation* **66**(suppl 2):236, 1982.

Andersen MP, Fredericksen J, Jurgensen HJ, et al: Effect of alprenolol on mortality among patients with definite or suspected acute myocardial infarction. *Lancet* **2**:865, 1979.

Andersen P, Arnesen H, Hjermann I: Hyperlipoproteinaemia and reduced fibrinolytic activity in healthy coronary high risk men. *Acta Med Scand* **209**:199, 1981.

Anderson JT, Lawler A, Keys A: Weight gain from simple overeating. II. Serum lipids and blood volume. *J Clin Invest* **36**:81, 1957.

Anderson JT, Grande F, Keys A: Hydrogenated fats in the diet and lipids in the serum of man. *J Nutr* **75**:388, 1961.

Anderson JT, Grande F, Keys A: Effect on man's serum lipids of two proteins with different amino acid composition. *Am J Clin Nutr* **24**:524, 1971.

Anderson JT, Grande F, Keys A: Cholesterol-lowering diets. *J Am Diet Assoc* **62**:133, 1973.

Anderson JT, Grande F, Keys A: Independence of the effects of cholesterol and degree of saturation of the fat in the diet on serum cholesterol in man. *Am J Clin Nutr* **29**:1184, 1976.

Anderson JT, Jacobs DR, Foster N, et al: Scoring systems for evaluation of dietary pattern effect on serum cholesterol. *Prev Med* **8**:525, 1979.

Angster H, Glonner R, Halhuber M: Risk factor modification in the framework of rehabilitation. *Adv Cardiol* **31**:176, 1982.

Annest JL, Sing CF, Biron P, et al: Familial aggregation of blood pressure and weight in adoptive families. *Am J Epidemiol* **110**:492, 1979.

Antihypertensive drugs, plasma lipids, and coronary disease, editorial. *Lancet* **2**:19, 1980.

Anturane Reinfarction Italian Study: Sulphinpyrazone in post-myocardial infarction. *Lancet* **1**:237, 1982.

Anturane Reinfarction Trial Research Group: Sulfinpyrazone in the prevention of cardiac death after myocardial infarction. *N Engl J Med* **298**:289, 1978.

Anturane Reinfarction Trial Research Group: Sulfinpyrazone in the prevention of sudden death after myocardial infarction. *N Engl J Med* **302**:250, 1980.

Archer M, Rinzler S, Christakis G: Social factors affecting participation in a study of diet and coronary heart disease. *J Health Soc Behav* **8**:22, 1967.

Areskog M: Oesophageal dysfunction and ischaemic heart disease as origin of chest pain in non-infarction coronary care unit patients and patients with myocardial infarction. *Acta Med Scand*, suppl 644, p. 69, 1981.

Ariga T, Oshiba S, Tamada T: Platelet aggregation inhibitor in garlic. *Lancet* **1**:150, 1981.

Armstrong A, Duncan B, Oliver MF, et al: Natural history of acute coronary heart attacks. A community study. *Br Heart J* **34**:67, 1972.

Armstrong ML: Regression of atherosclerosis. *Atherosclerosis Rev* **1**:137, 1976.

Armstrong ML, Warner ED, Connor WE: Regression of coronary atheromatosis in rhesus monkeys. *Circ Res* **27**:59, 1970.

Arntzenius AC, Strikwerda S, Kempen N, et al: Coronary lesions and serum lipids before and after 2 years diet in 22 patients. *Circulation* **66**(suppl 2):284, 1982.

Arntzenius AC, Kromhout D, Kempen N, et al: Effect of diet on total cholesterol/HDL-C ratio in patients of Leiden Regression Trial. *Circulation* **68**(suppl 3):226, 1983.

Aronow WS: Effect of passive smoking on angina pectoris. *N Engl J Med* **299**:21, 1978.

Aronson HB, Magora F, Schenker JG: Effect of oral contraceptives on blood viscosity. *Am J Obstet Gynecol* **110**:997, 1971.

Ashby P. Dalby AM, Millar JHD: Smoking and platelet stickiness. *Lancet* **2**:158, 1965.

Ashley FW, Kannell WB: Relation of weight change to changes in atherogenic traits: The Framingham Study. *J Chron Dis* **27**:103, 1974.

Ashley MJ: Alcohol consumption, ischemic heart disease and cerebrovascular disease. *J Stud Alcohol* **43**:869, 1982.

Askanas A, Udoshi M, Sadjadi SA: The heart in chronic alcoholism: A noninvasive study. *Am Heart J* **99**:9, 1980.

Aspirin after myocardial infarction, editorial. *Lancet* **1**:1172, 1980.

Auerbach O, Hammond EC, Garfinkel L: Smoking in relation to atherosclerosis of the coronary arteries. *N Engl J Med* **273**:775, 1965.

Australian National Blood Pressure Study: The Australian Therapeutic Trial in mild hypertension. *Lancet* **1**:1261, 1980.

Avogaro P. Cazzolato G, Bittolo B, et al: HDL-Cholesterol, apolipoproteins A1 and B. *Atherosclerosis* **31**:85, 1978.

Avogaro P, Bittolo BG, Gazzolato G, et al: Are apolipoproteins better discriminators than lipids for atherosclerosis? *Lancet* **1**:901, 1979.

Ayachi S: Increased dietary calcium lowers blood pressure in the spontaneously hypertensive rat. *Metabolism* **28**:1234, 1979.

Baba N, Basha WJ, Keller MD, et al: Pathology of atherosclerotic heart disease in sudden death. I. Organizing thrombosis and acute coronary vessel lesions. *Circulation* **52**(suppl 3):53, 1975.

Badeer HS: Biological significance of cardiac hypertrophy. *Am J Cardiol* **14**:133, 1964.

Bandura A: *Social Learning Theory*. Englewood Cliffs, NJ, Prentice-Hall, Inc, 1977.

Bandura A, Blanchard EB, Ritter B: The relative efficacy of desensitization and modeling approaches for inducing behavioral, affective, and attitudinal changes. *J. Pers Soc Psychol* **13**:173, 1969.

Bandura A, Simon KM: The role of proximal intentions in self-regulation of refractory behavior. *Cognitive Ther Res* **1**:177, 1977.

Bang HO, Dyerberg J: Plasma lipids and lipoproteins in Greenlandic West Coast eskimos. *Acta Med Scand* **192**:85, 1972.

Bang HO, Dyerberg J, Nielsen AB: Plasma lipid and lipoprotein pattern in Greenlandic West-Coast eskimos. *Lancet* **1**:1143, 1971.

Bang HO, Dyerberg J, Hjorn N: The composition of food consumed by Greenland eskimos. *Acta Med Scand* **200**:69, 1976.

Barber JM, Boyle DM, Chaturvedi NC, et al: Practolol in acute myocardial infarction. *Acta Med Scand*, suppl 587, p. 213, 1975.

Barboriak JJ, Rimm AA, Anderson AJ, et al: Coronary artery occlusion and alcohol intake. *Br Heart J* **39**:289, 1977.

Barboriak JJ: Alcohol and coronary-artery disease. *Lancet* **1**:1212, 1977.

Barnard RJ, Weber F, Weingarten W, et al: Effects on an intensive, short-term exercise and nutrition program on patients with coronary heart disease. *J. Cardiac Rehab* **1**:99, 1981.

Barnard RJ, Guzy PM, Rosenberg JM, et al: Effects of an intensive exercise and nutrition program on patients with coronary artery disease: 5-year follow-up. *J Cardiac Rehab* **3**:183, 1983.

Baroldi G: Different types of myocardial necrosis in coronary heart disease: A pathophysiologic review of their functional significance. *Am Heart J* **89**:742, 1975.

Baroldi G, Falzi G, Mariani F: Sudden coronary death. A postmortem study in 208 selected cases compared to 97 "control" subjects. *Am Heart J* **98**:20, 1979.

Barrett-Connor E, Suarez L, Criqui MH: Spouse concordance of plasma cholesterol and triglyceride. *J Chron Dis* **35**:333, 1982.

Barrow JG, Quinlan CB, Cooper GR, et al: Studies in atherosclerosis. III. An epidemiologic study of atherosclerosis in Trappist and Benedictine monks: A preliminary report. *Ann Intern Med* **52**:368, 1960.

Bashe WJ, Baba N, Keller MD, et al: Pathology of atherosclerotic heart disease in sudden death. II. The significance of myocardial infarction. *Circulation* **52**(suppl 3):63, 1975.

Bass C, Wade C: Type A behaviour: Not specifically pathogenetic? *Lancet* **2**:1147, 1982.

Baum RS, Alvarez H, Cobb LA: Survival after resuscitation from out-of-hospital ventricular fibrillation. *Circulation* **50**:1231, 1974.

Beaglehole R, Salmond CE, Hooper A, et al: Blood pressure and social interaction in Tokelauan migrants in New Zealand. *J. Chron Dis* **30**:803, 1977.

Beaglehole R, Prior I, Salmond C, et al: Coronary heart disease in Maoris: Incidence and case mortality. *NZ Med J* **88**:138, 1978.

Beaglehole R, La Rosa JC, Heiss G, et al: Serum cholesterol, diet, and the decline in coronary heart disease mortality. *Prev. Med.* **8**:538, 1979.

Beaglehole R, Bonita R, Jackson RT, et al: Decline in incidence of coronary heart disease in Auckland, New Zealand. *Am J Epidemiol* **120**:225, 1984.

Beard TC, Gray WR, Cooke HM, et al: Randomised controlled trial of a no-added-sodium diet for mild hypertension. *Lancet* **2**:455, 1982.

Becker MH: Sociobehavioral determinants of compliance, in Sacket DL, Haynes RB (eds): *Compliance with Therapeutical Regimes.* Baltimore, Johns Hopkins Univ Press, 1976, pp. 40–50.

Becker MH, Maiman LA: Sociobehavioral determinants of compliance with health and medical care recommendations. *Med Care* **13**:10, 1975.

Belfrage P, Berg B, Cronholm T, et al: Prolonged administration of ethanol to young, healthy volunteers: Effects on biochemical, morphological and neurophysiological parameters. *Acta Med Scand*, suppl 552, 1973.

Belizan JM, Villar J, Pineda O, et al: Reduction of blood pressure with calcium supplementation in young adults. *JAMA* **249**:1161, 1983.

Bellack AS: A comparison of self-reinforcement and self-monitoring in a weight reduction program. *Behav Ther* **7**:68, 1976.

Bennett W, Gurin J: *The Dieter's Dilemma.* New York, Basic Books, 1982.

Berenson GS, Blonde CV, Farris RP, et al: Cardiovascular disease risk factor variables during the first year of life. *Am J Dis Child* **133**:1049, 1979.

Berenson GS, Frank GC, Hunter S, et al: Cardiovascular risk factors in children. Should they concern the pediatrician? *Am J Dis Child* **136**:855, 1982.

Berg K, Borresen AL, Dahlen G: Effect of smoking on serum levels of HDL apoproteins. *Atherosclerosis* **34**:339, 1979.

Berglund G, Wilhelmsen L: Factors related to blood pressure in a general population sample of Swedish men. *Acta Med Scand* **198**:291, 1975.

Berglund G, Sannerstedt R, Andersson O, et al: Coronary heart-disease after treatment of hypertension. *Lancet* **1**:1, 1978.

Berkel J: *The Clean Life.* Amsterdam, Amsterdam Drukkerij Insulinde, 1979.

Berkman LF, Breslow L: *Health and Ways of Living: The Alameda County Study.* New York, Oxford University Press, 1983.

Berkman L, Syme SL: Social networks, host resistance, and mortality: A nine-year follow-up study of Alameda County residents. *Am J Epidemiol* **109**:186, 1979.

Berkson DM, Whipple IT, Shireman L, et al: Evaluation of an automated blood pressure measuring device intended for general public use. *Am J Public Health* **69**:473, 1979.

Berkson J: Are there two regressions? *J Am Stat Assoc* **45**:164, 1950.

Bertino M, Beauchamp GK, Engelman K: Long-term reduction in dietary sodium alters the taste of salt. *Am J Clin Nutr* **36**:1134, 1982.

Bertolasi CA, Tronge JE, Ricitelli MA, et al: Natural history of unstable angina with medical or surgical therapy. *Chest* **70**:596, 1976.

Beta Blocker Heart Attack Study Group: The Beta-Blocker Heart Attack Trial. *JAMA* **246**:2073, 1981.

Beta Blocker Heart Attack Trial Research Group: A randomized trial of propranolol in patients with acute myocardial infarction: I. Mortality results. *JAMA* **247**:1707, 1982.

Beta Blocker Heart Attack Trial Research Group: A randomized trial of propranolol in patients with acute myocardial infarction. II. Morbidity results. *JAMA* **250**:2814, 1983.

Beveridge JMR, Connell WF, Mayer Ga, et al: Plant sterols, degree of unsaturation, and hypocholesterolemic action of certain fats. *Can J Biochem Physiol* **36**:895, 1958.

Bierenbaum ML, Fleischman AI, Green DP, et al: The 5-year experience of modified fat diets on younger men with coronary heart disease. *Circulation* **42**:943, 1970.

Bjernulf A: Hemodynamic effects of physical training after myocardial infarction. *Acta Med Scand*, suppl 548, 1973.

Blacket RB, Leelarthaepin B, McGilchrist CA, et al: The synergistic effect of weight loss and changes in dietary lipids on the serum cholesterol of obese men with hypercholesterolaemia: Implications for Prevention of coronary heart disease. *Aust NZ J Med* **9**:521, 1979.

Blackwell B: Drug therapy: Patient compliance. *N Engl J Med* **289**:249, 1973.

Blair D, Habicht JP, Sims EA, et al: Evidence for an increased risk of hypertension with centrally located body fat and the effect of race and sex on the risk. *Am J Epidemiol* **119**:526, 1984.

Blaustein MP: Sodium ions, calcium ions, blood pressure regulation and hypertension: A reassessment and a hypothesis. *Am J Physiol* **232**:C165, 1977.

Blazer DG: Social support and mortality in an elderly community population. *Am J Epidemiol* **115**:684, 1982.

Block G: A review of validations of dietary assessment methods. *Am J Epidemiol* **115**:492, 1982.

Blonde CV, Webber LS, Foster TA, et al: Parental history and cardiovascular disease risk factor variables in children. *Prev Med* **10**:25, 1981.

Bloxham CA, Beevers DG, Walker JM: Malignant hypertension and cigarette smoking. *Br Med J* **1**:581, 1979.

Blumenthal JA, Williams RB, Kong Y, et al: Type A behavior pattern and coronary atherosclerosis. *Circulation* **58**:634, 1978.

Bordia A: Effect of garlic on human platelet aggregation in vitro. *Atherosclerosis* **30**:355, 1978.

Borgers D, Junge B: Thiocyanate as an indicator of tobacco smoking. *Prev Med* **8**:351, 1979.

Boulton TJC: Serum cholesterol in early childhood. *Acta Paediatr Scand* **69**:441, 1980.

Bounous EP, Wagner GS, Califf RM, et al: QRS score as prognosticator in coronary artery disease. *Circulation* **64**(suppl 4):41, 1981.

Boyer JL, Kasch FW: Exercise therapy in hypertensive men. *JAMA* **211**:1668, 1970.

Bradley DD, Wingerd J, Petitti DB, et al: Serum high-density-lipoprotein cholesterol in women using oral contraceptives, estrogens and progestins. *N Engl J Med* **299**:17, 1978.

Brain damage after open-heart surgery, editorial. *Lancet* **1**:1161, 1982.

Brand RJ, Paffenbarger RS, Sholtz RI, et al: Work activity and fatal heart attack studied by multiple logistic risk analysis. *Am J Epidemiol* **110**:52, 1979.

Braunwald E, Friedewald WT, Furberg CD (eds): Proceedings of the Workshop on Platelet-active Drugs in the Secondary Prevention of Cardiovascular Events. *Circulation* **62**(suppl 5):1, 1980.

Breddin K, Loew D, Lechnerk, et al: Secondary prevention of myocardial infarction. Comparison of acetylsalicylic acid, phenprocoumon and placebo. A multicenter two-year prospective study. *Thromb Haemos* **40**:225, 1979.

Brensike JF, Levy RI, Kelsey SF, et al: Effects of therapy with cholestyramine on progression of coronary arteriosclerosis: Results of the NHLBI Type II coronary intervention study. *Circulation* **69**:313, 1984.

Breslow L: Risk factor intervention for health maintenance. *Science* **200**:908, 1978.

Brown KA, Boucher CA, Okada RD, et al: Prognostic value of exercise thallium-201 imaging in patients presenting for evaluation of chest pain. *J Am Coll Cardiol* **1**:994, 1983.

Brownell KD: Exercise and obesity. *Bahav Med Update* **4**:7, 1982a.

Brownell KD: Obesity: Understanding and treating a serious, prevalent, and refractory disorder. *J Consult Clin Psychol* **50**:820, 1982b.

Brownell KD, Stunkard AJ: Exercise in the development and control of obesity, in Stunkard AJ (ed): *Obesity*. Philadelphia, WB Saunders Co, 1980.

Brownell KD, Bachorik PS, Ayerle RS: Changes in plasma lipid and lipoprotein levels in men and women after a program of moderate exercise. *Circulation* **65**:477, 1982.

Brownell KD, Heckerman CL, Westlake RJ, et al: The effect of couples training and partner co-operativeness in the behavioral treatment of obesity. *Behav Res Ther* **16**:323, 1978.

Bruschke A, Proudfit WL, Sones FM: Progress study of 590 consecutive non-surgical cases of coronary disease followed 5–9 years. *Circulation* **47**:1147, 1973.

Bruschke AVG, Wijers TS, Kolsters W, et al: The anatomic evolution of coronary artery disease demonstrated by coronary arteriography in 256 nonoperated patients. *Circulation* **63**:527, 1981.

Buja LM, Willerson JT: Clinicopathologic correlates of acute ischemic heart disease syndromes. *Am J Cardiol* **47**:343, 1981.

Burr ML, Sweetnam PM: Vegetarianism, dietary fiber, and mortality. *Am J Clin Nutr* **36**:873, 1982.

Burslem J, Schonfeld G, Howald MA, et al: Plasma apoprotein and lipoprotein lipid levels in vegetarians. *Metabolism* **27**:711, 1978.

Bush TL, Comstock GW: Smoking and cardiovascular mortality in women. *Am J Epidemiol* **118**:480, 1983.

Byington R, Dyer AR, Garside D, et al: Recent trends of major coronary risk factors and CHD mortality in the United States and other industrialized countries, in *Proceedings of the Conference on the Decline in Coronary Heart Disease Mortality*, publication 79–1610, US Dept of HEW, May 1979, p. 359.

Caggiula AW, Christakis G, Farrand M, et al: The Multiple Risk Factor Intervention Trial (MRFIT) IV. Intervention on blood lipids. *Prev Med* **10**:443, 1981.

Cambien F, Ducimetiere P, Richard J: Total serum cholesterol and cancer mortality in a middle-aged male population. *Am J Epidemiol* **112**:388, 1980.

Campbell MJ, Elwood PC, Abbas S, et al: Chest pain in women: a study of prevalence and mortality follow up in South Wales. *J Epidemiol Comm Health* **38**:17, 1984.

Canada Fitness Survey: *The Physically Active High School Graduate: An Endangered Species?* no 11, Aug 1983.

Canessa M, Adragna N, Solomon HS, et al: Increased sodium–lithium countertransport in red cells of patients with essential hypertension. *N Engl J Med* **302**:772, 1980.

Carlson LA, Bottiger LE: Ischemic heart disease in relation to fasting values of plasma triglycerides and cholesterol. *Lancet* **1**:865, 1972.

Carrol KK, Giovannetti PM, Huff MW, et al: Hypocholesterolemic effect of substituting soybean protein for animal protein in the diet of healthy young women. *Am J Clin Nutr* **31**:1312, 1978.

Carvalho ACA, Colman RW, Lees RS: Platelet function in hyperlipoproteinemia. *N Engl J Med* **290**:434, 1974.

Casper BA, Hayslip DE, Foree SB: The effect of nutrition education on dietary habits of fifth graders. *J Sch Health* **47**:475, 1977.

CASS principal investigators and associates: Coronary Artery Surgery Study (CASS): A randomized trial of coronary artery bypass surgery. Quality of life in patients randomly assigned to treatment groups. *Circulation* **68**:951, 1983a.

CASS principal investigators and associates: Coronary Artery Surgery Study (CASS): A randomized trial of coronary artery bypass surgery. Survival data. *Circulation* **68**:939, 1983b.

CASS principal investigators and associates: Coronary Artery Surgery Study (CASS): A randomized trial of coronary artery bypass surgery. Comparability of entry characteristics in randomized patients and nonrandomized patients meeting randomization criteria. *J Am Coll Cardiol* **3**:114, 1984a.

CASS principal investigators and associates: Myocardial infarction and mortality in the Coronary Artery Surgery Study (CASS) randomized trial. *N Engl J Med* **310**:750, 1984b.

Cassel J, Heyden S, Bartel AG, et al: Incidence of coronary heart disease by ethnic group, social class and sex. *Arch Intern Med* **128**:901, 1971.

Castelli WP, Gordon T, Hjortland MC, et al: Alcohol and blood lipids. *Lancet* **2**:153, 1977.

Castelli WP, Dawber TR, Feinleib M, et al: The filter cigarette and coronary heart disease: The Framingham Study. *Lancet* **2**:109, 1981.

Castelli WP, Abbott RD, McNamara PM: Summary estimates of cholesterol used to predict coronary heart disease. *Circulation* **67**:730, 1983.

Chafetz ME: Alcohol and the heart, in *Alcohol and Health*, publication (ADM) 75–212. Washington, DC, US Dept of Health, Education and Welfare, 1974, pp. 68–72.

Chamberlain DA, Julian DG, Boyle DMcC, et al: Oral mexiletine in high-risk patients after myocardial infarction. *Lancet* **2**:1324, 1980.

Chandra V, Szklo M, Goldberg R, et al: The impact of marital status on survival after an acute myocardial infarction: A population-based study. *Am J Epidemiol* **117**:320, 1983.

Chapman JM, Massey FJ: The interrelationship of serum cholesterol, hypertension, body weight and risk of coronary heart disease: Results of the first ten years follow-up in the Los Angeles Heart Study. *J Chron Dis* **17**:933, 1964.

Chiang BN, Perlman LV, Ostrander LD, et al: Relationship of premature systoles to coronary heart disease and sudden death in the Tecumseh epidemiologic study. *Ann Intern Med* **70**:1159, 1969.

Chiang BN, Perlman LV, Fulton M, et al: Predisposing factors in sudden cardiac death in Tecumseh, Michigan. A prospective study. *Circulation* **41**:31, 1970.

Choquette G, Ferguson RJ: Blood pressure reduction in "borderline" hypertensives following physical training. *Can Med Assoc J* **108**:699, 1973.

Clarke WR, Schrott HG, Leaverton PE, et al: Tracking of blood lipids and blood pressures in school age children: The Muscatine Study. *Circulation* **58**:626, 1978.

Clausen JP, Trap-Jensen J: Heart rate and arterial blood pressure during exercise in patients with angina pectoris. *Circulation* **53**:436, 1976.

Clausen JP, Larson OA, Trap-Jensen J: Physical training in the management of coronary artery disease. *Circulation* **40**:143, 1969.

Coates TJ, Jeffery RW, Slinkard LA: Heart, healthy eating and exercise: Introducing and maintaining changes in health behaviors. *Am J Public Health* **71**:15, 1981.

Cobb LA, Baum RS, Alvarez H, et al: Resuscitation from out-of-hospital ventricular fibrillation: 4 years follow-up. *Circulation* **52**(suppl 3):223, 1975.

Cobb LA, Werner JA, Trobaugh DB: Sudden cardiac death. I. A Decade's experience with out-of-hospital resuscitation. *Mod Concepts Cardiovasc Dis* **49**:31, 1980a.

Cobb LA, Werner JA, Trobaugh DB: Sudden cardiac death. II. Outcome of resuscitation. Management and future directions. *Mod Concepts Cardiovasc Dis* **49**:37, 1980b.

Coccheri S, Fiorentini P: Platelet adhesiveness and aggregation in hypertensive patients. *Acta Med Scand*, suppl 525, p. 273, 1971.

Cohen JB, Syme SL, Jenkins CD, et al: The cultural context of type A behavior and the risk of CHD. *Am J Epidemiol* **102**:434, 1975.

Cohen JB, Matthews KA, Waldron I: Coronary prone behavior: Developmental and cultural considerations, in Dembroski TM, Weiss SM, Shields JL (eds): *Coronary Prone Behavior*. New York, Springer Verlag, 1978, p. 188.

Cohen JD, Bartsch GE: A comparison between carboxyhemoglobin and serum thiocyanate determinations as indicators of cigarette smoking. *Am J Public Health* **70**:284, 1980.

Coll S, Castaner A, Betriu A, et al: Colesterol y severidad de la en fermedad coronaria. Su valor en el pronostico despues del infarto de miocardio. *Rev Espanola Cardiol* **36**:21, 1983.

Committee of Principal Investigators: A co-operative trial in the primary prevention of ischaemic heart disease using clofibrate. *Br Heart J* **40**:1069, 1978.

Committee of Principal Investigators, WHO Clofibrate Trial: Primary prevention of ischaemic heart disease: WHO coordinated cooperative trial. *Bull WHO* **57**:801, 1979.

Committee of Principal Investigators: WHO Cooperative trial on primary prevention of ischaemic heart disease using clofibrate to lower serum cholesterol: Mortality follow-up. *Lancet* **2**:379, 1980.

Committee on Youth: A new approach to teenage smoking. *Pediatrics* **57**:465, 1976.

Comstock GW: Fatal arteriosclerotic heart disease, water hardness at home, and socioeconomic characteristics. *Am J Epidemiol* **94**:1, 1971.

Connor WE: Cross-cultural studies of diet and plasma lipids and lipoproteins, in Lauer RM, Shekelle RB (eds): *Childhood Prevention of Atherosclerosis and Hypertension*. New York, Raven Press, 1980, p. 99.

Connor WE, Witiak DT, Stone DB, et al: Cholesterol balance and fecal neutral steroid and bile acid excretion in normal men fed dietary fats of different acid composition. *J. Clin Invest* **48**:1363, 1969.

Connor WE, Cerqueira MT, Connor RW, et al: The plasma lipids, lipoproteins and diet of the Tarahumara Indians of Mexico. *Am J Clin Nutr* **31**:1131, 1978.

Cooper KH: *The New Aerobics*. New York, Bantam Books, 1972.

Cooper KH, Pollock ML, Martin RP, et al: Physical fitness levels vs. selected coronary risk factors. *JAMA* **236**:166, 1976.

Cooper R, Stamler J, Dyer A, et al: The decline in mortality from coronary heart disease, USA 1968–1975. *J Chron Dis* **31**:709, 1978.

Cooper R, Soltero I, Liu K, et al: The association between urinary sodium excretion and blood pressure in children. *Circulation* **62**:97, 1980.

Corbett JR, Dehmer GJ, Lewis SE, et al: The prognostic value of submaximal exercise testing with radionuclide ventriculography before hospital discharge in patients with recent myocardial infarction. *Circulation* **64**:535, 1981.

Coronary Drug Project Research Group: Factors influencing long-term prognosis after recovery from myocardial infarction. Three-year findings of the Coronary Drug Project. *J Chron Dis* **27**:267, 1974.

Coronary Drug Project Research Group: Clofibrate and niacin in coronary heart disease. *JAMA* **231**:360, 1975.

Coronary Risk Calculator. Cincinnati, Ohio, Merrel Dow Pharmaceuticals, Inc, 1983.

Council on Scientific Affairs, American Medical Association: Sodium in processed foods. *JAMA* **249**:784, 1983.

Crawford MA, Stevens PA: Essential fatty acids, diet and heart disease, in Bazan NG, Paoletti R,

Iacono JM (eds): *New Trends in Nutrition, Lipid Research and Cardiovascular Disease.* New York, Alan R Liss, Inc, 1981, pp. 217–228.

Criqui MH, Wallace RB, Heiss G, et al: Cigarette smoking and plasma high-density lipoprotein cholesterol. *Circulation* **62**(suppl 4):70, 1980a.

Criqui MH, Barrett-Connor E, Holdbrook MJ, et al: Clustering of cardiovascular disease risk factors. *Prev Med* **9**:525, 1980b.

Criqui MH, Wallace RB, Mishkell M, et al: Alcohol consumption and blood pressure. *Hypertension* **3**:557, 1981.

Criqui MH, Mebane I, Wallace RB, et al: Multivariate correlate of adult blood pressures in nine North American populations: The Lipid Research Clinics Prevalence Study. *Prev Med* **11**: 391, 1982.

Croog SH, Richards NP: Health beliefs and smoking patterns in heart patients and their wives. *Am J Public Health* **67**:921, 1977.

Crouch M, Sallis JF, King A, et al: Personal and mediated health counseling for sustained dietary reduction of hypercholesterolemia. Submitted to *Prev Med* for publication.

Cruz-Coke R, Etcheverry R, Nagel R: Influence of migration on blood pressure of Easter-Islanders. *Lancet* **1**:697, 1964.

Dahl LK, Silver L, Christie RW: The role of salt in the fall of blood pressure accompanying the reduction of obesity. *N Engl J Med* **258**:1186, 1958.

Danaher BG: Research on rapid smoking: Interim summary and recommendations. *Addict Behav* **2**: 151, 1977.

Davidson DM, DeBusk RF: Prognostic value of a single exercise test 3 weeks after uncomplicated myocardial infarction. *Circulation* **61**:236, 1980.

Davis HT, DeCamilla J, Bayer LW, et al: Survivorship patterns in the posthospital phase of myocardial infarction. *Circulation* **60**:1252, 1979.

Dawber TR: *The Framingham Study. The Epidemiology of Atherosclerotic Disease.* Cambridge, Mass, Harvard University Press, 1980, p. 163.

Day JL, Simpson N, Metcalfe J, et al: Metabolic consequences of atenolol and propranolol in treatment of essential hypertension. *Br Med J* **1**:77, 1979.

Day N: *Alcohol and mortality. Separating the drink from the drinker*, doctorial thesis. Univ of California, Berkeley, 1979.

Dayton S, Pearce ML, Hashimoto S, et al: A controlled clinical trial of a diet high in unsaturated fat in preventing complications of atherosclerosis. *Circulation* **40**(suppl 2):1, 1969.

De Backer G, Kornitzer M, Kittel F, et al: Relation between coronary-prone behavior pattern, excretion of urinary catecholamines, heart rate, and heart rhythm. *Prev Med* **8**:14, 1979.

De Backer G, Rosseneu M, Deslypere JP: Discriminative value of lipids and apoproteins in coronary heart disease. *Atherosclerosis* **42**:197, 1982.

De Groot AP, Luyken R, Pikaar NR: Cholesterol-lowering effect of rolled oats. *Lancet* **2**:303, 1963.

Dembroski TM, MacDougall JM, Shields JL: Physiologic reaction to social challenge in persons evidencing the Type A coronary-prone behavior pattern. *J Human Stress* **3**:2, 1977.

Detre K, Hultgren H, Takaro T: Veterans Administration Cooperative Study of Surgery for Coronary Arterial Occlusive Disease. *Am J Cardiol* **40**:212, 1977.

Detre K, Peduzzi P, Murphy M, et al, and the V.A. Cooperative Study Group for Surgery for Coronary Arterial Occlusive Disease: Effects of bypass surgery on survival in patients in low- and high-risk subgroups delineated by the use of simple clinical variables. *Circulation* **63**: 1329, 1981.

Detry JM, Bruce RA: Effects of physical training on exertional S-T segment depression in coronary heart disease. *Circulation* **44**:390, 1971.

Detry JRM, Rousseau M, Vandenbroucke G, et al: Increased arteriovenous oxygen difference after physical training in coronary heart disease. *Circulation* **44**:109, 1971.

Deubner DC, Wilkinson WE, Helms MJ, et al: Logistic model estimation of the deaths attributable to risk factors for cardiovascular disease in Evans County, Ga. *Am J Epidemiol* **112**:135, 1980.

DeWardener HE: The natriuretic hormone. *Ann Clin Biochem* **19**:137, 1982.

Diamond GA, Forrester JS: Analysis of probability as an aid in the clinical diagnosis of coronary artery disease. *N Engl J Med* **300**:1350, 1979.

Dickey FF, Mattar ME, Chudzik GM: Pharmacist counselling increases drug regime compliance. *Hospitals* **49**:85, 1975.

Diehl H, Mannerberg D: Hypertension, hyperlipidaemia, angina and coronary disease, in Trowell HC, Burkitt DP (eds): *Western Diseases, Their Emergence and Prevention*. Cambridge, Mass, Harvard Univ Press, 1981, p. 392.

Dimsdale JE, Hackett TP, Catanzano DM, et al: The relationship between diverse measures for Type A personality and coronary angiographic findings. *J Psychosom Res* **23**:289, 1979.

Dishman RK: Compliance/adherence in health-related exercise. *Health Psychol* **1**:237, 1982.

Doba N, Abe H, Hayashida N, et al: Semi-supervised exercise training program for patients with coronary heart disease—its effectiveness and possible diagnostic implications for predicting their severity. *Jpn Circ J* **47**:735, 1983.

Dodge R: The effects of indoor pollution on Arizona children. *Arch Environ Health* **37**:151, 1982.

Donner A, Koval JJ: A multivariate analysis of family data. *Am J Epidemiol* **114**:149, 1981.

Dorso CR, Levin RI, Eldor A, et al: Chinese food and platelets. *N Engl J Med* **303**:756, 1980.

Doyle JT, Heslin AS, Hilleboe HE, et al: A prospective study of degenerative cardiovascular disease in Albany—I. Ischemic heart disease. *Am J Public Health* **47**(suppl 4):25, 1957.

Doyle JT, Dawber TR, Kannel WB, et al: Cigarette smoking and coronary heart disease. *New Engl J Med* **266**:796, 1962.

Dunbar JM, Agras WS: Compliance with medical instructions, In Ferguson JM, Taylor CB (eds): *The Comprehensive Handbook of Behavioral Medicine*. Vol 3, *Extended Applications and Issues*. New York, Spectrum, 1980, pp. 115–145.

Dunnigan MG, Harland WA: Seasonal incidence and mortality of ischemic heart disease. *Lancet* **2**:793, 1970.

Du Plessis JP, Vivier FS, De Lange DJ: The biochemical evaluation of the nutrition status of urban school children aged 7–15 years: Serum cholesterol and phospholipid levels and serum and urinary amylase activities. *S Afr Med J* **41**:1216, 1967.

Dwyer T, Hetzel B: A comparison of trends of coronary heart disease mortality in Australia, USA and England and Wales with reference to 3 major risk factors—hypertension, cigarette smoking and diet. *Int J Epidemiol* **9**:65, 1980.

Dyer AR, Stamler J, Paul O, et al: Alcohol consumption, cardiovascular risk factors, and mortality in two Chicago epidemiologic studies. *Circulation* **56**:1067, 1977.

Dyer AR, Stamler J, Paul O, et al: Alcohol consumption and 17-year mortality in the Chicago Western Electric Company Study. *Prev Med* **9**:78, 1980.

Dyer AR, Stamler J, Shekelle RB, et al: Relative weight and blood pressure in four Chicago epidemiologic studies. *J Chron Dis* **35**:897, 1982.

Dyerberg J, Bang O: Haemostatic function and platelet polyunsaturated fatty acids in Eskimos. *Lancet* **2**:433, 1979.

Dyerberg J, Bang HO, Stoffersen E: Eicosapentaenoic acid and prevention of thrombosis and atherosclerosis? *Lancet* **2**:117, 1978.

Ebers G: *Papyros Ebers, das Hermetische. Buch ueber die Arzneimittel der alten Aegypter in hieratischer Schrift*, vol 2. Leipzig, Engelman, 1875, pp. 37–38. Quoted by Leibowitz JO: *The History of Coronary Heart Disease*. London, Welcome Institute of the History of Medicine, 1970.

Ederer F, Leren P, Turpeinen O, et al: Cancer among men on cholesterol-lowering diets. *Lancet* **2**:203, 1971.

Ehnholm C, Huttunen JK, Pietinen P, et al: Effect of diet on serum lipoproteins in a population with a high risk of coronary heart disease. *N Engl J Med* **307**:850, 1982.

Eisenberg M, Bergner L, Hallstrom A: Paramedic programs and out-of-hospital cardiac arrest: I. Factors associated with successful resuscitation. *Am J Public Health* **69**:30, 1979a.

Eisenberg M, Bergner L, Hallstrom A: Paramedic programs and out-of-hospital cardiac arrest: II. Impact on community mortality. *Am J Public Health* **69**:39, 1979b.

Eisenberg MS, Hallstrom A, Bergner L: Long-term survival after out-of-hospital cardiac arrest. *N Engl J Med* **306**:1340, 1982.

El Lozy M: Dietary variability and its impact on nutritional epidemilogy. *J Chron Dis* **36**:237, 1983.

Elwood PC, Sweetnam PM: Aspirin and secondary mortality after myocardial infarction. *Circulation* **62**(suppl 5):53, 1980.

Elwood PC, Cochrane AL, Burr ML, et al: A randomized controlled trial of acetylsalicylic acid in the secondary prevention of mortality from myocardial infarction. *Brit Med J* **1**:436, 1974.

Ettinger PO, Wu CF, DeLa Cruz C, et al: Arrhythmias and the "Holiday Heart": Alcohol-associated cardiac rhythm disorders. *Am Heart J* **95**:555, 1978.

European Coronary Surgery Study Group: Prospective randomised study of coronary artery bypass surgery in stable angina pectoris. *Lancet* **2**:491, 1980.

European Coronary Surgery Study Group. Prospective randomized study of coronary artery by-pass surgery in stable angina pectoris: A progress report on survival. *Circulation* **65**(suppl 2):67, 1982.

Evans PH: Relation of longstanding blood-pressure levels to atherosclerosis. *Lancet* **1**:516, 1965.

Falkner B, Kushner H, Onesti G, et al: Cardiovascular characteristics in adolescents who develop essential hypertension. *Hypertension* **3**:521, 1981.

Farquhar JW: *The American Way of Life Need Not Be Hazardous to Your Health.* New York, WW Norton, 1978.

Farquhar JW, Wood PD, Breitrose H, et al: Community education for cardiovascular health. *Lancet* **1**:1192, 1977.

Farris RP, Frank GC, Webber LS, et al: Influence of milk source on serum lipids and lipoproteins during the first year of life, Bogalusa Heart Study. *Am J Clin Nutr* **35**:42, 1982.

Fehily AM, Burr ML, Phillips KM, et al: The effect of fatty fish on plasma lipid and lipoprotein concentrations. *Am J Clin Nutr* **38**:349, 1983.

Feinleib M, Labarthe D, Shekelle R, et al: Criteria for evaluation of automated blood pressure measuring devices for use in hypertensive screening programs. *Circulation* **49** (p. 6 at back of March 1974 edition).

Feinleib M, Kannel WB, Tedeschi CG, et al: The relation of antemortem characteristics to cardiovascular findings at autopsy. *Atherosclerosis* **34**:145, 1979.

Ferguson RJ, Cote P, Gauthier P, et al: Changes in exercise coronary sinus blood flow with training in patients with angina pectoris. *Circulation* **58**:41, 1978.

Fernandez D, Rosenthal JE, Cohen LS, et al: Alcohol-induced Prinzmetal variant angina. *Am J Cardiol* **32**:238, 1973.

Fisch IR, Frank J: Oral contraceptives and blood pressure. *JAMA* **237**:2499, 1977.

Fitness Profile of American Youth. A Report on 1981–83 Fitness Tests Involving more than 4 million Boys and Girls in over 10,000 Schools. East Hanover, NJ, Nabisco Brands, 1983.

Flaxman J: Quitting smoking now or later: Gradual, abrupt, immediate, and delayed quitting. *Behav Ther* **9**:260, 1978.

Fleischman AI, Justice D, Bierenbaum ML, et al: Beneficial effect of increased dietary linoleate upon in vivo platelet function in man. *J Nutr* **105**:1286, 1975.

Fleischman AI, Watson PB, Stier A, et al: Effect of increased dietary linoleate upon blood pressure, platelet function and serum lipids in hypertensive adult humans. *Prev Med* **8**:163, 1979.

Folsom AR, Luepker RV, Gillum RF, et al: Improvement in hypertension detection and control from 1973–74 to 1980–81. *JAMA* **250**:916, 1983.

Folstrom A, Gillum R, Prineas R, et al: Trends in out-of-hospital coronary heart disease deaths in a metropolitan community. *Circulation* **64**(suppl 4):213, 1981.

Forrester TE, Alleyne GAO: Sodium, potassium, and rate constants for sodium efflux in leucocytes from hypertensive Jamaicans. *Br Med J* **283**:5, 1981.

Foxx RM, Brown RA: Nicotine fading and self-monitoring for cigarette abstinence or controlled smoking. *J Appl Behav Anal* **12**:111, 1979.

Francis V, Korsch BM, Morris MJ: Gaps in doctor–patient communication: Patients' response to medical advice. *N Engl J Med* **280**:535, 1969.

Frank GC, Berenson GS, Webber LS: Dietary studies and the relationship of diet to cardiovascular disease risk factor variables in 10-year-old children. The Bogalusa Heart Study. *Am J Clin Nutr* **31**:328, 1978.

Frank K, Heller SS, Kornfeld DS, et al: Type A behavior pattern and coronary angiographic findings. *JAMA* **240**:761, 1978.

Fraser GE: Definite myocardial infarction in Auckland. *Aust NZ J Med* **8**:479, 1978a.

Fraser GE: Sudden death in Auckland. *Aust NZ J Med* **8**:490, 1978b.

Fraser GE, Swannell RJ: Diet and serum cholesterol in Seventh-day Adventists: A cross-sectional study showing significant relationships. *J Chron Dis* **34**:487, 1981.

Fraser GE, Upsdell M: Alcohol and other discriminants between cases of sudden death and myocardial infarction. *Am J Epidemiol* **114**:462, 1981.

Fraser GE, Jacobs DR, Anderson JT, et al: The effect of various vegetable supplements on serum cholesterol. *Am J Clin Nutr* **34**:1272, 1981.

Fraser GE, Anderson JT, Foster N, et al: The effect of alcohol on serum high density lipoprotein (HDL)—a controlled experiment. *Atherosclerosis* **46**:275, 1983a.

Fraser GE, Phillips RL, Harris R: Physical fitness and blood pressure in school children. *Circulation* **67**:405, 1983b.

Fraser GE, Schneider L, Kubo C, et al: Results of a long-term outpatient cardiac rehabilitation program to assess compliance and risk factor modification, 1984 (manuscript submitted for publication).

Fraser GE, Dysinger W, Best C: Coronary risk factors in middle-aged Seventh Day Adventist men and their neighbors. Manuscript in preparation.

Freis ED: Electrocardiographic changes in the course of antihypertensive treatment. *Am J Med* (suppl, Sept 26):111, 1983.

Frerichs RR, Srinivasan SR, Webber LS, et al: Serum cholesterol and triglyceride levels in 3,446 children from a biracial community. The Bogalusa Heart Study. *Circulation* **54**:302, 1976.

Frerichs RR, Srinivasan SR, Webber LS, et al: Serum lipids and lipoproteins at birth in a biracial population. The Bogalusa Heart Study. *Pediatr Res* **12**:858, 1978.

Frerichs RR, Webber LS, Voors AW, et al: Cardiovascular disease risk factor variables in children at two successive years—The Bogalusa Heart Study. *J Chron Dis* **32**:251, 1979.

Frick MH, Katila M: Hemodynamic consequences of physical training after myocardial infarction. *Circulation* **37**:192, 1968.

Friedman GD, Petitti DB, Bawol RD, et al: Mortality in cigarette smokers and quitters. *N Engl J Med* **304**:1407, 1981.

Friedman HS: Acute effects of ethanol on myocardial blood flow in the non-ischemic and ischemic heart. *Am J Cardiol* **47**:61, 1981.

Friedman M, Rosenman RH: Association of specific overt behavior pattern with blood and cardiovascular findings. *JAMA* **169**:1286, 1959.

Friedman M, Rosenman RH, Carroll V: Changes in serum cholesterol and blood clotting time in men subjected to cyclic variation of occupational stress. *Circulation* **17**:852, 1958.

Friedman M, Rosenman RH, Strauss R, et al: The relationship of behavior pattern A to the state of the coronary vasculature. *Am J Med* **44**:525, 1968.

Friedman M, Byers SO, Diamant J, et al: Plasma catecholamine response of coronary-prone subjects (type A) to a specific challenge. *Metabolism* **24**:205, 1975.

Frink RJ, Trowbridge JO, Rooney PA: Nonobstructive coronary thrombosis in sudden cardiac death. *Am J Cardiol* **42**:48, 1978.

Froelicher V, Jensen D, Atwood JE, et al: Cardiac rehabilitation: Evidence for improvement in myocardial perfusion and function. *Arch Phys Med Rehabil* **61**:517, 1980.

Fuster V, Chesebro JH, Frye RL, et al: Platelet survival and the development of coronary artery disease in the young adult: Effects of cigarette smoking, strong family history and medical therapy. *Circulation* **63**:546, 1981.

Fyfe T, Cochran KM, Baxter RH, et al: Plasma-lipid changes after myocardial infarction. *Lancet* **2**:997, 1971.

Galbraith WB, Connor WE, Stone DB: Serum lipid changes in obese subjects given reducing diets of varied cholesterol content. *Clin Res* **12**:352, 1964.

Galli G, Agradi E, Petroni A, et al: Modulation of prostaglandin production in tissues by dietary essential fatty acids. *Acta Med Scand*, suppl 642, p. 171, 1980.

Garay RP, Meyer P: A new test showing abnormal net Na$^+$ and K$^+$ fluxes in erythrocytes of essential hypertensive patients. *Lancet* 1:349, 1979.

Garcia MJ, McNamara PM, Gordon T, et al: Morbidity and mortality in diabetics in the Framingham population. *Diabetes* 23:105, 1974.

Garcia-Palmieri MR, Sorlie PD, Costas R, et al: An apparent inverse relationship between serum cholesterol and cancer mortality in Puerto Rico. *Am J Epidemiol* 114:29, 1981.

Garcia-Palmieri MR, Costas R, Cruz-Vidal M, et al: Increased physical activity: A protective factor against heart attacks in Puerto Rico. *Am J Cardiol* 50:749, 1982.

Garland C, Barrett-Connor E, Suarez L, et al: Isolated systolic hypertension and mortality after age 60 years. *Am J Epidemiol* 118:365, 1983.

Garn SM, Clarke DC: Trends in fatness and the origins of obesity. *Pediatrics* 57:443, 1976.

Garn SM, Larkin FA, Cole PE: The real problem with 1-day diet records. *Am J Clin Nutr* 31:1114, 1978.

Garn SM, Bailey SM, Higgins ITT: Effects of socioeconomic status, family line, and living together on fatness and obesity, in Lauer RM, Shekelle RB (eds): *Childhood Prevention of Atherosclerosis and Hypertension*. New York, Raven Press, 1980, p. 187.

Garrison RJ, Kannel WB, Feinleib M, et al: Cigarette smoking and HDL cholesterol. *Atherosclerosis* 30:17, 1978.

Garrison RJ, Castelli WP, Feinleib M, et al: The association of total cholesterol, triglycerides and plasma lipoprotein cholesterol levels in first degree relatives and spouse pairs. *Am J Epidemiol* 110:313, 1979.

Garrison RJ, Wilson PW, Castelli WP, et al: Obesity and lipoprotein cholesterol in the Framingham Offspring Study. *Metabolism* 29:1053, 1980.

Genton E: A perspective on platelet-suppressant drug treatment in coronary artery and cerebrovascular disease. *Circulation* 62(suppl 5):111, 1980.

Gentry DW: Psychosocial concerns and benefit in cardiac rehabilitation, in Pollock ML, Schmidt DH (eds): *Heart Disease and Rehabilitation*. Boston, Houghton-Mifflin, 1979, p. 697.

Gerrard JM, White JG, Krivit W: Labile aggregation stimulating substance, free fatty acids and platelet aggregation. *J Lab Clin Med* 87:73, 1976.

Gerstenblith G, Ouyang P, Achuff SC, et al: Nifedipine in unstable angina. A double-blind, randomized trial. *N Engl J Med* 306:885, 1982.

Gibbons LW, Blair SN, Cooper KH, et al: Association between coronary heart disease risk factors and physical fitness in healthy adult women. *Circulation* 67:977, 1983.

Gibson RS, Beller GA: Should exercise electrocardiographic testing be replaced by radioisotope methods? in Rahimtoola SH (ed): *Controversies in Coronary Artery Disease*. Philadelphia, FA Davis Co, 1983, p. 5.

Gibson RS, Watson DD, Craddock GB, et al: Predicting cardiac events after uncomplicated myocardial infarction: A prospective study comparing predischarge exercise thallium-201 scintigraphy and coronary angiography. *Circulation* 68:321, 1983.

Gifford RW, Borhani N, Krishan I, et al: The dilemma of "mild" hypertension. Another viewpoint of treatment. *JAMA* 250:3171, 1983.

Gillum RF: Pathology of hypertension in blacks and whites. *Hypertension* 1:468, 1979.

Gillum RF, Grant CT: Coronary heart disease in black populations. II. Risk factors. *Am Heart J* 104:852, 1982.

Gillum RF, Taylor HL, Brozek J, et al: Blood lipids in young men followed 32 years. *J Chron Dis* 35:635, 1982.

Gillum RF, Prineas RJ, Jeffrey RW, et al: Non-pharmacologic therapy of hypertension: The independent effects of weight reduction and sodium restriction in overweight borderline hypertensive patients. *Am Heart J* 105:128, 1983.

Gillum RF, Folsom AR, Blackburn H: Decline in coronary heart disease mortality. *Am J Med* 76:1055, 1984.

Gleiberman L: Blood pressure and dietary salt in human populations. *Ecology Food Nutr* 2:143, 1973.

Gluck Z, Baumgartner G, Weidmann P, et al: Increased ratio between serum β- and α-lipoproteins during diuretic therapy: An adverse effect? *Clin Sci Mol Med* 55:325s, 1978.

Glueck CJ: Detection of risk factors for coronary artery disease in children: Semmelweis revisited? *Pediatrics* 66:834, 1980.

Glueck CJ, Tsang RC: Pediatric familial type II hyperlipoproteinemia: Effects of diet on plasma cholesterol in the first year of life. *Am J Clin Nutr* 25:224, 1972.

Glueck CJ, Fallat RW, Tsang R, et al: Hyperlipidemia in progeny of parents with myocardial infarction before age 50. *Am J Dis Child* 127:70, 1974.

Glueck CJ, Taylor HL, Jacobs D, et al: Plasma high-density lipoprotein cholesterol: Association with measurements of body mass. *Circulation* 62(suppl 4):62, 1980.

Godfrey RC, Stenhouse NS, Cullen KJ, et al: Cholesterol and the child: Studies of the cholesterol levels of Busselton school children and their parents. *Aust Pediatr* 8:72, 1972.

Goldberg SJ, Allen HD, Friedman G, et al: Use of health education and attempted dietary change to modify atherosclerotic risk factors: A controlled trial. *Am J Clin Nutr* 33:1272, 1980.

Goldbourt U, Medalie JH, Neufeld H: Clinical myocardial infarction over a five-year period. III. A multivariate analysis of incidence. The Israel Ischemic Heart Disease Study. *J Chron Dis* 28:217, 1975.

Goldman AI, Steele BW, Schnaper HW, et al: Serum lipoprotein levels during chlorthalidone therapy. *JAMA* 244:1691, 1980.

Goldschlager N, Cohn K, Goldschlager A: Exercise-related ventricular arrhythmias. *Mod Concepts Cardiovasc Dis* 48:67, 1979.

Goldstein JL, Brown MS: Atherosclerosis: The low-density lipoprotein receptor hypothesis. *Metabolism* 26:1257, 1977.

Goldstein S: The necessity of a uniform definition of sudden coronary death: Witnessed death within 1 hour of the onset of acute symptoms. *Am Heart J* 103:156, 1982.

Goldstein S, Landis JR, Leighton R, et al: Characteristics of the resuscitated out-of-hospital cardiac arrest victim with coronary heart disease. *Circulation* 64:977, 1981.

Golubjatnikov R, Paskey T, Inhorn SL: Serum cholesterol levels of Mexican and Wisconsin schoolchildren. *Am J Epidemiol* 96:36, 1972.

Goodnight SH, Harris WS, Connor WE: The effects of dietary w3 fatty acids on platelet composition and function in man: A prospective, controlled study. *Blood* 58:880, 1981.

Gordis L, Markowitz M, Lilienfeld AM: Why patients don't follow medical advice. *J Pediatr* 75:957, 1969.

Gordon T, Kannel WB: Drinking habits and cardiovascular disease: The Framingham Study. *Am Heart J* 105:667, 1983.

Gordon T, Sorlie P, Kannel WB: Coronary heart disease, atherothrombotic brain infarction, intermittent claudication. A multivariate analysis of some factors related to their incidence: Framingham Study, 16-year follow-up, in Kannel WB, Gordon T (eds): *The Framingham Study. An Epidemiologic Investigation of Cardiovascular Disease*, section 27. Washington, DC, US Government Printing Office, 1971.

Gordon T, Kannel WB, McGee D: Death and coronary attacks in men after giving up cigarette smoking. *Lancet* 2:1345, 1974.

Gordon T, Kannel WB, Dawber TR, et al: Changes associated with quitting cigarette smoking: The Framingham Study. *Am Heart J* 90:322, 1975.

Gordon T, Castelli WP, Hjortland MC, et al: High-density lipoprotein as a protective factor against coronary heart disease. The Framingham Study. *Am J Med* 62:707, 1977a.

Gordon T, Castelli WP, Hjortland MC, et al: Predicting coronary heart disease in middle-aged and older persons. *JAMA* 238:497, 1977b.

Gordon T, Kagan A, Garcia-Palmieri M, et al: Diet and its relation to coronary heart disease and death in three populations. *Circulation* 63:500, 1981.

Gori GB: Summary of the Workshop on Carbon Monoxide and Cardiovascular Disease, Berlin, October 10–12, 1978. *Prev Med* 8:404, 1979.

Gotto AM: The plasma apolipoproteins: Regulation of the structure and function of the plasma lipoproteins. *Cardiovas Rev Rep* **3**:1032, 1982.

Grande F, Anderson JT, Keys A: Comparison of effects of palmitic and stearic acids in the diet on serum cholesterol in man. *Am J Clin Nutr* **23**:1184, 1970.

Grande F, Anderson JT, Keys A: Diets of different fatty acid composition producing identical serum cholesterol levels in man. *Am J Clin Nutr* **25**:53, 1972.

Grande F, Anderson JT, Keys A: Sucrose and various carbohydrate-containing foods and serum lipids in man. *Am J Clin Nutr* **27**:1043, 1974.

Green KG, Chamberlain DA, Fulton RM, et al: Reduction in mortality after myocardial infarction with long-term beta-adrenoceptor blockade. *Br Med J* **2**:419, 1977.

Green LH, Seroppian E, Handin RI: Platelet activation during exercise-induced myocardial ischemia. *N Engl J Med* **302**:193, 1980.

Greenberg G, Brennan PJ, Miall WE: Effects of diuretic and beta-blocker therapy in the Medical Research Council Trial. *Am J Med* **76**(2A):45, 1984.

Greenspon AJ, Schaal SF: The "holiday heart": Electrophysiologic studies of alcohol effects in alcoholics. *Ann Intern Med* **98**:135, 1983.

Greig M, Pemberton J, Hay I, et al: A prospective study of the development of coronary heart disease in a group of 1202 middle-aged men. *J Epidemiol Community Health* **34**:23, 1980.

Grim CE, Luft FC, Miller JZ, et al: Racial differences in blood pressure in Evans County, Georgia: Relationship to sodium and potassium intake and plasma renin activity. *J Chron Dis* **33**:87, 1980.

Grimm RH, Leon AS, Hunninghake DB, et al: Effects of thiazide diuretics on plasma lipids and lipoproteins in mildly hypertensive patients. *Ann Intern Med* **94**:7, 1981.

Grundy SM: Effect of polyunsaturated fats on lipid metabolism in patients with hypertriglyceridemia. *J Clin Invest* **55**:269, 1975.

Grundy SM: Dietary fats and sterols, in Levy RI, Rifkind BM, Dennis BH, et al (eds): *Nutrition, Lipids, and Coronary Heart Disease*. New York, Raven Press, 1979.

Haft JI: Role of blood platelets in coronary artery disease. *Am J Cardiol* **43**:1197, 1979.

Hagberg JM, Goldring D, Ehsani AA, et al: Effect of exercise training on the blood pressure and hemodynamic features of hypertensive adolescents. *Am J Cardiol* **52**:763, 1983.

Hagstrom RM, Federspiel CF, Ho YC: Incidence of myocardial infarction and sudden death from coronary heart disease in Nashville, Tennessee. *Circulation* **44**:884, 1971.

Halhuber MJ: Arguments for institutional rehabilitation after myocardial infarction. *Bull Eur Org Control Circ Dis* **2**:83, 1977.

Hall AJ: A lady from China's past. *National Geographic Magazine* **145**:660, 1974.

Hall EM, Olsen AY, Davis FE: Portal cirrhosis. Clinical and pathological review of 782 cases from 16,600 necropsies. *Am J Pathol* **29**:993, 1953.

Hames C, Heyden S, Tyroler H, et al: The combined effect of smoking and coffee drinking on LDL–HDL cholesterol. *Am J Cardiol* **41**:404, 1978.

Hamilton DV, Lea EJA, Jones SP: Dietary fatty acids and ischemic heart disease. *Acta Med Scand* **208**:337, 1980.

Hammerschmidt DE: Szechwan purpura. *N Engl J Med* **302**:1191, 1980.

Hammerschmidt DE: Platelets and the environment. *JAMA* **247**:345, 1982.

Hammond EC: Smoking in relation to the death rates of one million men and women, in Haenszel W (ed): *Epidemiologic Study of Cancer and Other Chronic Diseases*, monograph 19. Bethesda, Md, National Cancer Institute, 1966, pp. 127–204.

Hanley SP, Bevan J, Cockbill SR, et al: Differential inhibition by low-dose aspirin of human venous prostacyclin synthesis and platelet thromboxane synthesis. *Lancet* **1**:969, 1981.

Hansteen V, Moinichen E, Lorentsen E, et al: One year's treatment with propranolol after myocardial infarction: Preliminary report of Norwegian multicentre trial. *Br Med J* **1**:155, 1982.

Harburg E, Erfurt JC, Hauenstein LS, et al: Socio-ecological stress, suppressed hostility, skin color, and black–white male blood pressure: Detroit. *Psychosom Med* **35**:276, 1973.

Harburg E, Ozgoren F, Hawthorne VM, et al: Community norms of alcohol usage and blood pressure: Tecumseh, Michigan. *Am J Public Health* **70**:813, 1980.

Hardinge MG, Crooks H, Stare FJ: Nutritional studies of vegetarians' dietary and serum levels of cholesterol. *J Clin Nutr* **2**:83, 1954.

Hardinge MG, Crooks H, Stare FJ: Nutritional studies of vegetarians. IV. Dietary fatty acids and serum cholesterol levels. *Am J Clin Nutr* **10**:516, 1962.

Hardy RJ, Hawkins CM: The impact of selected indices of antihypertensive treatment on all-cause mortality. *Am J Epidemiol* **117**:566, 1983.

Harrel JP: Psychological factors and hypertension: Status report. *Psychol Bull* **87**:482, 1980.

Harris MB, Bruner CG: A comparison of a self-control and contract procedures for weight control. *Behav Res Ther* **9**:347, 1971.

Harris MB, Hallbauer ES: Self-directed weight control through eating and exercise. *Behav Res Ther* **11**:523, 1973.

Harris RD, Phillips RL, Williams PM, et al: The child–adolescent blood pressure study: I. Distribution of blood pressure levels in Seventh-day Adventist (SDA) and Non-SDA children. *Am J Public Health* **71**:1342, 1981.

Hartley LH, Sherwood J, Herd JA: Weight loss, serum lipid reduction, and lessening of exercise-induced ischemia by dietary restriction of lipids. *Circulation* **64**(suppl 4):83, 1981.

Hartung GH, Vlasek I: Effect of exercise training on subjects with initially elevated blood pressures. *Prev Med* **9**:435, 1980.

Hartung GH, Squires WG, Gotto AM: Effect of exercise training on plasma high-density lipoprotein cholesterol in coronary disease patients. *Am Heart J* **101**:181, 1981.

Haskell WL: Cardiovascular complications during exercise training of cardiac patients. *Circulation* **57**:920, 1978.

Haskell WL: Mechanisms by which physical activity may enhance the clinical status of cardiac patients, in Pollock ML, Schmidt DH (eds): *Heart Disease and Rehabilitation*. Boston, Houghton-Mifflin,1979, p. 276.

Haskell WL, Camargo C, Williams PT, et al: The effect of cessation and resumption of moderate alcohol intake on serum high density lipoprotein subfractions. *New Engl J Med* **310**:805, 1984.

Haut MJ, Cowan DH: The effect of ethanol on hemostatic properties of human blood platelets. *Am J Med* **56**:22, 1974.

Havlik RJ, Garrison RJ, Feinleib M, et al: Blood pressure aggregation in families. *Am J Epidemiol* **110**:304, 1979.

Hay CRM, Durber AP, Saynor R: Effect of fish oil on platelet kinetics in patients with ischaemic heart disease. *Lancet* **1**:1269, 1982.

Haynes RB: A critical review of the "determinants" of patient compliance with therapeutic regimes, in Sackett DL, Haynes RB (eds): *Compliance with Therapeutic Regimes*. Baltimore, Johns Hopkins Univ Press, 1976a, pp. 26–50.

Haynes RB: Strategies for improving compliance: A methodological analysis and review, in Sackett DL, Haynes RB (eds): *Compliance with Therapeutic Regimes*. Baltimore, Johns Hopkins Univ Press, 1976b, p. 75.

Haynes SG, Feinleib M: Women, work, and coronary heart disease: Prospective findings from the Framingham Study. *Am J Public Health* **70**:133, 1980.

Haynes SG, Feinleib M, Kannel WB: The relationship of psychosocial factors to coronary heart disease in the Framingham Study. III. Eight-year incidence of coronary heart disease. *Am J Epidemiol* **111**:37, 1980.

Haynes SG, Eaker E, Feinleib M: Spouse behavior and CHD: Results from a 10-year follow-up study in Framingham. *Cardiovasc Dis Epidemiol Newsletter* **31**:22, 1982.

Heath GW, Ehsani AA, Hagberg JM, et al: Exercise training improves lipoprotein lipid profiles in patients with coronary artery disease. *Am Heart J* **105**:889, 1983.

Heberden W: Some account of a disorder in the breast. *Med Trans Coll Physicians (Lond)* **2**:59, 1772.

Heinzelman F, Bagley RW: Response to physical activity programs and their effects on health behavior. *Public Health Rep* **85**:905, 1970.

Heiss G, Johnson NJ, Reiland S, et al: The epidemiology of plasma high-density lipoprotein cholesterol levels. The Lipid Research Clinics Program Prevalence Study summary. *Circulation* **62**(suppl 4):116, 1980a.

Heiss G, Haskell W, Mowery R, et al: Plasma high-density lipoprotein cholesterol and socioeconomic status. The Lipid Research Clinics Program Prevalence Study. *Circulation* **62**(suppl 4): 108, 1980b.

Helgeland A, Hjermann I, Leren P: High-density lipoprotein cholesterol and antihypertensive drugs: The Oslo Study. *Br Med J* **2**:403, 1978.

Heliovaara M, Karvonen MJ, Punsar S, et al: Importance of coronary risk factors in the presence or absence of myocardial ischemia. *Am J Cardiol* **50**:1248, 1982.

Hellerstein HK: Exercise therapy in coronary disease. *Bull NY Acad Med* **44**:1028, 1968.

Helmers C, Lundman T: Early and sudden deaths after myocardial infarction. *Acta Med Scand* **205**: 3, 1979.

Helsing KJ, Comstock GW, Szklo M: Causes of death in a widowed population. *Am J Epidemiol* **116**:524, 1982.

Hennekens CH, Rosner B, Cole DS: Daily alcohol consumption and fatal coronary heart disease. *Am J Epidemiol* **107**:196, 1978.

Hennekens CH, Lown B, Rosner B, et al: Ventricular premature beats and coronary risk factors. *Am J Epidemiol* **112**:93, 1980.

Hepner G, Fried R, St. Jeor S, et al: Hypocholesterolemic effect of yogurt and milk. *Am J Clin Nutr* **32**:19, 1979.

Heptinstall S, Mulley GP, Taylor PM, et al: Platelet release reaction in myocardial infarction. *Br Med J* **1**:80, 1980.

Heyden S, Bartel A, Hames CG, et al: Elevated blood pressure levels in adolescents, Evans County, Georgia: Seven year follow-up of 30 patients and 30 controls. *JAMA* **209**:1683, 1969.

Higano N, Robinson RW, Cohen WD: Increased incidence of cardiovascular disease in castrated women. *N Engl J Med* **268**:1123, 1963.

Higgins M, Keller J, Moore F, et al: Studies of blood pressure in Tecumseh, Michigan. *Am J Epidemiol* **111**:142, 1980.

Hinkle LE, Whihney LH, Lehman EW, et al: Occupation, education and coronary heart disease. *Science* **161**:238, 1968.

Hirai A, Hamazaki T, Terano T, et al: Eicosapentaenoic acid and platelet function in Japanese. *Lancet* **2**:1132, 1980.

Hirst AE, Hadley GG, Gore I: The effect of chronic alcoholism and cirrhosis of the liver on atherosclerosis. *Am J Med Sci* **249**:143, 1965.

Hitchcock NE, Gracey M: Diet and serum cholesterol. An Australian family study. *Arch Dis Child* **52**:790, 1977.

Hjalmarson A, Herlitz J: Limitation of infarct size by beta blockers and its potential role for prognosis. *Circulation* **67**(suppl 1):68, 1983.

Hjalmarson A, Herlitz J, Malek I, et al: Effect on mortality of metoprolol in acute myocardial infarction. *Lancet* **2**:823, 1981.

Hjermann I, Holme I, Velve Byre K, et al: Effect of diet and smoking intervention on the incidence of coronary heart disease. *Lancet* **2**:1303, 1981.

Hognestad J, Teisberg P: Heart pathology in chronic alcoholism. *Acta Pathol Microbiol Scand* **81**: 315, 1973.

Holly JMP, Evans SJW, Goodwin FJ, et al: Re-analysis of data in two *Lancet* papers on the effect of dietary sodium and potassium on blood pressure. *Lancet* **2**:1384, 1981.

Holme I, Helgeland A, Hjermann I, et al: Four and two-thirds years incidence of coronary heart disease in middle-aged men: The Oslo Study. *Am J Epidemiol* **112**:149, 1980.

Holmes TH, Rahe RH: The social readjustment rating scale. *J Psychosom Res* **11**:213, 1967.

Horan MJ, Kennedy HL: Characteristics and prognosis of apparently healthy patients with frequent and complex ventricular ectopy: Evidence for a relatively benign new syndrome with occult myocardial and/or coronary disease. *Am Heart J* **102**:809, 1981.

Horie T, Sekiguchi M, Hirosawa K: Coronary thrombosis in pathogenesis of acute myocardial infarction. *Br Heart J* **40**:153, 1978.

Hornstra G, Chait A, Karvonen J, et al: Influence of dietary fat on platelet function in men. *Lancet* **1**:1155, 1973.

House JS, Robbins C, Metzner HL: The association of social relationships and activities with mortality: Prospective evidence from the Tecumseh Community Health Study. *Am J Epidemiol* **116**:123, 1982.

Howard AN, Marks J: Hypocholesterolaemic effect of milk. *Lancet* **2**:255, 1977.

Howell WL, Manion WC: The low incidence of myocardial infarction in patients with portal cirrhosis of the liver: A review of 639 cases of cirrhosis of the liver from 17,731 autopsies. *Am Heart J* **60**:341, 1960.

Hulley S, Ashman P, Kuller L, et al: HDL cholesterol levels in the Multiple Risk Factor Intervention Trial (MRFIT) by the MRFIT Research Group. *Lipids* **14**:119, 1979.

Hulley SB, Rosenman RH, Bawol RD, et al: Epidemiology as a guide to clinical decisions. The association between triglyceride and coronary heart disease. *N Engl J Med* **302**:1383, 1980.

Humphries JO, Kuller L, Ross RS, et al: Natural history of ischemic heart disease in relation to arteriographic findings. *Circulation* **49**:489, 1974.

Hurd PD, Johnson CA, Pechacek T, et al: Prevention of cigarette smoking in seventh-grade students. *J Behav Med* **3**:15, 1980.

Hyatt KH, Kamenetsky LG, Smith WM: Extravascular dehydration as an etiologic factor in postrecumbency orthostatism. *Aerospace Med* **40**:644, 1969.

Hypertension Detection and Follow-up Program Cooperative Group: Blood pressure studies in 14 communities. *JAMA* **237**:2385, 1977a.

Hypertension Detection and Follow-up Program Cooperative Group: Race, education and prevalence of hypertension. *Am J Epidemiol* **106**:351, 1977b.

Hypertension Detection and Follow-up Program Cooperative Group: Variability of blood pressure and the results of screening in the HDFP program. *J Chron Dis* **31**:651, 1978.

Hypertension Detection and Follow-up Program Cooperative Group: Five-year findings of the Hypertension Detection and Follow-up Program. *JAMA* **242**:2562, 1979a.

Hypertension Detection and Follow-up Program Cooperative Group: Therapeutic control of blood pressure in the Hypertension Detection and Follow-up Program. *Prev Med* **8**:2, 1979b.

Hypertension Detection and Follow-up Program Cooperative Group: *Presentation of 5-Year Results*. Bethesda, Md, US Dept of Health and Human Services, 1980, p. 6.

Hypertensive Detection and Follow-up Program Cooperative Group: Effect of antihypertensive medication on left ventricular hypertrophy. *Am J Epidemiol* **116**:579, 1982.

Hypertension in blacks and whites, editorial. *Lancet* **2**:73, 1980.

Iacono JM, Marshall MW, Dougherty RM, et al: Reduction in blood pressure associated with high polyunsaturated fat diets that reduce blood cholesterol in man. *Prev Med* **4**:426, 1975.

Iimura O, Kijima T, Kikuchi K, et al: Studies on the hypotensive effect of high potassium intake in patients with essential hypertension. *Clin Sci* **61**:77s, 1981.

Ikeda Y, Kikuchi M, Toyama K, et al: Inhibition of human platelet functions by verapamil. *Thromb Haemost* **45**:158, 1981.

Insel PM, Fraser GE, Phillips R, et al: Psychosocial factors and blood pressure in children. *J Psychosomat Res* **25**:505, 1981.

International Collaborative Group: Circulating cholesterol level and risk of death from cancer in men aged 40 to 69 years. *JAMA* **248**:2853, 1982.

Ishikawa T, Fidge N, Thelle DS, et al: The Tromso Heart Study: Serum apolipoprotein A1 concentration in relation to future coronary heart disease. *Eur J Clin Invest* **8**:179, 1978.

Isles C, Brown JJ, Cumming AMM, et al: Excess smoking in malignant-phase hypertension. *Br Med J* **1**:579, 1979.

Jacobs DR, Barrett-Connor E: Retest reliability of plasma cholesterol and triglyceride. *Am J Epidemiol* **116**:878, 1982.

Jacobs DR, Anderson JT, Blackburn H: Diet and serum cholesterol. Do zero correlations negate the relationship? *Am J Epidemiol* **110**:77, 1979.

Jakubowski JA, Ardlie NG: Modification of human platelet function by a diet enriched in saturated or polyunsaturated fat. *Atherosclerosis* **31**:335, 1978.

Janis IL: The role of social support in adherence to stressful decisions. *Am Psychol* **38**:143, 1983.

Janis IL, Hoffman E: Effective partnerships in a clinic for smokers, in Janis IL (ed): *Counselling on Personal Decisions: Theory and Research on Short-term Helping Relationships.* New Haven, Conn, Yale Univ Press, 1982.

Jenkins CD: Recent evidence supporting psychologic and social risk factors for coronary disease (first of two parts). *N Engl J Med* **294**:987, 1976a.

Jenkins CD: Recent evidence supporting psychologic and social risk factors for coronary disease (second of two parts). *N Engl J Med* **294**:1033, 1976b.

Jenkins CD: A comparative review of the interview and questionnaire methods in the assessment of the coronary-prone behavior pattern, in Dembroski TM, Weiss SM, Shields JL, et al (eds): *Coronary-Prone Behavior.* New York, Springer Verlag, 1978, p. 71.

Jenkins CD, Rosenman RH, Zyzanski SJ: Prediction of clinical coronary heart disease by a test for the coronary-prone behavior pattern. *N Engl J Med* **290**:1271, 1974.

Jenkins CD, Zyzanski SJ, Rosenman RH: Risk of new myocardial infarction in middle-aged men with manifest coronary heart disease. *Circulation* **53**:342, 1976.

Jenkins DJA, Newton C, Leeds AR, et al: Effect of pectin, guar gum, and wheat fibre on serum-cholesterol. *Lancet* **1**:1116, 1975.

Jesse MJ, Cohen MM, Cunningham N, et al: Task force 1: The physician and children (pediatric and adolescent practice and the school). *Am J Cardiol* **47**:741, 1981.

Johnson KG, Yano K, Kato H: Coronary heart disease in Hiroshima, Japan: A report of a six-year period of surveillance, 1958–1964. *Am J Public Health* **58**:1355, 1968.

Johnson H: Effects by nifedipine (Adalat) on platelet function in vitro and in vivo. *Thromb Res* **21**: 523, 1981.

Joint International Society and Federation of Cardiology/World Health Organization (WHO) Task Force on Standardization of Clinical Nomenclature: Nomenclature and criteria for diagnosis of ischemic heart disease. *Circulation* **59**:607, 1979.

Joint National Committee on Detection, Evaluation, and Treatment of High Blood Pressure: The 1984 report of the Joint National Committee on Detection, Evaluation, and Treatment of High Blood Pressure. *Arch Intern Med* **144**:1045, 1984.

Joossens JV: Salt and hypertension, water hardness and cardiovascular death rate. *Triangle* **12**:9, 1973.

Joseph JG, Prior IAM, Salmond CE, et al: Elevation of systolic and diastolic blood pressure associated with migration: The Tokelau Island Migrant Study. *J. Chron Dis* **36**:507, 1983.

Joyce CRB, Caple G, Mason M, et al: Quantitative study of doctor–patient communication. *Q J Med* **38**:183, 1969.

Julian DG, Prescott RJ, Jackson FS, et al: Controlled trial of sotalol for one year after myocardial infarction. *Lancet* **1**:1142, 1982.

Kagan A, Harris BR, Winkelstein W, et al: Epidemiologic studies of coronary heart disease and stroke in Japanese men living in Japan, Hawaii and California: Demographic, physical, dietary and biochemical characteristics. *J Chron Dis* **27**:345, 1974.

Kagan A, Gordon T, Rhoads GG, et al: Some factors related to coronary heart disease incidence in Honolulu Japanese men: The Honolulu Heart Study. *Int J Epidemiol* **4**:271, 1975.

Kagan AR, Uemura K, Vihert AM, et al: Atherosclerosis of the aorta and coronary arteries in five towns. *Bull WHO* **53**:485, 1976.

Kagan A, McGee DL, Yanok K, et al: Serum cholesterol and mortality in a Japanese–American population—The Honolulu Heart Program. *Am J Epidemiology* **114**:11, 1981.

Kahn HA, Medalie JH, Neufeld HN, et al: Serum cholesterol: Its distribution and association with dietary and other variables in a survey of 10,000 men. *Isr J Med Sci* **5**:1117, 1969.

Kallio V: Rehabilitation programs as secondary prevention: A community approach. *Adv Cardiol* **31**:120, 1982.

Kallio V, Hamalainen H, Hakkila J, et al: Reduction in sudden deaths by a multifactorial intervention programme after acute myocardial infarction. *Lancet* **2**:1091, 1979.

Kambara H, Kawashita K, Yoshida A, et al: Identification of patients with coronary artery disease using a scoring system of coronary risk factors, electrocardiography and myocardial perfusion imaging. *Jpn Circ J* **46**:235, 1982.

Kannel WB: Role of blood pressure in cardiovascular disease: The Framingham Study. *Angiology* **26**:1, 1975.

Kannel WB: Recent highlights from the Framingham Study. *Aust NZ J Med* **6**:373, 1976.

Kannel WB: High-density lipoproteins: Epidemiologic profile and risks of coronary artery disease. *Am J Cardiol* **52**:93, 1983a.

Kannel WB: Prevalence and natural history of electrocardiographic left ventricular hypertrophy. *Am J Med* **75**:4, 1983b.

Kannel WB, Gordon T: *An Epidemiological Investigation of Cardiovascular Disease. The Framingham Study.* Section 5, Bivariate correlations among some characteristics of the Framingham cohort at Exam. 2 by sex and age. Washington, DC, US Dept of Health, Education and Welfare, US Public Health Service, 1968.

Kannel WB, Gordon T: *An Epidemiological Investigation of Cardiovascular Disease. The Framingham Study.* Section 24, Diet and regulation of serum cholesterol, publication 20.2002:F84. Washington, DC, US Dept of Health, Education and Welfare, US Public Health Service, 1970.

Kannel WB, Gordon T: *The Framingham Study. An Epidemiologic Investigation of Cardiovascular Disease.* Coronary heart disease, atherothrombotic brain infarction intermittent claudication—A multivariate analysis of some factors related to their incidence: 16 year followup. Appendix B. US Government Printing Office, Washington, DC, 1971.

Kannel WB, Feinleib M: Natural history of angina pectoris in the Framingham Study. *Am J Cardiol* **29**:154, 1972.

Kannel WB, Gordon T: *The Framingham Study. An Epidemiologic Investigation of Cardiovascular Disease.* Section 30, Some characteristics related to the incidence of cardiovascular disease and death: 18-Year follow-up, publication 74–599. Washington, DC, US Government Printing Office, 1974.

Kannel WB, McGee DL: Diabetes and cardiovascular disease. The Framingham Study. *JAMA* **241**:2035, 1979.

Kannel WB, Sorlie P: Some health benefits of physical activity. The Framingham Study. *Arch Intern Med* **139**:857, 1979.

Kannel WB, Gordon T: The search for an optimum serum cholesterol. *Lancet* **2**:374, 1982.

Kannel WB, Brand N, Skinner JJ, et al: The relation of adiposity to blood pressure and development of hypertension. The Framingham Study. *Ann Intern Med* **67**:48, 1967a.

Kannel WB, LeBauer EJ, Dawber TR, et al: Relation of body weight to development of coronary heart disease. *Circulation* **35**:734, 1967b.

Kannel WB, Schwartz MJ, McNamara PM: Blood pressure and risk of coronary heart disease: The Framingham Study. *Dis Chest* **56**:43, 1969.

Kannel WB, Castelli WP, Gordon T, et al: Serum cholesterol, lipoproteins, and the risk of coronary heart disease. *Ann Intern Med* **74**:1, 1971.

Kannel WB, Sorlie P, McNamara PM: Prognosis after initial myocardial infarction: The Framingham Study. *Am J Cardiol* **44**:53, 1979.

Kannel WB, Sorlie P, Castelli WP, et al: Blood pressure and survival after myocardial infarction: The Framingham Study. *Am J Cardiol* **45**:326, 1980a.

Kannel WB, Dawber TR, McGee DC: Perspectives on systolic hypertension. *Circulation* **61**:1179, 1980b.

Kaplan BH, Cassel JC, Tyroler HA, et al: Occupational mobility and coronary heart disease. *Arch Intern Med* **128**:938, 1971.

Kark JD, Smith AH, Hames CG: The relationship of serum cholesterol to the incidence of cancer in Evans County, Georgia. *J Chron Dis* **33**:311, 1980.

Karoly P, Kanfer FH (eds): *Self-Management and Behavior Change: From Theory to Practice.* New York, Pergamon Press, 1982.

Kasch FW, Boyer JL: Changes in maximum work capacity resulting from six months training in patients with ischemic heart disease. *Med Sci Sports* **1**:156, 1969.

Katch FI, McArdle WD: *Nutrition, Weight Control and Exercise.* Boston, Houghton-Mifflin, 1977.

Kato H, Tillotson J, Nichaman MZ, et al: Epidemiologic studies of coronary heart disease and stroke in Japanese men living in Japan, Hawaii and California. Serum lipids and diet. *Am J Epidemiol* **97**:372, 1973.

Kay RM, Truswell AS: Effect of citrus pectin on blood lipids and fecal steroid excretion in man. *Am J Clin Nutr* **30**:171, 1977.

Kay RM, Strasberg SM: Origin, chemistry, physiological effects and clinical importance of dietary fibre. *Clin Invest Med* **1**:9, 1978.

Kay RM, Jacobs M, Rotstein OD: Sustained alterations in lipoprotein cholesterol concentrations dependent on the daily distribution of lipid intake. *Atherosclerosis* **47**:63, 1983.

Kelsay JL, Behall KM, Prather ES: Effect of fiber from fruits and vegetables on metabolic responses of human subjects. *Am J Clin Nutr* **31**:1149, 1978.

Kempner W: Treatment of hypertensive vascular disease with rice diet. *Am J Med* **4**:545, 1948.

Kennedy CC, Spiekerman RE, Lindsay MI, et al: One-year graduated exercise program for men with angina pectoris. *Mayo Clin Proc* **51**:231, 1976.

Kentala E: Physical fitness and feasibility of physical rehabilitation after myocardial infarction in men of working age. *Ann Clin Res* **4**(suppl 9):1, 1972.

Kesteloot H, Geboers J: Calcium and blood pressure. *Lancet* **1**:813, 1982.

Kesteloot H, Lee CS, Park HM, et al: A comparative study of serum lipids between Belgium and Korea. *Circulation* **65**:795, 1982.

Keys A (ed): Coronary heart disease in seven countries. *Circulation* **41**(suppl 1):1, 1970.

Keys A: Alpha lipoprotein (HDL) cholesterol in the serum and the risk of coronary heart disease and death. *Lancet* **2**:603, 1980a.

Keys A: *Seven Countries. A Multivariate Analysis of Death and Coronary Heart Disease.* Cambridge, Mass, Harvard Univ Press, 1980b.

Keys A, Anderson JT, Grande F: Prediction of serum-cholesterol responses of man to changes in fats in the diet. *Lancet* **2**:959, 1957.

Keys A, Anderson JT, Grande F: Effect on serum cholesterol in man of monoene fatty acid (oleic acid) in the diet. *Proc Soc Exp Biol Med* **98**:387, 1958a.

Keys A, Kimura N, Kusukawa A, et al: Lessons from serum cholesterol studies in Japan, Hawaii and Los Angeles. *Ann Intern Med* **48**:83, 1958b.

Keys A, Anderson JT, Grande F: Diet-type (fats constant) and blood lipids in man. *J Nutr* **70**:257, 1960.

Keys A, Taylor HL, Blackburn H, et al: Coronary heart disease among Minnesota business and professional men followed 15 years. *Circulation* **28**:381, 1963.

Keys A, Anderson JT, Grande F: Serum cholesterol response to changes in the diet. III. Differences among individuals. *Metabolism* **14**:766, 1965a.

Keys A, Anderson JT, Grande F: Serum cholesterol response to changes in the diet. II. The effect of cholesterol in the diet. *Metabolism* **14**:759, 1965b.

Keys A, Anderson JT, Grande F: Serum cholesterol response to changes in the diet. IV. Particular saturated fatty acids in the diet. *Metabolism* **14**:776, 1965c.

Keys A, Aravanis C, Blackburn H, et al: Probability of middle-aged men developing coronary heart disease in five years. *Circulation* **45**:815, 1972.

Keys A, Aravanis C, van Buchem FSP, et al: The diet and all-causes death rate in the Seven Countries Study. *Lancet* **2**:58, 1981.

Khaw KT, Peart WS: Blood pressure and contraceptive use. *Br Med J* **2**:403, 1982.

Khaw KT, Thom S: Randomized double-blind cross-over trial of potassium on blood pressure in normal subjects. *Lancet* **2**:1127, 1982.

King AC, Frederiksen LW: Low-cost strategies for increasing exercise behavior: Relapse prevention training and social support. *Behav Modif* **8**:3, 1984.

Kirkendall W, Burton AC, Epstein FH, et al: *Recommendations for Human Blood Pressure Determination by Sphygmomanometers*. Dallas, Texas, American Heart Association, 1976.

Kirscht JP, Rosenstock IM. Patients' problems in following recommendations of health experts, in Stone GC, Cohen F, Adler NE (eds): *Health Psychology*—a handbook. San Francisco, Jossey-Bass, 1979, pp. 189–216.

Kittel F, Kornitzer M, Zyzanski SJ, et al: Two methods of assessing the Type A coronary-prone behavior pattern in Belgium. *J Chron Dis* **31**:147, 1978.

Kittner SJ, Garcia-Palmieri MR, Costas R, et al: Alcohol and coronary heart disease in Puerto-Rico. *Am J Epidemiol* **117**:538, 1983.

Klatsky AL, Friedman GD, Siegelaub AB, et al: Alcohol consumption and blood pressure. *N Engl J Med* **296**:1194, 1977.

Klatsky AL, Friedman GD, Siegelaub AS: Alcohol use, myocardial infarction, sudden cardiac death and hypertension. *Alcoholism: Clin Exp Res* **3**:33, 1979.

Klatsky AL, Friedman GD, Siegelaub AB: Alcohol and mortality. A ten-year Kaiser-Permanente experience. *Ann Intern Med* **95**:139, 1981.

Kleinman JC, Feldman JJ, Monk MA: Trends in smoking and ischemic heart disease mortality, in Havlik RJ, Feinleib M (eds): *Proceedings of the Conference on the Decline in Coronary Heart Disease Mortality*, publication 79–1610. Bethesda, Md, National Institutes of Health, 1979, pp. 202, 204.

Klimov AN, Glueck CJ, Gartside PS, et al: Cord blood high-density lipoproteins: Leningrad and Cincinnati. *Pediatr Res* **13**:208, 1979.

Klissouras VJ: Heritability of adaptive variation. *J Appl Physiol* **31**:338, 1971.

Klissouras VJ, Pirnay F, Petit J: Adaptation to maximal effort: Genetics and age. *J Appl Physiol* **35**:288, 1973.

Knuiman JT, Hermus RJJ, Hautvast JGAJ: Serum total and high-density lipoprotein (HDL) cholesterol concentrations in rural and urban boys from 16 countries. *Atherosclerosis* **36**:529, 1980.

Kobayashi S, Hirai A, Terano T, et al: Reduction in blood viscosity by eicosapentaenoic acid. *Lancet* **2**:197, 1981.

Kokubu T, Itoh I, Kurita H, et al: Effect of prazosin on serum lipids. *J Cardiovasc Pharmacol* **4**(suppl 2):S228, 1982.

Konig K: Organization of rehabilitation centres. *Adv Cardiol* **24**:136, 1978.

Koplan JP, Powell KE, Sikes RK, et al: An epidemiologic study of the benefits and risks of running. *JAMA* **248**:3118, 1982.

Kornitzer M, Dramaix M, Thilly C, et al: Belgian Heart Disease Prevention Project: Incidence and mortality results. *Lancet* **1**:1066, 1983.

Korsch BM, Negrete VF: Doctor–patient communication. *Sci Am* **227**:66, 1972.

Koskenvuo M, Kaprio J, Kesaniemi A, et al: Differences in mortality from ischemic heart disease by marital status and social class. *J Chron Dis* **33**:95, 1980.

Kosowsky BD, Taylor J, Lown B, et al: Long-term use of procaine amide following acute myocardial infarction. *Circulation* **47**:1204, 1973.

Kotchen JM, Kotchen TA, Schwertman NC, et al: Blood pressure distributions of urban adolescents. *Am J Epidemiol* **99**:315, 1974.

Kozarevic D, McGee D, Vojvodic N, et al: Serum cholesterol and mortality. The Yugoslavia Cardiovascular Disease Study. *Am J Epidemiol* **114**:21, 1981.

Kozarevic DJ, Vojvodic N, Dawber T, et al: Frequency of alcohol consumption and morbidity and mortality: The Yugoslavia Cardiovascular Disease Study. *Lancet* **1**:613, 1980.

Kozarevic D, Vojvodic N, Gordon T, et al: Drinking habits and death. *Int J Epidemiol* **12**:145, 1983.

Kozlowski LT, Herman CP, Frecker RC: What researchers make of what cigarette smokers say: Filtering smokers' hot air. *Lancet* **1**:699, 1980.

Kramer JR, Kitazume H, Proudfit WL, et al: Segmental analysis of the rate of progression in patients with progressive coronary atherosclerosis. *Am Heart J* **106**:1427, 1983.

Kramer K, Kuller L, Fisher R: The increasing mortality attributed to cirrhosis and fatty liver, in Baltimore (1957–1966). *Ann Intern Med* **69**:273, 1968.

Krasemann ED, Jungmann H: Return to work after myocardial infarction. *Cardiology* **64**:190, 1979.

Kraus AS, Lilienfeld AM: Some epidemiologic aspects of the high mortality rate in the young widowed group. *J Chron Dis* **10**:207, 1959.

Kraus JF, Borhani ND, Franti CE: Socioeconomic status, ethnicity and risk of coronary heart disease. *Am J Epidemiol* **111**:407, 1980.

Krauss RM, Lindgren FT, Wood PT, et al: Differential increases in plasma high-density lipoprotein subfractions and apolipoproteins (APO-LP) in runners. *Circulation* **55**(suppl 3):4, 1977.

Krueger DE, Ellenberg SS, Bloom S, et al: Fatal myocardial infarction and the role of oral contraceptives. *Am J Epidemiol* **111**:655, 1980.

Kuller L, Cooper M, Perper J: Epidemiology of sudden death. *Arch Intern Med* **129**:714, 1972.

Kuller LH: Prodromata of sudden death and myocardial infarction. *Adv Cardiol* **25**:61, 1978.

Kuller LH: Natural history of coronary heart disease, in Pollock ML, Schmidt DG (eds): *Heart Disease and Rehabilitation*. Boston, Houghton-Mifflin, 1979.

Kuller LH, Cooper M, Perper J, et al: Myocardial infarction and sudden death in an urban community. *Bull NY Acad Med* **49**:532, 1973.

Kuller L, Neaton J, Caggiula A, et al: Primary prevention of heart attacks: The Multiple Risk Factor Intervention Trial. *Am J Epidemiol* **112**:185, 1980.

Kumpuris AG, Luchi RJ, Waddell CC, et al: Production of circulating platelet aggregates by exercise in coronary patients. *Circulation* **61**:62, 1980.

Lambert CA, Netherton DR, Finison LJ, et al: Risk factors and life style: A statewide health-interview survey. *N Engl J Med* **306**:1048, 1982.

Lando HA: Successful treatment of smokers with a broad spectrum behavioral approach. *J Consult Clin Psychol* **45**:361, 1977.

Lando HA, McGovern PG: Three-year data on a behavioral treatment for smoking: A follow-up note. *Addict Behav* **7**:177, 1982.

Langford HG, Watson RL: Electrolytes, environment and blood pressure. *Clin Sci Mol Med* **45**: 111S, 1973.

LaPorte RE, Cresanta JL, Kuller LH: The relationship of alcohol consumption to atherosclerotic heart disease. *Prev Med* **9**:22, 1980.

Lasser NL, Grandits G, Caggiula AW, et al: Effects of antihypertensive therapy on plasma lipids and lipoproteins with Multiple Risk Factor Intervention Trial. *Am J Med* **76**(2A):52, 1984.

Lauer RM, Connor WE, Leaverton PE, et al: Coronary heart disease risk factors in school children: The Muscatine Study. *J Pediatr* **86**:697, 1975.

Leibowitz JO: *The History of Coronary Heart Disease*. London, Wellcome Institute of the History of Medicine, 1970.

Lemon FR, Walden RT: Death from respiratory system disease among Seventh-day Adventist men. *JAMA* **198**:117, 1966.

Leon AS, Blackburn H: The relationship of physical activity to coronary heart disease and life expectancy. *Ann NY Acad Sci* **301**:561, 1977.

Leon AS, Conrad J, Hunninghake DB, et al: Effects of a vigorous walking program on body composition and carbohydrate and lipid metabolism of obese young men. *Am J Clin Nutr* **32**: 1776, 1979.

Leren P: The Oslo Diet–Heart Study. Eleven-year report. *Circulation* **42**:935, 1970.

Leren P, Helgeland A, Holme I, et al: Effect of propranolol and prazosin on blood lipids. *Lancet* **2**: 4, 1980.

Letac B, Cribier A, Desplanches JF: A study of left ventricular function in coronary patients before and after physical training. *Circulation* **56**:375, 1977.

Letcher RL, Chien S, Pickering TG, et al: Direct relationship between blood pressure and blood viscosity in normal and hypertensive subjects. *Am J Med* **70**:1195, 1981.

Leventhal H, Singer R, Jones S: The effects of fear and specificity of recommendations on attitudes and behavior. *J Pers Soc Psychol* **2**:20, 1965.

Levi GF, Quadri A, Ratti S, et al: Preclinical abnormality of left ventricular function in chronic alcoholics. *Br Heart J* **39**:35, 1977.

Levine PH: An acute effect of cigarette smoking on platelet function. *Circulation* **48**:619, 1973.

Levine RS, Hennekens CH, Klein B, et al: A longitudinal evaluation of blood pressure in children. *Am J Public Health* **69**:1175, 1979.

Levine SP, Lindenfeld JA, Ellis JB, et al: Increased plasma concentrations of platelet factor 4 in coronary artery disease. *Circulation* **64**:626, 1981.

Levy RI, Brensike JF, Epstein SE, et al: The influence of changes in lipid values induced by cholestyramine and diet on progression of coronary artery disease: Results of the NHLBI Type II coronary intervention study. *Circulation* **69**:325, 1984.

Lewis HD, Davis JW, Archibald DG, et al: Protective effects of aspirin against acute myocardial infarction and death in men with unstable angina. *N Engl J Med* **309**:396, 1983.

Lewis RP, Boudoulas H: Catecholamines, cigarette smoking, arrhythmias and acute myocardial infarction. *Am Heart J* **88**:526, 1974.

Ley P: Psychological studies of doctor–patient communications, in Rachman S (ed): *Contributions to Medical Psychology*, vol 1. New York, Pergamon Press, 1977, pp. 9–42.

Liard R, Perdrizet S, Reinert P: Wheezy bronchitis in infants and parents' smoking habits. *Lancet* **1**:334, 1982.

Liberthson RR, Nagel EL, Hirschman JC, et al: Pathophysiologic observations in prehospital ventricular fibrillation and sudden cardiac death. *Circulation* **49**:790, 1974.

Liberthson R, Nagel EL, Hirschman JC, et al: Prehospital ventricular defibrillation. *N Engl J Med* **291**:317, 1976.

Lichstein E, Morganroth J, Harrist R, et al: Effect of propranolol on ventricular arrhythmia. The Beta Blocker Heart Attack Trial experience. *Circulation* **67**(suppl 1):5, 1983.

Lichtenstein E, Rodrigues MR: Long-term effects of rapid smoking treatment for dependent cigarette smokers. *Addict Behav* **2**:109, 1977.

Lie JT, Titus JL: Pathology of the myocardium and the conduction system in sudden coronary death. *Circulation* **52**(suppl 3):41, 1975.

Lifsic AM: Alcohol consumption and atherosclerosis, in "Atherosclerosis of the Aorta and Coronary Arteries in Five Towns." *Bull WHO* **53**:623, 1976.

Lilienfeld AM: The humean fog: Cancer and cholesterol. *Am J Epidemiol* **114**:1, 1981.

Linder CW, DuRant RH: Exercise, serum lipids and cardiovascular disease—Risk factors in children. *Pediatr Clin N Am* **29**:1341, 1982.

Lipid Research Clinics Program Epidemiology Committee: Plasma lipid distributions in selected North American populations: The Lipid Research Clinics Program Prevalence Study. *Circulation* **60**:427, 1979.

Lipid Research Clinics Study Group: *The Lipid Research Clinics Population Studies Data Book*. vol 1, *The Prevalence Study*, NIH publication 80–1527. Bethesda, Md, US Dept of Health and Human Services, 1980.

Lipid Research Clinics Program: The Lipid Research Clinics Coronary Primary Prevention Trial results. I. Reduction in incidence of coronary heart disease. *JAMA* **251**:351, 1984a.

Lipid Research Clinics Program. The Lipid Research Clinics Coronary Primary Prevention Trial results. II. The relationship of reduction in incidence of coronary heart disease to cholesterol lowering. *JAMA* **251**:365, 1984b.

Liu K, Cooper R, McKeever P, et al: Assessment of the association between habitual salt intake and high blood pressure: Methodological problems. *Am J Epidemiol* **110**:219, 1979.

Londe S, Goldring D: High blood pressure in children: Problems and guidelines for evaluation and treatment. *Am J Cardiol* **37**:650, 1976.

London Research Group: Low-fat diet in myocardial infarction. A controlled trial. *Lancet* **2**:501, 1965.

Long AR: Cardiovascular renal disease: Report of a case of 3000 years ago. *Arch Pathol* **12**:92, 1931.

Lopez SA, Vial R, Balart L, et al: Effect of exercise and physical fitness on serum lipids and lipoproteins. *Atherosclerosis* **20**:1, 1974.

Lorenz R, Spengler U, Fischer S, et al: Platelet function, thromboxane formation and blood pressure control during supplementation of the Western diet with cod liver oil. *Circulation* **67**: 505, 1983.

Lovell RH: Arrhythmia prophylaxis: Long-term suppressive medication. *Circulation* **52**(suppl 3): 236, 1975.

Lown B: Sudden cardiac death—1978. *Circulation* **60**:1593, 1979.

Lown B, De Silva RA: Roles of psychologic stress and autonomic nervous system changes in provocation of ventricular premature complexes. *Am J Cardiol* **41**:979, 1978.

Lown B, Verrier R, Corbalan R: Psychologic stress and threshold for repetitive ventricular response. *Science* **182**:834, 1973.

Lown B, De Silva RA, Reich P, et al: Psychophysiologic factors in sudden cardiac death. *Am J Psychiatry* **137**:1325, 1980.

Lozy ME: Dietary variability and its impact on nutritional epidemiology. *J Chron Dis* **36**:237, 1983.

Luft FC, Weinberger MH, Grim CE: Sodium sensitivity and resistance in normotensive humans. *Am J Med* **72**:726, 1982.

Luria MH, Knoke JD, Wachs JS, et al: Survival after recovery from acute myocardial infarction. *Am J Med* **67**:7, 1979.

Maccoby N, Farquhar JW: Communication for health: Unselling heart disease. *J Commun* **25**:114, 1975.

Maccoby N, Farquhar JW, Wood PD, et al: Reducing the risk of cardiovascular disease: Effects of a community-based campaign on knowledge and behavior. *J Community Health* **3**:100, 1977.

Maciejko JJ, Holmes DR, Kottke BA, et al: Apolipoprotein A-1 as a marker of angiographically assessed coronary artery disease. *N Engl J Med* **309**:385, 1983.

Magnus K, Matroos A, Strackee J: Walking, cycling, or gardening, with or without seasonal interruption, in relation to acute coronary events. *Am J Epidemiol* **110**:724, 1979.

Mahoney MJ: Self-reward and self-monitoring techniques for weight control. *Behav Ther* **5**:48, 1974.

Mahoney MJ, Mahoney K: *Permanent Weight Control.* New York, WW Norton, 1976.

Mahoney MJ, Moura NG, Wade TC: The relative efficacy of self-reward, self-punishment and self-monitoring techniques for weight loss. *J Consult Clin Psychol* **40**:404, 1973.

Makheja AN, Vanderhoek JY, Bailey JM: Inhibition of platelet aggregation and thromboxane synthesis by onion and garlic. *Lancet* **1**:781, 1979.

Malinow MR: Regression of atherosclerosis in humans: Fact or myth? *Circulation* **64**:1, 1981.

Malmros H: The relation of nutrition to health. *Acta Med Scand*, suppl 246, p. 137, 1950.

Mann GV: A factor in yogurt which lowers cholesterolemia in man. *Atherosclerosis* **26**:335, 1977.

Mann GV, Pearson G, Gordon T, et al: Diet and cardiovascular disease in the Framingham Study. I. Measurement of dietary intake. *Am J Clin Nutr* **11**:200, 1962.

Mann JI, Inman WHW, Thorogood M: Oral contraceptive use in older women and fatal myocardial infarction. *Br Med J* **2**:445, 1976.

Marcus ML, Mueller TM, Gascho JA, et al: Effects of cardiac hypertrophy secondary to hypertension on the coronary circulation. *Am J Cardiol* **44**:1023, 1979.

Marenah CB, Lewis B, Hassal D, et al: Hypocholesterolaemia and non-cardiovascular disease: Metabolic studies on subjects with low plasma cholesterol concentrations. *Br Med J* **286**: 1603, 1983.

Margolis JR, Kannel WB, Feinleib M, et al: Clinical features of unrecognized myocardial infarction—silent and symptomatic. *Am J Cardiol* **32**:1, 1973.

Mark AL, Lawton WJ, Abboud FM, et al: Effects of high and low sodium intake on arterial pressure and forearm vascular resistance in borderline hypertension. *Circ Res*, suppl 36, pp. 1–194, 1975.

Marlatt GA, Gordon JR: Determinants of relapse: Implications for the maintenance of behavior change, in Davidson PO, Davidson SM (eds): *Behavioral Medicine: Changing Health Lifestyles.* New York, Brunner/Mazel, 1980.

Marmot MG, Syme SL, Kagan A, et al: Epidemiologic studies of CHD and stroke in Japanese men living in Japan, Hawaii and California. Prevalence of coronary and hypertensive heart disease and associated risk factors. *Am J Epidemiol* **102**:514, 1975.

Martin JE, Dubbert PM: Exercise applications and promotion in behavioral medicine: Current status and future directions. *J Consult Clin Psychol* **50**:1004, 1982.

Maseri A: The revival of coronary spasm. *Am J Med* **70**:752, 1981.

Mathews JD: Alcohol use, hypertension and coronary heart disease. *Clin Sci Mol Med* **51**:661S, 1976.

Mathur KS, Kahn MA, Sharma RD: Hypocholesterolaemic effect of Bengal gram: A long-term study in man. *Br Med J* **1**:30, 1968.

Matova EE, Vihert AM: Atherosclerosis and hypertension, in "Atherosclerosis of the Aorta and Coronary Arteries in Five Towns." *Bull WHO* **53**:539, 1976.

Matta RJ, Lawler JE, Lown B: Ventricular electrical instability in the conscious dog: Effects of psychologic stress and beta-adrenergic blockade. *Am J Cardiol* **38**:594, 1976.

Matter S, Weltman A, Stamford BA: Body fat content and serum lipid levels. *J Am Diet Assoc* **77**: 149, 1980.

Matthews DK, Fox EL: *The Physiological Basis of Physical Education and Athletics.* Philadelphia, WB Saunders Co, 1976, p. 446.

Matthews KA, Glass DC, Rosenman RH, et al: Competitive drive, pattern A, and coronary heart disease: A further analysis of some data from the Western Collaborative Group Study. *J Chron Dis* **30**:489, 1977.

Matthews KA, Krantz DS, Dembroski TM, et al: Unique and common variance in structured interview and Jenkins Activity Survey Measures of the Type A behavior pattern. *J Pers Soc Psychol* **42**:303, 1982.

Mayer J: *Overweight: Causes, Cost and Control.* Englewood Cliffs, NJ. Prentice-Hall, Inc, 1968.

Mayou RA: A controlled trial of early rehabilitation after myocardial infarction. *J Cardiac Rehab* **3**:397, 1983.

Mazzuca SA: Does patient education in chronic disease have therapeutic value? *J Chron Dis* **35**:521, 1982.

McAlister A, Perry C, Killen J, et al: Pilot study of smoking, alcohol and drug abuse prevention. *Am J Public Health* **70**:719, 1980.

McCarron DA: Low serum concentrations of ionized calcium in patients with hypertension. *N Engl J Med* **307**:226, 1982.

McCarron DA: Calcium and magnesium nutrition in human hypertension. *Ann Intern Med* **98**(part 2):800, 1983.

McCarron DA, Morris CD, Cole C: Diet calcium in human hypertension. *Science* **217**:267, 1982.

McDonough JR, Garrison GE, Hames CG: Blood pressure and hypertensive disease among negroes and whites. *Ann Intern Med* **61**:208, 1964.

McGandy RB, Hall B, Ford C, et al: Dietary regulation of blood cholesterol in adolescent males: A pilot study. *Am J Clin Nutr* **25**:61, 1972.

McGill HC: Potential mechanisms for the augmentation of atherosclerosis and atherosclerotic disease by cigarette smoking. *Prev Med* **8**:390, 1979.

McGill HC: Morphologic development of the atherosclerotic plaque, in Lauer RM, Shekell RB (eds): *Childhood Prevention of Atherosclerosis and Hypertension.* New York, Raven Press, 1980, p. 41.

McGregor GA, Best FE, Cam JM, et al: Double-blind randomised crossover trial of moderate sodium restriction in essential hypertension. *Lancet* **1**:351, 1982a.

McGregor GA, Smith SJ, Markandu ND, et al: Moderate postasium supplementation in essential hypertension. *Lancet* **2**:567, 1982b.

McKee PA, Castelli WP, McNamara PM, et al: The natural history of congestive heart failure: The Framingham Study. *N Engl J Med* **285**:1441, 1971.

McNeilly RH, Pemberton J: Duration of last attack in 998 fatal cases of coronary artery disease and its relation to possible cardiac resuscitation. *Br Med J* **3**:139, 1968.

McPherson BD, Paivio A, Yuhasz MS: Psychological effects of an exercise program for post-infarct and normal adult men. *J Sports Med Phys Fitness* **7**:95, 1967.

Meade TW, Chakrabarti R, Haines AP, et al: Characteristics affecting fibrinolytic activity and plasma fibrinogen concentrations. *Br Med J* 1:153, 1979.

Medalie JH, Goldbourt U: Unrecognized myocardial infarction: Five-year incidence, mortality, and risk factors. *Ann Intern Med* 84:526, 1976a.

Medalie JH, Goldbourt U: Angina pectoris among 10,000 men. II. Psychosocial and other risk factors as evidenced by a multivariate analysis of a five-year incidence study. *Am J Med* 60:910, 1976b.

Medalie JH, Kahn HA, Neufeld HN, et al: Five-year myocardial infarction incidence—II. Association of single variables to age and birth place. *J Chron Dis* 26:329, 1973a.

Medalie JH, Snyder M, Groen JJ, et al: Angina pectoris among 10,000 men. 5-Year incidence and univariate analysis. *Am J Med* 55:583, 1973b.

Medical Research Council Research Committee: Controlled trial of soy-bean oil in myocardial infarction. *Lancet* 2:693, 1968.

Mehta J: Platelets and prostaglandins in coronary artery disease. *JAMA* 249:2818, 1983.

Mehta J, Mehta P: Platelet function in hypertension and effect of therapy. *Am J Cardiol* 47:331, 1981a.

Mehta J, Mehta P: Role of blood platelets and prostaglandins in coronary artery disease. *Am J Cardiol* 48:366, 1981b.

Mehta J, Mehta P: Significance of platelet function and thromboxane B$_2$ levels across the human myocardial vascular bed in man. *Acta Med Scand*, suppl 651, p. 111, 1981c.

Mehta J, Mehta P: Effects of propranolol therapy on platelet release and prostaglandin generation in patients with coronary heart disease. *Circulation* 66:1294, 1982.

Mehta P, Mehta J, Pepine CJ, et al: Platelet aggregation across the myocardial vascular bed in man: I. Normal versus diseased coronary arteries. *Thromb Res* 14:423, 1979.

Mendoza S, Contreras G, Ineichen E, et al: Lipids and lipoproteins in Venezuelan and American schoolchildren: Within and cross-cultural comparisons. *Pediatr Res* 14:272, 1980.

Messerli FH: Cardiovascular effects of obesity and hypertension. *Lancet* 1:1165, 1982.

Messerli FH, Glade LB, Elizardi DG, et al: Cardiac rhythm, arterial pressure and urinary catecholamines in hypertension with and without left ventricular hypertrophy. *Am J Cardiol* 47:480, 1981.

Meyer AJ, Henderson JB: Multiple risk factor reduction in the prevention of cardiovascular disease. *Prev Med* 3:225, 1974.

Miall WE: Implications of the relation between blood pressure and age. *Milbank Mem Fund Q* 47:107, 1969.

Miall WE, Lovell HG: Relation between change of blood pressure and age. *B Med J* 2:660, 1967.

Miall WE, Bell RA, Lovell HG: Relation between change in blood pressure and weight. *Br J Prev Soc Med* 22:73, 1968.

Mild hypertension: No more benign neglect, editorial.—*N Engl J Med* 302:293, 1980.

Miller NE, Hammett F, Saltissi S, et al: Relation of angiographically defined coronary artery disease to plasma lipoprotein subfractions and apolipoproteins. *Br Med J* 282:1741, 1981.

Miller PB, Johnson RL, Lamb LE: Effect of moderate physical exercise during four weeks of bed rest on circulatory function in man. *Aerospace Med* 36:1077, 1965.

Mitchell JRA: Secondary prevention of myocardial infarction—The present state of the art. *Br Med J* 1:1128, 1980.

Moreyra AE, Kostis JB, Passannante AJ, et al: Acute myocardial infarction in patients with normal coronary arteries after acute ethanol intoxication. *Clin Cardiol* 5:425, 1982.

Morgan P, Gildiner M, Wright G: Smoking reduction in adults who take up exercise: A survey of a running club for adults. *J Can Assoc Health Phys Educ* 42:39, 1976.

Morgan T, Myers JB: Hypertension treated by sodium restriction. *Med J Aust* 2:396, 1981.

Morgan T, Gillies A, Morgan G, et al: Hypertension treated by salt restriction. *Lancet* 1:227, 1978.

Morris JN, Crawford MD: Coronary heart disease and physical activity of work. Evidence of a national necropsy survey. *Br Med J* 2:1485, 1958.

Morris JN, Heady JA, Raffle PAB: Physique of London busmen. The epidemiology of uniforms. *Lancet* 2:569, 1956.

Morris JN, Heady JA, Raffle PAB, et al: Coronary heart-disease and physical activity of work. *Lancet* **2**:1053, 1953.

Morris JN, Marr JW, Heady JA, et al: Diet and plasma cholesterol in 99 bank men. *Br Med J* **1**:571, 1963.

Morris JN, Kagan A, Pattison DC, et al: Incidence and prediction of ischaemic heart-disease in London busmen. *Lancet* **2**:553, 1966.

Morris JN, Marr JW, Clayton DG: Diet and heart: A postscript. *Br Med J* **2**:1307, 1977.

Morris JN, Pollard R, Everitt MG, et al: Vigorous exercise in leisure-time: Protection against coronary heart disease. *Lancet* **2**:1207, 1980.

Morris JN, Everitt MG, Pollard R, et al: Exercise and the heart. *Lancet* **1**:267, 1981.

Morrison JA, Kelly K, Mellies M, et al: Cigarette smoking, alcohol intake, and oral contraceptives: Relationships to lipids and lipoproteins in adolescent school-children. *Metabolism* **28**:1166, 1979.

Morrison JA, Larsen R, Glatfelter L, et al: Interrelationships between nutrient intake and plasma lipids and lipoproteins in schoolchildren aged 6–19: The Princeton School District Study. *Pediatrics* **65**:727, 1980.

Morrison JA, Khoury P, Mellies M, et al: Lipid and lipoprotein distributions in black adults. *JAMA* **245**:939, 1981.

Morrison LM: Diet in coronary atherosclerosis. *JAMA* **173**:884, 1960.

Moss AJ, Davis HT, De Camilla J, et al: Ventricular ectopic beats and their relation to sudden and nonsudden cardiac death after myocardial infarction. *Circulation* **60**:998, 1979.

Mudge GH, Grossman W, Mills RM, et al: Reflex increase in coronary vascular resistance in patients with ischemic heart disease. *N Engl J Med* **295**:1333, 1976.

Mulcahy R: Influence of cigarette smoking on morbidity and mortality after myocardial infarction. *Br Heart J* **49**:410, 1983.

Mulcahy R, Hickey N, Graham IM, et al: Factors affecting the 5-year survival rate of men following acute coronary heart disease. *Am Heart J* **93**:556, 1977.

Multicenter Postinfarction Research Group: Risk stratification and survival after myocardial infarction. *N Engl J Med* **309**:331, 1983.

Multiple Risk Factor Intervention Trial Research Group: Multiple risk factor intervention trial. *JAMA* **248**:1465, 1982.

Multiple Risk Factor Intervention Trial Research Group: Exercise electrocardiogram and coronary heart disease mortality in the Multiple Risk Factor Intervention Trial. *Am J Cardiol* **55**:16, 1985.

Murchison LE, Fyfe T: Effects of cigarette smoking on serum-lipids, blood-glucose, and platelet adhesiveness. *Lancet* **2**:182, 1966.

Murphy M, Hultgren HN, Detre K, et al: Treatment of chronic stable angina. *N Engl J Med* **297**:621, 1977.

Mustard JF, Murphy EA: Effect of smoking on blood coagulation and platelet survival in man. *Br Med J* **1**:846, 1963.

Myocardial Infarction Community Register. Copenhagen, World Health Organization, Regional Office for Europe, 1976.

Nadler JL, Velasco JS, Hortan R: Cigarette smoking inhibits prostacyclin formation. *Lancet* **1**:1248, 1983.

Nagakawa Y, Orimo H, Harasawa M, et al: Effect of eicosapentaenoic acid on the platelet aggregation and composition of fatty acid in man. *Atherosclerosis* **47**:71, 1983.

National Cancer Institute: *For Good. A Guide to Living as a Nonsmoker*, NIH publication 83–2494. Bethesda, Md, US Dept of Health and Human Services, 1983.

National Cooperative Study Group: Unstable angina pectoris: National Cooperative Study Group to compare surgical and medical therapy. *Am J Cardiol* **42**:839, 1978.

National Health Survey 1971–74. *Vital Health Stat (11)* 203, 1978.

National Heart and Lung Institute Task Force on Cardiovascular Rehabilitation: *Needs and Opportunities for Rehabilitating the Coronary Heart Disease Patient*, NIH publication 79–750. Bethesda, Md, US Dept of Health, Education and Welfare, 1974.

National Heart, Lung and Blood Institute: *Fiscal Year 1983 Fact Book*. Bethesda, Md, National Institutes of Health, 1983a.

National Heart, Lung and Blood Institute: *Recommendations for Treatment of Mild Hypertension*. Bethesda, Md, National Institutes of Health, 1983b.

Neaton JD, Broste S, Cohen L. et al: The Multiple Risk Factor Intervention Trial (MRFIT). VII. A comparison of risk factor changes between the two study groups. *Prev Med* 10:519, 1981.

Nestel PJ, Havenstein N, Whyte HM, et al: Lowering of plasma cholesterol and enhanced sterol excretion with consumption of polyunsaturated ruminant fats. *N Engl J Med* 288:379, 1973.

Nestal PJ, Havenstein N, Homma Y, et al: Increased sterol excretion with polyunsaturated-fat high-cholesterol diets. *Metabolism* 24:189, 1975.

Nestel PJ, Poyser A, Boulton TJC: Changes in cholesterol metabolism in infants in response to dietary cholesterol and fat. *Am J Clin Nutr* 32:2177, 1979.

Nichols AB, Ravenscroft C, Lamphiear DE, et al: Daily nutritional intake and serum lipid levels. The Tecumseh Study. *Am J Clin Nutr* 29:1384, 1976.

Nizankowska-Blaz T, Abramowicz T: Effects of intensive physical training on lipids and lipoproteins. *Acta Pediatr Scand* 72:357, 1983.

Noppa H, Bengtsson C, Wedel H, et al: Obesity in relation to morbidity and mortality from cardiovascular disease. *Am J Epidemiol* 111:682, 1980.

Nora JJ: Identifying the child at risk for coronary disease as an adult: A strategy for prevention. *J. Pediatr* 97:706, 1980.

Nordoy A, Rodset JM: Platelet function and platelet phospholipids in patients with hyperbetalipoproteinemia. *Acta Med Scand* 189:385, 1971.

Norris RM, Agnew TM, Brandt PW, et al: Coronary surgery after recurrent myocardial infarction: Progress of a trial comparing surgical with nonsurgical management for asymptomatic patients with advanced coronary disease. *Circulation* 63:785, 1981.

Norwegian Multicenter Study Group: Timolol-induced reduction in mortality and reinfarction in patients surviving acute myocardial infarction. *N Engl J Med* 304:801, 1981.

Oalmann MC, Malcom GT, Toca VT, et al: Community pathology of atherosclerosis and coronary heart disease: Post mortem serum cholesterol and extent of coronary atherosclerosis. *Am J Epidemiol* 113:396, 1981.

O'Brien JR, Etherington MD, Jamieson S, et al: Effect of a diet of polyunsaturated fats on some platelet-function tests. *Lancet* 2:995, 1976.

Office of Cancer Communications: *The Smoking Digest. Progress on a Nation Kicking the Habit*. Bethesda, Md, National Cancer Institute, US Dept of Health, Education and Welfare, 1977.

Office of Cancer Communications: *Clearing the Air*. Bethesda, Md, National Cancer Institute, US Dept of Health, Education and Welfare, 1982.

Oldridge NB, Wicks JR, Hanley C, et al: Noncompliance in an exercise rehabilitation program for men who have suffered a myocardial infarction. *Canad Med Assoc J* 118:361, 1978.

Oldridge NB, Donner AP, Duck CW, et al: Predictors of dropout from cardiac exercise rehabilitation. *Am J Cardiol* 51:70, 1983.

Oliva PB: Pathophysiology of acute myocardial infarction, 1981. *Ann Intern Med* 94:236, 1981.

Ornish D, Scherwitz LW, Doody RS, et al: Effects of stress management training and dietary changes in treating ischemic heart disease. *JAMA* 249:54, 1983.

Ostfeld AM, Lebovits BZ, Shekelle RB, et al: A prospective study of the relationship between personality and coronary heart disease. *J Chron Dis* 17:265, 1964.

Ostrander LD, Lamphiear DE, Block WD, et al: Oral contraceptives and physiological variables. *JAMA* 244:677, 1980.

Packham MA, Mustard JF: Pharmacology of platelet-affecting drugs. Circulation 62(suppl 5):26, 1980.

Paffenbarger RS, Thorne MC, Wing AL: Chronic disease in former college students. VIII. Characteristics in youth predisposing to hypertension in later years. *Am J Epidemiol* 88:25, 1968.

Paffenbarger RS, Wing AL, Hyde RT: Physical activity as an index of heart attack risk in college alumni. *Am J Epidemiol* 108:161, 1978.

Paffenberger RS, Wing AL, Hyde RT, et al: Physical activity and incidence of hypertension in college alumni. *Am J Epidemiol* **117**:245, 1983.

Page LB: Dietary sodium and blood pressure: Evidence from human studies, in Lauer RM, Shekelle RB (eds): *Childhood Prevention of Atherosclerosis and Hypertension.* New York, Raven Press, 1980, p. 291.

Page LB, Damo A, Moellering RC: Antecedents of cardiovascular disease in six Solomon Island societies. *Circulation* **49**:1132, 1974.

Page LB, Vandevert D, Nader K, et al: Blood pressure, diet, and body form in traditional nomads of the Qash'qai tribe, southern Iran. *Acta Cardiol* **33**:102, 1978.

Parijs J, Joossens JV, Van der Linden L, et al: Moderate sodium restriction and diuretics in the treatment of hypertension. *Am Heart J* **85**:22, 1973.

Parkes CM, Benjamin B, Fitzgerald RG: Broken heart: A statistical study of increased mortality among widowers. *Br Med J* **1**:740, 1969.

Pearson TA, Bulkley BH, Achuff SC, et al: The association of low Levels of HDL cholesterol and arteriographically defined coronary artery disease. *Am J Epidemiol* **109**:285, 1979.

Pell S, D'Alonzo CA: Immediate mortality and five-year survival of employed men with a first myocardial infarction. *N Engl J Med* **270**:915, 1964.

Pell S, D'Alonzo CA: A five-year mortality study of alcoholics. *J Occup Med* **15**:120, 1973.

Pennington JAT, Church HN: *Bowes and Church's Food Values of Portions Commonly Used.* Philadelphia, JB Lippincott Co, 1980.

Perry C, Killen J, Telch M, et al: Modifying smoking behavior of teenagers: A school-based intervention. *Am J Public Health* **70**:722, 1980.

Peter T, Ross D, Duffield A, et al: Effect on survival after myocardial infarction of long-term treatment with phenytoin. *Br Heart J* **40**:1356, 1978.

Peters RK, Cady LD, Bischoff DP, et al: Physical fitness and subsequent myocardial infarction in healthy workers. *JAMA* **249**:3052, 1983.

Petitti DB, Wingerd J, Pellegrin F, et al: Risk of vascular disease in women. *JAMA* **242**:1150, 1979.

Phillips RL, Lemon FR, Beeson WL, et al: Coronary heart disease mortality among Seventh-day Adventists with differing dietary habits: A preliminary report. *Am J Clin Nutr* **31**:S191, 1978.

Phillips RL, Garfinkel L, Kuzma JW, et al: Mortality among Californian Seventh-day Adventists for selected cancer sites. *JNCI* **65**:1097, 1980.

Pirie P. Elias W, Wackman D, et al: Characteristics of participation in a community risk factor screening. *Circulation* **66**(suppl 2):115, 1982.

Poikolainen K: Inebriation and mortality. *Int J Epidemiol* **12**:151, 1983.

Pollock ML, Schmidt DH: *Heart Disease and Rehabilitation.* Boston, Houghton-Mufflin, 1979.

Pooling Project Research Group: Relationships of blood pressure, serum cholesterol, smoking habit, relative weight and ECG abnormalities to incidence of major coronary events: Final report of the Pooling Project. *J Chron Dis* **31**:201, 1978.

Poplawski A, Skorulska M, Niewiarowski S: Increased platelet adhesiveness in hypertensive cardiovascular disease. *J Atherosclerosis Res* **8**:721, 1968.

Portal RW: Alcoholic heart disease. *Br Med J* **283**:1202, 1981.

Poston L, Sewell RB, Williams R, et al: The effect of (1) a low molecular weight natriuretic substance and (2) plasma from hypertensive patients on the sodium transport of leukocytes from normal subjects, in Zumkley H, Losse H (eds): *Intracellular Electrolytes and Arterial Hypertension.* Stuttgart, Georg Thieme, 1980, pp. 93–95.

Poston L, Sewell RB, Wilkinson SP, et al: Evidence for a circulating sodium transport inhibitor in essential hypertension. *Br Med J* **282**:847, 1981.

Potter JF, Beevers DG: Pressor effect of alcohol in hypertension. *Lancet* **1**:119, 1984.

Powell DR, McCann BS: The effects of a multiple treatment program and maintenance procedures on smoking cessation. *Prev Med* **10**:104, 1981.

Pozen M: Pre-hospital coronary care: The current case for a paramedic strategy. *Am J Public Health* **69**:13, 1979.

President's Council on Physical Fitness and Sports: The physically underdeveloped child, publication 0-239-894. Washington, DC, US Government Printing Office, 1977.

Prineas RJ, Crow RS, Blackburn H: The Minnesota Code Manual of Electrocardiographic Findings. Boston, John Wright Publishing, Inc, 1982.

Prior I, Tasman-Jones C: New Zealand Maori and Pacific Polynesians, in Trowell HC, Burkitt DP (eds): *Western Diseases: Their Emergence and Prevention.* Cambridge, Mass, Harvard Univ Press, 1981, p. 227.

Prior IAM: Cardiovascular epidemiology in New Zealand and the Pacific. *NZ Med J* **80**:245, 1974.

Prior IAM, Evans JG, Harvey HPB, et al: Sodium intake and blood pressure in two Polynesian populations. *N Engl J Med* **279**:515, 1968.

Prognosis after myocardial infarction, editorial. *Br Med J* **2**:1311, 1979.

Pugh B, Platt MR, Mills JL, et al: Unstable angina pectoris. A randomized study of patients treated medically and surgically. *Am J Cardiol* **41**:1291, 1978.

Puska P, Tuomilehto J, Salonen J, et al: Changes in coronary risk factors during comprehensive five-year community programme to control cardiovascular diseases (North Karelia Project). *Br Med J* **2**:1173. 1979.

Puska P, Vartiainen E, Pallonen U, et al: The North Karelia Youth Project: Evaluation of two years of intervention on health behavior and CVD risk factors among 13- to 15-year-old children. *Prev Med* **11**:550, 1982.

Puska P, Nissinen A, Vartiainen E, et al: Controlled, randomised trial of the effect of dietary fat on blood pressure. *Lancet* **1**:1, 1983a.

Puska P, Salonen JT, Nissinen A, et al: Change in risk factors for coronary heart disease during 10 years of a community intervention programme (North Karelia Project). *Br Med J* **287**:1840, 1983b.

Pyorala K, Reunane A, Laakso M: Cardiovascular and coronary heart disease mortality of diabetics and non-diabetics—Impact of risk factors. Presented at 32nd Annual Scientific Session. American College of Cardiology, New Orleans, La, March 1983.

Pyszka RH, Ruggels WL, Janowicz LM: *Health Behavior Change: Smoking Cessation.* Stanford, Calif, Stanford Research Institute, 1973.

Rabkin SW, Mathewson FAL, Tate RB: Relationship of ventricular ectopy in men without apparent heart disease to occurrence of ischemic heart disease and sudden death. *Am Heart J* **101**: 135, 1981.

Rabkin SW, Mathewson FAL, Tate RB. Relationship of blood pressure in 20- to 39-year-old men to subsequent blood pressure and incidence of hypertension over a 30-year observation period. *Circulation* **65**:291, 1982.

Rahimtoola SH: Coronary bypass surgery for chronic angina—1981. A perspective. *Circulation* **65**: 225, 1982.

Ramsdale DR, Bray CL, Beton DC, et al: Serum lipids as indicators of occult coronary disease assessed by angiography. *Am Heart J* **107**:811, 1984.

Rasanen L, Wilska M, Kantero RL, et al: Nutrition survey of Finnish rural children. IV. Serum cholesterol values in relation to dietary variables. *Am J Clin Nutr* **31**:1050, 1978.

Rautaharju PM, Warren JW, Jain U, et al: Cardiac infarction injury score: An electrocardiographic coding scheme for ischemic heart disease. *Circulation* **64**:249, 1981.

Rechnitzer PA: The effects of training: Reinfarction and death—an interim report. *Med Sci Sports* **11**:382, 1979.

Rechnitzer PA, Cunningham DA, Andrew GM, et al: Relation of exercise to recurrence rate of myocardial infarction in men. Ontario Exercise–Heart Collaborative Study. *Am J Cardiol* **51**:65, 1983.

Redwood DR, Rosing DR, Epstein SE: Circulatory and symptomatic effects of physical training in patients with coronary-artery disease and angina pectoris. *N Engl J Med* **286**:959, 1972.

Reed D, McGee D, Cohen J, et al: Acculturation and coronary heart disease among Japanese men in Hawaii. *Am J Epidemiol* **115**:894, 1982.

Reed D, McGee D, Yano K, et al: Social networks and coronary heart disease among Japanese men in Hawaii. *Am J Epidemiol* **117**:384, 1983.

Regan TJ, Haider B: Ethanol abuse and heart disease. *Circulation* **64** (suppl 3):14, 1981.

Regan TJ, Levinson GE, Oldewurtel HA, et al: Ventricular function in noncardiacs with alcoholic fatty liver: Role of ethanol in the production of cardiomyopathy. *J Clin Invest* **48**:397, 1969.

Regan TJ, Wu CF, Weisse AB, et al: Acute myocardial infarction in toxic cardiomyopathy without coronary obstruction. *Circulation* **51**:453, 1975.

Reichenbach DD, Moss NS, Meyer E: Pathology of the heart in sudden cardiac death. *Am J Cardiol* **39**:865, 1977.

Reid DD, Hamilton PJS, McCartney P, et al: Smoking and other risk factors for coronary heart-disease in British civil servants. *Lancet* **2**:979, 1976.

Reisin E, Abel R, Modan M, et al: Effect of weight loss without salt restriction on the reduction of blood pressure in overweight hypertensive patients. *N Engl J Med* **298**:1, 1978.

Reisin E, Frohlich ED, Messerli FH, et al: Cardiovascular changes after weight reduction in obesity hypertension. *Ann Intern Med* **98**:315, 1983.

Relman AS: Sulfinpyrazone after myocardial infarction: No decision yet. *N Engl J Med* **303**:1476, 1980.

Renaud S, Morazain R, Godsey F, et al: Platelet functions in relation to diet and serum lipids in British farmers. *Br Heart J* **46**:562, 1981.

Rengo F, Trimarco B, Chiariello M, et al: Incidence of sudden death among patients with premature ventricular contractions. *Jpn Heart J* **20**:385, 1979.

Rhoads GG, Gulbrandsen CL, Kagan A: Serum lipoproteins and coronary heart disease in a population study of Hawaii Japanese men. *N Engl J Med* **294**:293, 1976.

Rhoads GG. Blackwelder WC, Stemmerman GN, et al: Coronary risk factors and autopsy findings in Japanese-American men. *Lab Invest* **38**:304, 1978.

Rinzler SH: Primary prevention of coronary heart disease by diet. *Bull NY Acad Med* **44**:936, 1968.

Rissanen V: Coronary and aortic atherosclerosis in chronic alcoholics. *Z Rechtsmed* **75**:183, 1974.

Robbins SL, Cotran RS: Blood vessels, in Robbins SL, Coltran RS (eds): *Pathologic Basis of Disease*. Philadelphia, WB Saunders Co, 1979, p. 593.

Robert WC, Jones AA: Quantitation of coronary arterial narrowing at necropsy in sudden coronary death. *Am J Cardiol* **44**:39, 1979.

Robertson J, Brydon WG, Tadesse K, et al: The effect of raw carrot on serum lipids and colon function. *Am J Clin Nutr* **32**:1889, 1979.

Robertson WB, Strong JP: Atherosclerosis in persons with hypertension and diabetes mellitus. *Lab Invest* **18**:538, 1968.

Robinson D, Williams P: High-density lipoprotein in the Masai of East Africa: A cautionary note. *Br Med J* **1**:1249, 1979.

Roman O, Camuzzi AL, Villalon E, et al: Physical training program in aterial hypertension. *Cardiology* **67**:230, 1981.

Romanczyk RG: Self-monitoring in the treatment of obesity: Parameters of reactivity. *Behav Ther* **5**:531, 1974.

Romo M. Factors related to sudden death in acute ischaemic heart disease. *Acta Med Scand*, suppl 547, p. 30, 1972.

Rose GA: The diagnosis of ischaemic heart pain and intermittent claudication in field surveys. *Bull WHO* **27**:645, 1962.

Rose G: Cold weather and ischemic heart disease. *Br J Prev Soc Med* **20**:97, 1966.

Rose GA, Blackburn H: Cardiovascular Survey Methods. Monograph 56, WHO, Geneva, 1968.

Rose G, Shipley MJ: Plasma lipids and mortality: Source of error. *Lancet* **1**:523, 1980.

Rose GA, Marmot MG: Social class and coronary heart disease. *Br Heart J* **45**:13, 1981.

Rose GA, Thomson WB, Williams RT: Corn oil in treatment of ischaemic heart disease. *Br Med J* **1**:1531, 1965.

Rose G, Prineas RJ, Mitchell JRA: Myocardial infarction and the intrinsic calibre of coronary arteries. *Br Heart J* **29**:548, 1967.

Rose GA, Blackburn H, Keys A, et al: Colon cancer and blood-cholesterol. *Lancet* **1**:181, 1974.

Rose GA, McCartney P, Reid DD: Self-administration of a questionnaire on chest pain and intermittent claudication. *Br J Prev Soc Med* **31**:42, 1977.

Rose GA, Blackburn H, Gillum RF, et al: *Cardiovascular Survey Methods*. Geneva, World Health Organization, 1982.

Rose SP: *Group Therapy: A Behavioral Approach*. Englewood Cliffs, NJ, Prentice-Hall, Inc, 1977.

Rosenberg L, Armstrong B, Jick H: Myocardial infarction and estrogen therapy in post-menopausal women. *N Engl J Med* 294:1256, 1976.

Rosenberg L, Shapiro S, Kaufman DW, et al: Cigarette smoking in relation to the risk of myocardial infarction in young women. *Int J Epidemiol* 9:57, 1980a.

Rosenberg L, Slone D, Shapiro S, et al: Non-contraceptive estrogens and myocardial infarction in young women. *JAMA* 244:339, 1980b.

Rosenman RH, Friedman M, Jenkins CD, et al: Clinically unrecognized myocardial infarction in the Western Collaborative Group Study. *Am J Cardiol* 19:776, 1967.

Rosenman RH, Brand RJ, Jenkins CD, et al: Coronary heart disease in the Western Collaborative Group Study. Final follow-up experience of $8\frac{1}{2}$ years. *JAMA* 233:872, 1975.

Rosner B, Hennekens CH, Kass EH, et al: Age-specific correlation analysis of longitudinal blood pressure data. *Am J Epidemiol* 106:306, 1977.

Ross R: Platelets, smooth muscle proliferation and atherosclerosis. *Acta Med Scand*, suppl 642, p. 49, 1980.

Ross R: Lipoproteins, endothelial injury and atherosclerosis. *Cardiovasc Rev Rep* 3:1026, 1982.

Ross R, Glomset JA: The pathogenesis of atherosclerosis (first of two parts). *N Engl J Med* 295:369, 1976a.

Ross R, Glomset JA: The pathogenesis of atherosclerosis (second of two parts). *N Engl J Med* 295:420, 1976b.

Ross RK, Paganini-Hill A, Mack TM, et al: Menopausal oestrogen therapy and protection from death from ischaemic heart disease. *Lancet* 1:858, 1981.

Rossouw JE, Burger EM, Van der Vyver P, et al: The effect of skim milk, yoghurt, and full cream milk on human serum lipids. *Am J Clin Nutr* 34:351, 1981.

Rothrock DW, Phillipson BE, Illingworth DR, et al: The comparative effects of dietary fish oils vs. vegetable oils in normals and hyperlipidemic subjects. *Circulation* 66(suppl 2):159, 1982.

Rouse JL, Beilin LJ, Armstrong BK, et al: Blood pressure-lowering effect of a vegetarian diet: Controlled trial in normotensive subjects. *Lancet* 1:5, 1983.

Rowe JW. Systolic hypertension in the elderly. *N Engl J Med* 309:1246, 1983.

Rowlands DB, Clover DR, Ireland MA, et al: Assessment of left ventricular mass and its response to antihypertensive treatment. *Lancet* 1:467, 1982.

Royal College of General Practitioners Oral Contraception Study Group: Mortality among oral-contraceptive users. *Lancet* 2:727, 1977.

Rozensky RH: The effect of timing of self-monitoring behavior on reducing cigarette consumption. *J Behav Ther Exp Psychiat* 5:301, 1974.

Ruberman W, Weinblatt E, Goldberg JD, et al: Psychosocial influences on mortality after myocardial infarction. *New Engl J Med* 311:552, 1984.

Rubin E, Katz AM, Lieber CS, et al: Muscle damage produced by chronic alcohol consumption. *Am J Pathol* 83:499, 1976.

Ruys J, Hickie JB: Serum cholesterol and triglyceride levels in Australian adolescent vegetarians. *Br Med J* 2:87, 1976.

Sackett DL, Gibson ES, Taylor DW, et al: Randomised clinical trial of strategies for improving medication compliance in primary hypertension. *Lancet* 1:1205, 1975.

Sacks FM, Castelli WP, Donner A, et al: Plasma lipids and lipoproteins in vegetarians and controls. *N Engl J Med* 292:1148, 1975.

St. Leger AS, Cochrane AL, Moore F: Factors associated with cardiac mortality in developed countries with particular reference to the consumption of wine. *Lancer* 1:1017, 1979.

Salonen JT: Oral contraceptives, smoking and risk of myocardial infarction in young women. *Acta Med Scand* 212:141, 1982a.

Salonen JT: Primary prevention of sudden coronary death: A community-based program in North Karelia, Finland. *Ann NY Acad Sci* 382:423, 1982b.

Salonen JT: Socioeconomic status and risk of cancer, cerebral stroke, and death due to coronary heart disease and any disease: A longitudinal study in eastern Finland. *J Epidemiol Community Health* **36**:294, 1982c.

Salonen JT, Puska P: A community program for rehabilitation and secondary prevention for patients with acute myocardial infarction as part of a comprehensive community program for control of cardiovascular diseases (North Karelia Project). *Scand J Rehabil Med* **12**:33, 1980.

Salonen JT, Puska P, Kottke TE, et al: Changes in smoking, serum cholesterol and blood pressure levels during a community-based cardiovascular disease prevention program—the North Karelia Project. *Am J Epidemiol* **114**:81, 1981.

Salonen JT, Puska P, Kottke TE, et al: Decline in mortality from coronary heart disease in Finland from 1969 to 1979. *Br Med J* **286**:1857, 1983.

Saltin B, Blomqvist G, Mitchell JH, et al: Response to exercise after bed rest and after training. *Circulation* **37**(suppl 7):1, 1968.

Sandison AT: Degenerative vascular disease in the Egyptian mummy. *Med Hist* **6**:77, 1962.

Sato A, Taneichi Y, Sekine I, et al: Prinzmetal's variant angina induced only by alcohol ingestion. *Clin Cardiol* **4**:193, 1981.

Savage DD, Drayer JIM, Henry WL, et al: Echoardiographic assessment of cardiac anatomy and function in hypertensive subjects. *Circulation* **59**:623, 1979.

Schaffer WA, Cobb LA: Recurrent ventricular fibrillation and modes of death in survivors of out-of-hospital ventricular fibrillation. *N Engl J Med* **293**:259, 1975.

Schatzkin A, Cupples LA, Heeren T, et al: The epidemiology of sudden unexpected death: Risk factors for men and women in the Framingham Heart Study. *Am Heart J* **107**:1300, 1984.

Schiffer F, Hartley LH, Schulman CL, et al: Evidence for emotionally-induced coronary arterial spasm in patients with angina pectoris. *Br Heart J* **44**:62, 1980.

Schlant RC, Forman S, Stamler J, et al: The natural history of coronary heart disease: Prognostic factors after recovery from myocardial infarction in 2789 men. *Circulation* **66**:401, 1982.

Schmidt W, de Lint J: Causes of death in alcoholics. *Q J Stud Alcohol* **33**:171, 1972.

Schroll M: A longitudinal epidemiological survey of relative weight at age 25, 50 and 60 in the Glostrup population of men and women born in 1914. *Dan Med Bull* **28**:106, 1981.

Schrott HG, Clarke WR, Wiebe DA, et al: Increased coronary mortality in relatives of hypercholesterolemic schoolchildren: The Muscatine Study. *Circulation* **59**:320, 1979.

Schwartz PJ, Brown AM, Malliani A, et al: *Neural Mechanisms in Cardiac Arrhythmias.* New York, Raven Press, 1978.

Selden R, Neill WA, Ritzmann W, et al: Medical versus surgical therapy for acute coronary insufficiency. *N Engl J Med* **293**:1329, 1975.

Seltzer CC: Effect of smoking on blood pressure. *Am Heart J* **87**:558, 1974.

Sever PS, Peart WS, Gordon D, et al: Blood-pressure and its correlates in urban and tribal Africa. *Lancet* **2**:60, 1980.

Shapiro S, Rosenberg L, Slone D, et al: Oral contraceptive use in relation to myocardial infarction. *Lancet* **1**:743, 1979.

Shaw LW: Effects of a prescribed supervised exercise program on mortality and cardiovascular morbidity in patients after a myocardial infarction. *Am J Cardiol* **48**:39, 1981.

Shekelle RB: Status inconsistency, mobility and CHD. *J Health Soc Behav* **17**:83, 1976.

Shekelle RB, Ostfeld AM, Paul O: Social status and incidence of coronary heart disease. *J Chron Dis* **22**:381, 1969.

Shekelle RB, Schoenberger JA, Stamler J: Correlates of the JAS Type A behavior pattern score. *J Chron Dis* **29**:381, 1976.

Shekelle RB, Shryock AM, Paul O, et al: Diet, serum cholesterol, and death from coronary heart disease. The Western Electric Study. *N Engl J Med* **304**:65, 1981.

Shekelle R, Hulley S, Neaton J, et al: Type A behavior and risk of coronary death in MRFIT. *Cardiovasc Dis Epidemiol Newslett* **33**:34, 1983.

Shephard RJ: Cardiac rehabilitation in prospect, in Pollock ML, Schmidt DH (eds): *Heart Disease and Rehabilitation.* Boston, Houghton-Mifflin, 1979, p. 521.

Shmarak KL: Reduce your broken appointment rate: How one child and youth project reduced its broken appointment rate. *Am J Public Health* **61**:2400, 1971.

Shulman RS, Herbert PN, Capone RJ, et al: Effects of propranolol on blood lipids and lipoproteins in myocardial infarction. *Circulation* **67** (suppl 1):19, 1983.

Siervogel RM, Roche AF, Chumlea WC: Body composition effects on blood pressure. *Circulation* **62**(suppl 3):223, 1980.

Siess W, Scherer B, Boehlig B, et al: Platelet-membrane fatty acids, platelet aggregation, and thromboxane formation during a mackerel diet. *Lancet* **1**:441, 1980.

Siltanen P, Sundberg S, Hytonen I: Impact of a mobile coronary care unit on the sudden coronary mortality in a community. *Acta Med Scand* **205**:195, 1979.

Silverman KJ, Becker LC, Bulkley BH, et al: Value of early thallium-201 scintigraphy for predicting mortality in patients with acute myocardial infarction. *Circulation* **61**:996, 1980.

Sim DN, Neill WA: Investigation of the physiological basis for increased exercise threshold for angina pectoris after physical conditioning. *J Clin Invest* **54**:763, 1974.

Simmons RT: The blood group genetics of Easter Islanders (Pascuenfe) and other Polynesians, in Heyerdahl T, Ferdon EN (eds): *Reports of the Norwegian Archeological Expedition to Easter Island and the East Pacific*, vol 2, report 15, Chicago, Rand McNally, 1965.

Simon AB, Durham NC, Alonzo AA: Sudden death in nonhospitalized cardiac patients. *Arch Intern Med* **132**:163, 1973.

Simoons M, Lap C, Pool J: Heart rate levels and ventricular ectopic activity during cardiac rehabilitation. *Am Heart J* **100**:9, 1980.

Simpson HRC, Barker K, Carter RD, et al: Low dietary intake of linoleic acid predisposes to myocardial infarction. *Br Med J* **285**:683, 1982.

Simpson MT, Olewine DA, Jenkins CD, et al: Exercise-induced catecholamines and platelet aggregation in the coronary-prone behavior pattern. *Psychosom Med* **36**:476, 1974.

Singer K, Lundberg WB: Ventricular arrhythmias associated with the ingestion of alcohol. *Ann Intern Med* **77**:247, 1972.

Sive PH, Medalie JH, Kahn HA, et al: Distribution and multiple regression analysis of blood pressure in 10,000 Israeli men. *Am J Epidemiol* **93**:317, 1971.

Smith JB: Prostaglandins and platelet aggregation. *Acta Med Scand*, suppl 651, p. 91, 1981.

Smith JB, Araki H, Lefer AM: Thromboxane A2, prostacyclin and aspirin: Effects on vascular tone and platelet aggregation. *Circulation* **62**(suppl 5):19, 1980.

Smith JW: Mortality after recovery from myocardial infarction. *J Chron Dis* **33**:1, 1980.

Smitherman TC, Lewis HD, Archibald DG, et al: Diagnosis of new myocardial infarction by Minnesota Code with serial electrocardiagrams after unstable angina. *Circulation* **64**(suppl 4):42, 1981.

Sneiderman C, Heyden S, Heiss G, et al: Predictors of blood pressure over a 16-year follow-up of 163 youths. *Circulation* **54**(suppl 2):24, 1976.

Some consensus on coronary bypass surgery, editorial. *JAMA* **245**:550, 1981.

Sorlie PD, Garcia-Palmieri MR, Castillo-Staab MI, et al: The relation of antemortem factors to atherosclerosis at autopsy. *Am J Pathol* **103**:345, 1981.

Spain DM, Bradess VA: Occupational physical activity and the degree of coronary atherosclerosis in "normal" men. A postmortem study. *Circulation* **22**:239, 1960.

Spain DM, Bradess VA: Sudden death from coronary heart disease. Survival time, frequency of thrombi and cigarette smoking. *Chest* **58**:107, 1970.

Sparrow D, Dawber TR, Colton T: The influence of cigarette smoking on prognosis after a first myocardial infarction. *J Chron Dis* **31**:425, 1978.

Spicer J, McLeod WR, O'Brien KP, et al: Psychosomatic patterns of coronary risk in a community sample of New Zealand men. *J Chron Dis* **34**:271, 1981.

Spikerman RE, Brandenburg JT, Achor RWP, et al: The spectrum of coronary heart disease in a community of 30,000. *Circulation* **25**:57, 1962.

Spodick DH, Pigott VM, Chirife R: Preclinical cardiac malfunction in chronic alcoholism. *N Engl J Med* **287**:677, 1972.

Stadel BV: Oral contraceptives and cardiovascular disease. *N Engl J Med* **305**:612, 1981.

Stamler J: *Lectures on Preventive Cardiology.* New York, Grune & Stratton, 1967, p. 90.

Stamler JG: Public health aspects of optimal serum lipid–lipoprotein levels. *Prev Med* **8**:733, 1979.

Stamler J, Farinaro E, Mojonnier LM, et al: Prevention and control of hypertension by nutritional–hygienic means. *JAMA* **243**:1819, 1980.

Staniloff H, Diamond G, Forrester J, et al: Prediction of death, infarction, and worsening chest pain with exercise electrocardiography and thallium scintigraphy. *Am J Cardiol* **49**:967, 1982.

Starling MR, Crawford MH, Kennedy GT, et al: Exercise testing early after myocardial infarction: Predictive value for subsequent unstable angina and death. *Am J Cardiol* **46**:909, 1980.

Steinberg JD, Hayden MT: Prevalence of clinically occult cardiomyopathy in chronic alcoholism. *Am Heart J* **101**:461, 1981.

Stern MP, Gaskill SP: Secular trends in ischemic heart disease and stroke mortality from 1970 to 1976 in Spanish-surnamed and other white individuals in Bexar County, Texas. *Circulation* **58**:537, 1978.

Stern MP, Farquhar JW, Maccoby N, et al: Results of a two-year health education campaign on dietary behavior. The Stanford Three-Community Study. *Circulation* **54**:826, 1976.

Stolley PD: Epidemiologic studies of coronary heart disease: Two approaches. *Am J Epidemiol* **112**:217, 1980.

Stone GC: Patient compliance and the role of the expert. *J Soc Issues* **35**:34, 1979.

Story JA, Kritchevsky D: Comparison of the binding of various bile acids and bile salts in vitro by several types of fiber. *J Nutr* **106**:1292, 1976.

Strauer BE: Myocardial oxygen consumption in chronic heart disease: Role of wall stress, hypertrophy and coronary reserve. *Am J Cardiol* **44**:730, 1979.

Strauer BE: *Hypertensive Heart Disease.* New York, Springer Verlag, 1980.

Strong JP, Richards ML: Cigarette smoking and atherosclerosis in autopsied men. *Atherosclerosis* **23**:451, 1976.

Strong JP, Dalmann MC, Newman WP, et al: Coronary heart disease in young black and white males in New Orleans: Community Pathology Study. *Am Heart J* **108**:747, 1984.

Strong JP, McGill HC, Richards ML, et al: Relationship between cigarette smoking habits and coronary atherosclerosis in autopsied males (*P*). *Circulation* **33**(suppl 3):31, 1966.

Strong JP, Solberg LA, Restrepo C: Atherosclerosis in persons with coronary heart disease. *Lab Invest* **18**:527, 1968.

Stuart RB, Davis B: *Slim chance in a fat world: Behavioral control of obesity.* Champaign, Ill, Research Press, 1972.

Stuart RB, Mitchell C, Jensen JA: Therapeutic options in the management of obesity, in Prokop CK, Bradley LA (eds): *Medical Psychology: Contributions to Behavioral Medicine.* New York, Academic Press, 1981, pp. 321–353.

Syme SL, Hyman MM, Enterline PE: Some social and cultural factors associated with the occurrence of CHD. *J Chron Dis* **17**:277, 1964.

Syme SL, Borhani NO, Beuchley RW: Cultural mobility and coronary heart disease in an urban area. *Am J Epidemiol* **82**:334, 1966.

Takaro T, Hultgren HN, Lipton MJ, et al: The V.A. Cooperative Randomized Study of surgery for coronary arterial occlusive disease. *Circulation* **54**:(suppl 3):107, 1976.

Takaro T, Peduzzi P, Detre KM, et al: Survival in subgroups of patients with left main coronary artery disease. *Circulation* **66**:14, 1982.

Tarazi RC: Regression of left ventricular hypertrophy by medical treatment: Present status and possible implications. *Am J Med* **75**(suppl):80, 1983.

Taylor HL, Jacobs DR, Schucker B, et al: A questionnaire for the assessment of leisure time physical activities. *J Chron Dis* **31**:741, 1978.

Tejada C, Strong JP, Montenegro MR, et al: Distribution of coronary and aortic atherosclerosis by geographic location, race and sex. *Lab Invest* **18**:509, 1968.

Thelle DS, Shaper AG, Whitehead TP, et al: Blood lipids in middle-aged British men. *Br Heart J* **49**:205, 1983.

Theroux P, Waters DD, Halphen C, et al: Prognostic value of exercise testing soon after myocardial infarction. *N Engl J Med* **301**:341, 1979.

Thomas G, Haider B, Oldewurtel HA, et al: Progression of myocardial abnormalities in experimental alcoholism. *Am J Cardiol* **46**:233, 1980.

Thompson PD, Funk EJ, Carleton RA, et al: Incidence of death during jogging in Rhode Island from 1975 through 1980. *JAMA* **247**:2535, 1982.

Thorsen RD, Jacobs DR, Grimm RH, et al: Preventive cardiology in practice: A device for risk estimation and counseling in coronary disease. *Prev Med* **8**:548, 1979.

Tibbling L: Angina-like chest pain in patients with oesophageal dysfunction. *Acta Med Scand*, suppl 644, p. 56, 1981.

Toor M, Katchalsky A, Agmon J, et al: Serum-lipids and atherosclerosis among Yemenite immigrants in Israel. *Lancet* **1**:1270, 1957.

Tracy RE: Sex difference in coronary disease: Two opposing views. *J Chron Dis* **19**:1248, 1966.

Trowell H: Ischemic heart disease and dietary fiber. *Am J Clin Nutr* **25**:926, 1972.

Trowell H: Dietary fibre, ischaemic heart disease and diabetes mellitus. *Proc Nutr Soc* **32**:151, 1973.

Truswell AS: Food fibre and blood lipids. *Nutr Rev* **35**:51, 1977.

Truswell AS, Kay RM: Bran and blood-lipids. *Lancet* **1**:367, 1976.

Tsang RC, Glueck CJ: Perinatal cholesterol metabolism. *Clin Perinatol* **2**:275, 1975.

Tuck ML, Sowers J, Dornfeld L, et al: The effect of weight reduction on blood pressure, plasma renin activity, and plasma aldosterone levels in obese patients. *N Engl J Med* **304**:930, 1981.

Tuomilehto J, Salonen JT, Nissinen A, et al: Community programme for control of hypertension in North Karelia, Finland. *Lancet* **2**:900, 1980.

Turpeinen O, Karvonen MJ, Pekkarinen M, et al: Dietary prevention of coronary heart disease: The Finnish Mental Hospital Study. *Int J Epidemiol* **8**:99, 1979.

Tyroler HA, Heyden S, Bartel A, et al: Blood pressure and cholesterol as coronary heart disease risk factors. *Arch Intern Med* **128**:907, 1971.

Tyroler HA, Hames CG, Krishan I, et al: Black–white differences in serum lipids and lipoproteins in Evans County. *Prev Med* **4**:541, 1975.

Tyroler HA, Heiss G, Heyden S, et al: Family follow-up study of serum cholesterol in Evans County, Georgia. *J Chron Dis* **33**:323, 1980a.

Tyroler HA, Heiss G, Schonfeld G, et al: Apolipoprotein A-I, A-II and C-II in black and white residents of Evans County. *Circulation* **62**:249, 1980b.

US Public Health Service: *Teenage Smoking—National Patterns of Cigarette Smoking, Ages 12–18, in 1972 and 1974*, DHEW publication (NIH) 76–931. Washington, DC, US Government Printing Office, 1976.

US Select Committee on Nutrition and Human Needs, US Senate: *Dietary Goals for the United States*. Washington, DC, US Government Printing Office, 1977, pp. 4–5.

Uusitupa M, Pyorala K, Raunio H, et al: Sensitivity and specificity of Minnesota Code Q–QS abnormalities in the diagnosis of myocardial infarction verified at autopsy. *Am Heart J* **106**:753, 1983.

V.A. Cooperative Study Group on Antihypertensive Agents: Effects of treatment on morbidity in hypertension. I. Results in patients with diastolic blood pressures averaging 115 through 129 mm Hg. *JAMA* **202**:1028, 1967.

V.A. Cooperative Study Group on Antihypertensive Agents: Effects of treatment on morbidity in hypertension. II. Results in patients with diastolic blood pressure averaging 90 through 114 mm Hg. *JAMA* **213**:1143, 1970.

V.A. Cooperative Study Group on Antihypertensive Agents: Serum lipoprotein level during chlorthalidone therapy. *JAMA* **244**:1691, 1980.

Van Durme JP, Bogaert MG: Prevention of sudden death: The role of antiarrhythmic therapy, in Kulbertus HE, Wellens HJJ (eds): *Sudden Death*. The Hague, Martinus Nijhoff Publishers, 1980, p. 324.

Vedin A, Wilhelmsson C, Tibblin G, et al: The post-infarction clinic in Göteborg, Sweden. *Acta Med Scand* **200**:453, 1976.

Velasco M, Silva H, Morillo J, et al: Effect of prazosin on blood lipids and on thyroid function in hypertensive patients. *J Cardiovasc Pharmacol* **4**(suppl 2):S225, 1982.

Verani MS, Hartung GH, Hoepfel-Harris J, et al: Effects of exercise training on left ventricular performance and myocardial perfusion in patients with coronary artery disease. *Am J Cardiol* **47**:797, 1981.

Vihert AM: High and low atherosclerosis groups, in Kagan A (ed): "Atherosclerosis of the aorta and coronary arteries in five towns." *Bull WHO* **53**:519, 1976.

Vogt TM, Selvin S, Hulley SB: Comparison of biochemical and questionnaire estimates of tobacco exposure. *Prev Med* **8**:23, 1979.

Von Lossonczy TO, Ruites A, Bronsgeest-Schoute HC, The effect of fish diet on serum lipids in healthy human subjects. *Am J Clin Nutr* **31**:1340, 1978.

Voors AW, Foster TA, Frerichs RR, et al: Studies of blood pressures in children, ages 5–14 years, in a total biracial community. *Circulation* **54**:319, 1976.

Waaler HT, Hjort PF: Low mortality among Norwegian Seventh-day Adventists 1960–77: A message on lifestyle and health? *Tidsskr Nor Laegeforen* **11**:623, 1981.

Wagner GS, Freye CJ, Palmeri ST, et al: Evaluation of a QRS scoring system for estimating myocardial infarct size. *Circulation* **65**:342, 1982.

Walden RT, Schaefer LE, Lemon FR, et al: Effect of environment on the serum cholesterol–triglyceride distribution among Seventh-day Adventists. *Am J Med* **36**:269, 1964.

Waldron I, Zyzanski S, Shekelle RB, et al: The coronary-prone behavior pattern in employed men and women. *J Human Stress* **3**:2, 1977.

Walker WJ: Relationship of adiposity to serum cholesterol and lipoprotein levels and their modification by dietary means. *Ann Intern Med* **39**:705, 1953.

Wallace RB, Hoover J, Barrett-Connor E, et al: Altered plasma lipid and lipoprotein levels associated with oral contraceptive and oestrogen use. *Lancet* **2**:111, 1979.

Wallace RB, Hunninghake DB, Reiland S, et al: Alterations of plasma high-density lipoprotein cholesterol levels associated with consumption of selected medications. *Circulation* **62**(suppl 4): 77, 1980.

Waller BF, Roberts WC: Sudden death while running in conditioned runners aged 40 years or over. *Am J Cardiol* **45**:1292, 1980.

Ward SD, Melin JR, Lloyd FP, et al: Determinants of plasma cholesterol in children—A family study. *Am J Clin Nutr* **33**:63, 1980.

Warnick GR, Albers JJ: Physiological and analytic variation in cholesterol and triglycerides. *Lipids* **11**:203, 1976.

Watson RL, Langford HG, Abernethy J, et al: Urinary electrolytes, body weight, and blood pressure. *Hypertension* **2**(suppl 1):93, 1980.

Webb CR, Ritter G, Goldstein S: Sudden cardiac death due to coronary artery disease: Prediction and prevention. *Cardiovasc Rev Rep* **2**:695, 1981.

Webb WR, Degerli IU: Ethyl alcohol and the cardiovascular system. Effects on coronary blood flow. *JAMA* **191**:1055, 1965.

Webber SA, Voors AW, Srinivasan SR, et al: Occurrence in children of multiple risk factors for coronary artery disease: The Bogalusa Heart Study. *Prev Med* **8**:407, 1979.

Weidman WH, Elveback LR, Nelson RA, et al: Nutrient intake and serum cholesterol level in normal children 6–16 years of age. *Pediatrics* **61**:354, 1978.

Weidman W, Kwiterovich P, Jesse MJ, et al: Diet in the healthy child. Task Force Committee of the Nutrition Committee and the Cardiovascular Disease in the Young Council of the American Heart Association. *Circulation* **67**:1411A, 1983.

Weinblatt E, Shapiro S, Frank CW: Prognosis of women with newly diagnosed coronary heart disease—A comparison with course of disease among men. *Am J Public Health* **63**:577, 1973.

Weinblatt E, Ruberman W, Goldberg et al: Relation of education to sudden death after myocardial infarction. *N Engl J Med* **299**:60, 1978.

Weir RJ, Briggs E, Mack A, et al: Blood-pressure in women after one year of oral contraception. *Lancet* **1**:467, 1971.

Weir RJ, Briggs E, Mack A, et al: Blood pressure in women taking oral contraceptives. *Br Med J* **1**: 533, 1974.

Weissler AM, O'Neill WW, Sohn YH, et al: Prognostic significance of systolic time intervals after recovery from myocardial infarction. *Am J Cardiol* **48**:995, 1981.

Weksler BB, Pett SB, Alonso D, et al: Differential inhibition by aspirin of vascules and platelet prostaglandin synthesis in atherosclerotic patients. *New Engl J Med* **308**:800, 1983.

Welborn TA, Cumpston GN, Cullen KJ, et al: The relevance of coronary heart disease and associated risk factors in an Australian rural community. *Am J Epidemiol* **89**:521, 1969.

Wenger NK: *Coronary Care: Rehabilitation After Myocardial Infarction.* Dallas, Texas, American Heart Association, 1973.

Wenger NK: *Coronary Care: Rehabilitation of the Patient with Symptomatic Coronary Atherosclerotic Heart Disease.* Dallas, Texas, American Heart Association, 1981.

West RO, Hayes OB: Diet and serum cholesterol levels. A comparison between vegetarians and nonvegetarians in a Seventh-day Adventist group. *Am J Clin Nutr* **21**:853, 1968.

Whelton PK: Systemic hypertension, diuretic drugs, arrhythmias and death. *Am J Cardiol* **55**:221, 1985.

Whelton PK, Thompson SG, Barnes GR, et al: Evaluation of the Vita-Stat automatic blood pressure recorder. *Am J Epidemiol* **117**:46, 1983.

White CW, Wright CB, Doty DB, et al: Does visual interpretation of the coronary angiogram predict the physiologic importance of a coronary stenosis. *New Engl J Med* **310**:819, 1984.

Whyte HM, Yee IL: Serum cholesterol levels of Australians and natives of New Guinea from birth to adulthood. *Aust Ann Med* **7**:336, 1958.

Wiklund O, Fager G, Craig IH, et al: Alphalipoprotein cholesterol levels in relation to acute myocardial infarction and its risk factors. *Scand J Clin Lab Invest* **40**:239, 1980.

Wilens SL: The relationship of chronic alcoholism to atherosclerosis. *JAMA* **135**:1136, 1947a.

Wilens SL: The resorption of arterial atheromatous deposits in wasting disease. *Am J Pathol* **23**: 793, 1947b.

Wilhelmsen L, Wedel H, Tibblin G: Multivariate analysis of risk factors for coronary heart disease. *Circulation* **48**:950, 1973.

Wilhelmsen L, Sanne H, Elmfeldt D, et al: A controlled trial of physical training after myocardial infarction. *Prev Med* **4**:491, 1975.

Wilhelmsen L, Elmfeldt D, Wedel H: Cause of death in relation to social and alcoholic problems among Swedish men aged 35–44 years. *Acta Med Scand* **213**:263, 1983.

Wilhelmsson C, Wilhelmsen L, Vedin JA, et al: Reduction of sudden deaths after myocardial infarction by treatment with alprenolol. *Lancet* **2**:1157, 1974.

Wilhelmsson C, Elmfeldt D, Vedin JA, et al: Smoking and myocardial infarction. *Lancet* **1**:415, 1975.

Williams PT, Wood PD, Haskell WL, et al: The effects of running mileage and duration on plasma lipoprotein levels. *JAMA* **247**:2674, 1982.

Williams PT, Wood PD, Krauss RM, et al: Does weight loss cause the exercise-induced increase in plasma high-density lipoproteins? *Atherosclerosis* **47**:173, 1983.

Williams RB, Haney TL, Lee KL, et al: Type A behavior, hostility and coronary atherosclerosis. *Psychosom Med* **42**:539, 1980.

Williams BR, Sorlie PD, Feinleib M, et al: Cancer incidence by levels of cholesterol. *JAMA* **245**: 247, 1980.

Williams RS, Miller H, Koisch FP Jr, et al: Guidelines for unsupervised exercise in patients with ischemic heart disease. *J Cardiac Rehabil* **1**:213, 1981.

Williams RS, Logue EE, Lewis JL, et al: Physical conditioning augments the fibrinolytic response to venous occlusion in healthy adults. *N Engl J Med* **302**:987, 1980.

Wilson D, Wood G, Johnston N, et al: Randomized clinical trial of supportive follow-up for cigarette smokers in a family practice. *Can Med Assoc J* **126**:127, 1982.

Winett RA: Parameters of deposit contracts in the modification of smoking. *Psychol Rec* **23**:49, 1973.

Wing RR, Jeffrey RW: Outpatient treatments of obesity: A comparison of methodology and clinical results. *Int J Obes* **3**:261, 1979.

Wingard DL, Suarez L, Barrett-Connor E: The sex differential in mortality from all causes and ischemic heart disease. *Am J Epidemiol* **117**:165, 1983.

Wissler RW, Vesselinovitch D: Development of the arteriosclerotic plaque, in Braunwald E (ed): *The Myocardium: Failure and Infarction.* New York, HP Publishing Co, Inc, 1974, p. 155.

Wissler RW, Vesselinovitch D: Regression of atherosclerosis in experimental animals and man. *Mod Concepts Cardiovasc Dis* **46**:27, 1977.

Wolf RN, Grundy SM: Influence of weight reduction on plasma lipoproteins in obese patients. *Arteriosclerosis* **3**:160, 1983.

Wolf RN, Grundy SM: Effects of caloric restriction on plasma lipids and lipoproteins. *Clin. Res.* **28**: 55A, 1980.

Wollam GL, Hall WD, Porter VD, et al: Time course of regression of left ventricular hypertrophy in treated hypertensive patients. *Am J Med*, suppl September 26, p. 100, 1983.

Woo KS, Norris RM: Bundle branch block after myocardial infarction—A long-term follow-up. *Aust NZ J Med* **9**:411, 1979.

Wood PD, Klein H, Lewis S, et al: Plasma lipoprotein concentrations in middle-aged male runners. *Circulation* **50**(suppl 3):115, 1974.

Wood PD, Haskell W, Klein H, et al: The distribution of plasma lipoproteins in middle-aged male runners. *Metabolism* **25**:1249, 1976.

Wood PD, Haskell WL, Blair SN, et al: Increased exercise level and plasma lipoprotein concentrations: A one-year, randomized, controlled study in sedentary, middle-aged men. *Metabolism* **32**:31, 1983.

Working Group on Arteriosclerosis of the National Heart, Lung and Blood Institute: *Arteriosclerosis 1981*, vol 1, NIH publication 81-2034. Bethesda, Md, US Dept of Health and Human Services, 1981a.

Working Group on Arteriosclerosis of the National Heart, Lung and Blood Institute: *Arteriosclerosis 1981*, vol 2, NIH publication 82-2035. Bethesda, Md, US Dept of Health and Human Services, 1981b.

Workshop on Cholesterol and Noncardiovascular Disease Mortality: *Summary.* National Heart, Lung and Blood and National Cancer Institutes, Bethesda, Md, May 11–12, 1981.

World Health Organization (WHO): Cardiovascular diseases, annual statistics 1955–1964 by sex and ages. *Epidemiol Vital Stat Rep* **20**:539, 1967.

World Health Organization European Collaborative Group: Multifactorial trial in the prevention of coronary heart disease: I, Recruitment and initial findings. *Eur Heart J* **1**:73, 1980.

World Health Organization European Collaborative Group: Multifactorial trial in the prevention of coronary heart disease: II. Risk factor changes at two and four years. *Eur Heart J* **3**:184, 1982.

World Health Organization European Collaborative Group: Multifactorial trial in the prevention of coronary heart disease: III. Incidence and mortality results. *Eur Heart J* **4**:141, 1983.

World Health Organization (WHO) Working Party Report: *Ischaemic Heart Disease Register*, part 2, May 12–14, 1969, Copenhagen.

Worth RM, Kato H, Rhoads GG, et al: Epidemiologic studies of CHD and stroke in Japanese men living in Japan, Hawaii, and California: Mortality. *Am J Epidemiol* **102**:481, 1975.

Wu M, Ware JH, Feinleib M: On the relation between blood pressure change and initial value. *J Chron Dis* **33**:637, 1980.

Wynder EL, Lemon FR, Bros IJ: Cancer and coronary artery disease among Seventh-day Adventists. *Cancer* **12**:1016, 1959.

Wynn V, Godsland I, Niththyananthan R, et al: Comparison of effects of different combined oral-contraceptive formulations on carbohydrate and lipid metabolism. *Lancet* **1**:1045, 1979.

Wysocki T, Hall G, Iwata B, et al: Behavioral management of exercise: Contracting for aerobic points. *J Appl Behav Anal* **12**:55, 1979.

Yano K, Rhoads GG, Kagan A: Coffee, alcohol and risk of coronary heart disease among Japanese men living in Hawaii. *N Engl J Med* **297**:405, 1977.

Yano K, Rhoads GG, Kagan A, et al: Dietary intake and the risk of coronary heart disease in Japanese men living in Hawaii. *Am J Clin Nutr* **31**:1270, 1978.

Yano K, Blackwelder WC, Kagan A, et al: Childhood cultural experience and the incidence of CHD in Hawaii Japanese men. *Am J Epidemiol* **109**:440, 1979.

Yarbrough P, Klonglan GE: Adoption and diffusion of innovations: Research findings, in Tait J, Goodrich J (eds): *Community Dental Health—Organizing for Action*, society report 113, Dept of Sociology and Anthropology. Ames, Ia, Iowa State Univ, 1974, pp. 27–28.

Zanchetti A: Summary of prazocin lipid studies. *Am J Med* 76(2A):122, 1984.

Zyzanski SJ, Jenkins CD, Ryan TJ, et al: Psychological correlates of coronary angiographic findings. *Arch Intern Med* 136:1234, 1976.

Index